The Healthy Socialist Life in Maoist China, 1949–1980

The Healthy Socialist Life in Maoist China, 1949–1980

Renée Krusche

LEXINGTON BOOKS
Lanham • Boulder • New York • London

Published by Lexington Books
An imprint of The Rowman & Littlefield Publishing Group, Inc.
4501 Forbes Boulevard, Suite 200, Lanham, Maryland 20706
www.rowman.com

86-90 Paul Street, London EC2A 4NE

British Library Cataloguing in Publication Information Available

Library of Congress Cataloging-in-Publication Data

Names: Krusche, Renée, author.
Title: The healthy socialist life in Maoist China, 1949–1980 / Renée Krusche.
Description: Lanham : Lexington Books, [2022] | Revision of Author's PhD thesis: "Living a Healthy Socialist Life—Cures for Maoist China", FAU, Germany, 2020. | Includes bibliographical references and index.
Identifiers: LCCN 2022035367 (print) | LCCN 2022035368 (ebook) | ISBN 9781793654557 (cloth) | ISBN 9781793654564 (ebook)
Subjects: LCSH: Medical policy—China—History—20th century. | Public health—China—History—20th century. | Medical care—China—History—20th century.
Classification: LCC RA395.C6 K78 2022 (print) | LCC RA395.C6 (ebook) | DDC 362.1095109045—dc23/eng/20220727
LC record available at https://lccn.loc.gov/2022035367
LC ebook record available at https://lccn.loc.gov/2022035368

For my parents, Meike and Norbert.

Contents

Acknowledgments

Writing a book is never easy and cannot be done by one person alone and it always has to take place while life happens around us. This book is the revised and partly rewritten version of my PhD thesis, which I handed in in 2020 at FAU, Germany. Back then it was titled "Living a Healthy Socialist Life—Cures for Maoist China." I first and foremost have to thank the two men who made this dissertation project possible: my doctoral supervisor, Marc Matten, and my husband, Roman, for their support, encouragement, and never-ending advice. Without Marc Matten's academic guidance, his input, and regular discussion sessions this piece would never have taken its form and I would not have benefitted and learned as much as I did over the past years. My husband I have to thank for his generous patience and willingness to listen and talk through issues that came up during the reading and writing process. I am also eternally indebted to my family, who always supported my academic endeavours and who made my first contact with China possible, which woke interest and passion for the faraway country back when I was in high school. A very special thank you goes out to my father who will never read this piece but who left his mark on it all the same. I thank my family-in-law for their suggestions on the final draft and their support throughout.

Furthermore, no book is written without scholarly exchange and input from colleagues. I thank my colleagues at the Chinese Studies Institute at FAU, Erlangen, who were with me throughout this project, especially Federico Brusadelli for talking me through some tough spots, Anne Schmiedl for commenting on my presentations, Michael Höckelmann for our weekly chats about our latest findings, and Henrike Rudolph for her helpful tips, kindness, and understanding. Without the discussions with experts such as Marta Hanson, Amanda Shuman and her curiosity about my topic, Lei Hsiang-lin and Chu Ping-yi from the Academia Sinica in Taibei, Li Xuetao at Beiwai, and many others, my ideas and understanding of the Chinese history of health would not have come to fruition. My thanks also go to Ben Young and his helpful comments in the last draft of the final manuscript, the anonymous peer reviewer for pointing me toward some weaknesses of the early draft, and to the different student assistants who helped at different stages of the project and contributed actively to the finished piece.

And last, but not least, this would not be a text of acknowledgment from me if I forgot the one who helped me through this time but who will never read this text herself. Nevertheless, she was eager to listen when I discussed difficult passages or problems; a huge thank you to my horse Macuca and her patience and gentleness with me.

Introduction

HEALTH IN A MODERN WORLD

In 1956, Shu Xincheng 舒新城 (1893–1960)[1] published a handbook entitled *How I Regained Health* (*Wo zenme huifu jiankangde* 我怎么恢复健康的), containing a comprehensive collection of health tips as well as details of the author's own health history. The first edition of this small book had been published in 1947, but it was reworked and reprinted after the founding of the People's Republic of China (PRC) in 1949. Shu Xincheng had been spurred to write it by his personal health history, for he was not a medical expert; in fact he was an educationalist who had published mainly on the Chinese education system and its reforms since the late 1920s.[2] His book, as the title promises, gives a comprehensive introduction to daily health practices. Shu claimed to have been very sick between 1942 and 1943. According to his record, he had grown up in the countryside and had never been seriously ill or a patient of a medical professional. At the outbreak of the Pacific War in 1941, however, Shu had been immersed in the social unrest that was part of everyday life in the Republic of China. Several changes in his place of residence, and the demands of frequent urgent meetings with editors and other intellectuals had made his life stressful, and after he turned 50 his health worsened. To illustrate this point, Shu includes entries on his daily habits taken from the diary kept by his wife, Liu Jiqun 刘济群, telling of irregular sleep, loss of appetite, unrest, and loss of vigor.[3] This discomfort drove Shu to search for a remedy, and hence led him to immerse himself in the research on health and then to share his results with a bigger audience. The handbook depicts how he himself became a health expert, implying that anybody might follow his example.

How Health Became an Issue for China

Between the nineteenth and twentieth centuries, huge political, economic, and social changes took place in the region that today is called China. The transformation of the Qing empire[4] into the Republic of China and then the founding of the People's Republic was not brought about solely by internal political and social tensions and confrontations, but was in part shaped by foreign forces. The colonial aggression of the European powers and Japan resulted in a national trauma that has been broached by many scholars over the years, and out of which emerged the idea of the Sick Man of East Asia. This image of China as a weak, frail old man, tormented by famine and opium, and lacking in physical strength and powers of organization, was first taken up by Western powers when they started to divide the Qing empire among themselves. It pathologized a politically weak state and applied the contemporary fashionable Darwinian world view to a situation that greatly benefited the foreign powers themselves. This metaphor, in the end, was shared among and internalized by the Qing reformers and their successors.[5] The stigma held so much national shame that programs to annihilate it went on well into the twentieth century. This makes it central to the motivations behind the discussion of health and the body that this book engages in. National objectives always included the improvement of the physical state of the Chinese people, as discussions of nutrition science and domestic management in the Republic of China have already demonstrated.[6]

The Republic of China pursued what the Qing reformers had initiated: the modernization of China to create a democratic nation. To achieve this the leadership leaned heavily on input from the outside, including the import of natural sciences, among which was biomedicine.[7] Different aspects of life were affected by the effort to lessen the impact of epidemics, raise health standards, and adapt medicine to local needs. The arrival of natural sciences and biomedicine influenced not only knowledge production in the twentieth century but also how the world was perceived. It changed the way the population was governed and how policies were conducted. The access to biomedicine and science made it possible to battle fiends that could not be defeated before, such as tuberculosis, the bubonic plague, and general issues of hygiene, as well as to face other diseases that were suddenly found to have cures.[8]

In the middle of the twentieth century, the health discourse became central to the rhetoric of nation building and revolution espoused by the Chinese Communist Party (CCP) on the way to establishing the *New China*. This manifested primarily in the mass movements for hygiene and health that were called the Patriotic Health Campaign.[9] Their specific rhetoric included the idea of class struggle and the narrative of exploitation by class enemies.

Both concepts influenced the way the body's energy sources were considered. While exploitation, according to the CCP, had been resolved in 1949 by the ousting of the old and oppressive system, class struggle was still a constant condition against which the body had to hold up, and for which a healthy and strong body was required. The common reference to Engels and his claim that "labour created man himself"[10] assigns absolute priority to labor and production as the basis for New China. The ambition to build a strong and rich nation was embodied in propaganda posters depicting the economic reconstruction and establishment of a new society. They display the socialist dream of a prosperous and strong nation standing in defiance of the old, so-called feudal, society and nefarious external influences. To attain this ideal, the Chinese state aimed for an increase in production to raise general living standards, and an expansion of knowledge production and dissemination to reach everybody in the population and to educate everyone about healthy living. This also included extensive education reforms and literacy campaigns to ensure the population was able to read and understand the necessary scientific knowledge.[11]

Since the CCP, and hence the Chinese state, assumed an air of omnipresence and omnipotence in all of this, it has often been accused of ruthless persuasion and coercion on its path to power. With the ultimate goal of Communism in mind, it has been described as totalitarian in its governmental practices, and as desirous of controlling every aspect of life.[12] Since the ultimate goal was the rebirth of the Chinese nation as a strong and able collective body, the PRC attempted to control and regulate the population.[13]

The introduction of medical knowledge helped in these regulatory endeavors, and brought about a changed perception of the physical body. Discussions about the presence or absence of health in the body raised one of the most pressing issues of the time: the question of the visibility of diseases. The general population's perception of health at the time was rather practical, involving the notion that if one could go about one's daily business then one was well, and it was difficult to convince them otherwise. Invisible diseases thus went unnoticed, which could result in chronic issues, the spreading of bacteria and viruses, and in the end the infringement of bodily functions. The mass campaigns against snail fever (schistosomiasis) are an example of a fight against a disease that was not seen as such, as well as an example of the fight to educate the population on health matters, as demonstrated in detail by Miriam Gross. Through a widespread campaign including visual materials, talks, and health classes, the rural population was convinced to give up their practically oriented view of health and inquire deeper into the biomedical conditions of the body in order to stop epidemic diseases such as snail fever.[14]

These campaigns highlight the divide between the understanding of the individual body and the wider governmental goal. On the one side, there is the unwitting person whose livelihood depends on being able to work; on the other, the authorities worried about the physical state of the population and its ability to keep up with the fast pace of modernization. This shows the changing understanding of the body in a society that suddenly came to be governed by scientific principles. By teaching the population about diseases, new habits were ingrained and a new scientific understanding of hygiene was fostered. The state of the body was to be assessed by experts in order to generate reliable evidence for its cure and improvement. To be able to do that, and to justify these previously unknown measures and secure the public's trust in them, the authorities had to spread health knowledge among the population.

GOVERNING KNOWLEDGE AND PEOPLE

Returning, then, to Shu's search for health, this sketch of the historical background allows us see that his quest was by no means exceptional in the context of the health tips literature of twentieth-century China; rather, it falls within the major struggle for physical strength to bolster national growth and prowess. When I initially embarked on my research on health in China, I asked myself what this sought-after "health" might have comprised. Much has already been written on the topics of public health, epidemics, Chinese Medicine, diseases in China, and *weisheng* 卫生, the principle of guarding life, which in the transition from the nineteenth to the twentieth century was commonly translated as hygiene of any kind;[15] but none of these terms corresponds to the conception of health for which I was searching. In her 2004 book *Hygienic Modernity*, Ruth Rogaski examines how the term *weisheng* (hygiene) evolved. A change in physical awareness was introduced to treaty-port China at a time when the Japanese aspired to gain more influence on the mainland. Through the power relations between colonizers, local population, and government in this knowledge exchange, the native term *weisheng* was redefined and restructured as a biomedical concept, bringing about an awareness of governmental responsibility to provide for the population. To achieve this, even in a colony, knowledge of the coveted improvements was spread and enforced for the benefit of public health.[16] The issue of naming hygiene practices and behaviors is central to another approach to *weisheng* undertaken by Lei Hsiang-lin, who focuses on local hygiene practices that were also called *weisheng* but did not belong to the imported idea of public hygiene described above. Instead, they were "personal hygiene" practices including eating habits and mental hygiene. Lei observes that a sense of shame was evoked by outsiders' critical attitude to a Chinese populace declared to be dirty and unhygienic. This generated a preoccupation with cleanliness, the opposite extreme, so as to avoid this dirty state. This adds another layer to the concept of hygiene that sets it apart from the later concept of *jiankang*.[17]

Jiankang 健康—health—does not have a direct connection to institutionalized colonial practices that are politicized and used to degrade the subject population, as was the case with *weisheng*; rather, it is a favored physical condition that is aspired to both by the collective and the individual, and which can be arrived at through various means. It has rarely been the subject of research, and the historical scholarship has not paid much attention to explaining it. This may be a consequence of the simple fact that defining health is tricky and raises questions that have no straightforward answer. It was my recognition of this that prompted the central questions of this book to change. Thus, I now came to ask: What health practices were there in socialist China? How was a healthy life led? What part did the Chinese state play in the health of the population? And in what way was a return to health, as Shu termed it, managed by the state as well as the individual? Since the socialist state sought to penetrate every level of the daily life of the population at the time, it stands to reason that health practices were also heavily impacted by it. I also came to include in the inquiry the question of how socialist health practices might differ from those that had existed earlier or those from across the borders. These questions appear even more pressing given that a thorough reading of the secondary literature on the history of medicine and the history of the PRC reveals that this time period has been underresearched so far.

The question of what health is can be approached from a wider frame of reference: thus, the 1948 WHO constitution[18] states that "health is a state of complete physical, mental and social well-being and not merely the absence of disease or infirmity."[19] This expression may seem straightforward and widely applicable, but it raises more questions than it answers: What is well-being? What is disease? What happens if one feels well despite being sick? Does that count as being sick or not?

Plügge and Kohn (1959) offer an interesting definition of the state of well-being, writing that "well-being is 'in general, synonymous with my noticing nothing about my body.'"[20] In socialist China's medical journals, physical education newspapers, and other similar sources that were used for this study, the healthy body is mainly "absent," that is, there is no thought about the healthy body, but rather the body is felt as soon as there is a change in this state and pain or discomfort emerges. Most of these body-related articles discuss deviations from the healthy state—namely diseases or injuries and how to fix them—not the state of health itself. This fixing involves a return to the state that is considered the norm, or health. This absence of the body—and thus absence of awareness of its health status—is a concept Drew Leder elaborates on in his book entitled *The Absent Body*: this "absence" not only describes a state of being "not ill," but also of being "not consciously" felt at the moment. Leder goes into detail about the process of thematizing parts of the body and thus establishing a new awareness,[21] because "in order to perceive any explicit object I must make use of means, clues, and information that are themselves unthematized and of which I have little or no direct awareness."[22]

Despite the difficulties in perception, and its newness to the Chinese language as a term that had entered from Japan, *jiankang* became an essential attribute for identifying strong and vigorous bodies in the socialist context of the PRC, and for making visible the deficiencies of other bodies. It describes an ideal and aspirational status of health. To introduce this new concept into the discourse of medicine and daily life it would have been preferable to build on previously existing knowledge, but as Nathan Sivin pointed out in 1987, "There is in fact no single word in traditional medicine that corresponds exactly to 'health.'"[23] In the existing medical tradition there was the notion of equilibrium and harmony, which can be related to *jiankang*. This harmonious state does not connote the black-and-white dichotomy of sick or healthy, but is rather a spectrum of conditions. Chinese medical treatment aims for the restoration of internal harmony to the body, as described by Ralph C. Croizier: "Since disease arises out of a disequilibrium in the human organism, the basic cure is in restoring harmony."[24]

Jiankang was not only attached to medicine but also to politics and to the nation-building process. It marked a turning point in the narrative of national shame and the negative self-image of the Sick Man of East Asia. *Jiankang* became the norm in Chinese health literature against which bodies were measured. The emerging practices and strategies to achieve the coveted state of health in the fight for revolution and the Chinese socialist nation are central to this book. I concentrate on socialist China's attempts (beginning in 1949) to improve the "national body," and I pursue these developments into the first decade after the beginning of the economic reform process, that is the mid-1980s, which gives me the opportunity to examine the degree of stability and continuity in health concepts and practices.

The effort to improve the health of the Chinese population was not peculiar to socialist China, but was ongoing throughout the twentieth century,[25] and included the fight against snail fever as well as the constant struggle against tuberculosis.[26] The continuing efforts toward optimal health in modern China show a continuing fascination with the subject of health and disease.[27] I argue that this continuity of medical thought and practice bolstered the development of a strong and stable health discourse, one that was linked to the global discourse but was almost impervious to external ruptures.

Health was pursued in the PRC through the establishment of institutional and governmental structures. Health practices were adapted to the socialist labor environment and were integrated into daily life by directly involving the broader population. The health care system was established by the authorities and built to simplify the governing of the population through monitoring and manipulating their physical health. The health care system represents the underlying framework I use for my observations;[28] my focus, however, is on the distribution of health knowledge as intended to educate the population on the idea of the "healthy body,' concerning both the individual and the collective.

Knowledge transfer, production, and dissemination led to the establishment of the health discourse among the population and the experts, and introduced among them biomedical concepts such as anatomy, physiology, or the metabolism as well as ideological output related to physical well-being. This included issues of labor security and other social and political discussions linked to health. The questions that need to be asked in connection with these processes concern the scope of governmental and individual health decisions, and hence to what degree the party-state (which in the Mao era relied heavily on political pressure and persecution when transforming social classes and cultural identities) could actually influence individual health behavior. How complex and hierarchical actually was the health and disease discourse governing the body in the PRC? Apart from the centralized establishment and development of healthy habits, the intervention and negotiation strategies between the state and its subjects also emerge from this study, and can be observed. In this context, I detail how state-building was pursued by forming and educating the individual body, while facing considerable limits to accessing it. These limits are a crucial part of my observations with regard to the often-assumed omnipotence of the party-state. The discussion of something as intangible and flexible as health leads to insights into governance (and its limits), self-care, and the opening of decision-making spaces for individual persons. In this process, the actors involved—both institutional and individual—are mapped out and the structures of the health discourse emerge. I do not employ a purely top-down approach toward understanding the findings, but rather seek to depict how governmental directives were expressed, passed down, and sometimes changed in response to feedback from the audience and the experts—and, in the case of "civilization diseases," by the physiological reaction of the population to new living standards. Here the patterns of reaction and interaction between the state-funded institutions and the experts become apparent.

In order to identify how a healthy body was defined, identified, and then created, various actors were involved ranging from state institutions to medical experts, from bureaucrats to persons at the grassroots level. The sources used provide deep insights into the processes of knowledge production and publication that shaped the understanding of health in this era.[29] They are mainly concerned with medical and hygiene approaches to the body, and derive from both traditional and scientific systems. The "new" biomedical knowledge takes center stage in many scientific publications, but it is not the only medical system that is intertwined in this discussion. The traditional Chinese medical system has long been the center of interest in Chinese medical history and historiography. In the twentieth century we witness the parallel existence and a state-fostered merging of the traditional Chinese system with the biomedical system, resulting in a body of knowledge called *New Medicine* (*xin yixue* 新医学). While I focus mainly on the biomedical discussion of health and practical health advice, I make sporadic references to the traditional knowledge system, references which later become more pronounced in the treatment of civilization diseases. There is, however, no systematic discussion of this knowledge by the primary sources. Instead of asking whether it is useful to maintain the dichotomy of "Chinese versus Western medicine," or rather whether it makes more sense to treat all medical knowledge equally, I aim to show the negotiations and reconciliations that took place between the premodern and rather implicit medical knowledge, and the newly imported biomedicine.[30]

At the same time, the knowledge production process includes tacit and expert knowledge, and earlier knowledge at times becomes more visible as a result of later developments. The different knowledge systems involved all belong to the discourse of health and form an almost organic and growing structure that evolves through exchange. The knowledge I look at is highly interconnected with transnational networks and phenomena.[31] I thus identify the crucial ideas and origins of this knowledge in order to show how the PRC corpus of health knowledge was constructed. The analysis allows similarities and differences in health practices to come to light, and shows how the public discussion of health was shaped by three main physiological needs and anthropological problems that had to be resolved in order to sustain the population: food, physical movement, and sleep. These needs are interconnected in a web of daily ritual and social exchanges that form the basic structure of socialist life against the backdrop of labor and revolution. They are behaviors that are observed transnationally, independent of locality or culture. Problems that occur in relation to these three activities are universal and have to be resolved globally as well as on a local level, since too much stress and too little sleep are problems in not only China but also in the rest of the world.

To better understand the impact this new knowledge had on life and its regulation, I identify the actors involved and the ensuing hierarchy between population, state, and experts, as well as the creation of networks for the circulation of knowledge. In this way, the changes that influence the health discourse can be uncovered. William Sewell's 1992 approach to structures and actors in the social sciences can help us to understand this dynamic frame of health practices. In Sewell's view, structures are dynamic entities that can change depending on the actors within and around them, as well as on their resources, their depth, and their overlaps with other structures.[32] Sewell opens up a framework which can illuminatingly be applied to multiple different areas of interest. It serves this study well to display the interconnected actors and the underlying cycle of knowledge production. In the case of China, knowledge production and policy are often seen as top-down processes where the central authority governs all outlets. While on the surface this may be the case, in the "deep structures," as Sewell puts it, it becomes clear that reciprocity is actually rather common. Actors exchange knowledge and opinions, and these actors are not just individuals, but include the state and its institutions as well. At the same time, one can identify different structures within this framework, which all build on each other. This engages with Bourdieu's idea of *habitus*,[33] which emerges as a result of "temporally durable structures."[34] The establishment of a health routine is nothing more than the building of *habitus*, a new structure that is approved by the state and incorporated into the national structures, thus setting new requirements for the other actors involved. The PRC established visible structures in the form of institutions, which at times also themselves become actors within the discourse of health, so that not only individual persons but also institutions such as universities and research facilities could "act" within this context.

How to Govern Bodies: Theoretical Concepts in the Quest for *Jiankang*

Governance and control over a population was famously analyzed at length by Michel Foucault, two of whose concepts need to be introduced here to understand how the PRC government dictated the health discourse to the Chinese nation, and how far its policymaking could reach: these concepts are *biopower* and *governmentality*. Foucault understood biopower as a mode of government that attempts to provide rational solutions to the problems a population faced on a daily basis: these problems included matters of health and hygiene, but also birth, longevity, and race.[35] In their account of the harsh and invasive methods of the One Child Policy, Susan Greenhalgh and Edwin Winckler observe that "*biopower* is the calculated power over human life, especially at the level of the population. Biopower is aimed at the administration of the vital characteristics of human populations and exercised in the name of optimizing individual or collective life, health, and welfare. Biopower entails the increased ordering of life at all levels."[36] The One Child Policy is a prime example of direct manipulation and forced behavior in the population, drastically invading women's privacy and bodies through enforced abortions and sterilizations, while at the same time, within the discourse of health and health practices, increased state activity can be detected on the educational and institutional level. While biopower is rooted in the ability for persuasion possessed by the executive power, for the purposes of this book it is more appropriate to work with Foucault's concept of governmentality, which denotes a mode of government that is not as heavily power-laden or prone to harsh coercion or penalties as biopower, but instead seeks to nudge and direct the individual toward the sanctioned ideal of health. Governmentality, understood in the Foucauldian sense, is concerned with the government of populations, and concentrates on their management and optimization.[37] The ideas in health literature which are meant to optimize and improve the nation's body operate on a much smaller scale and with less violent means than birth planning and reproductive limitations. Where the biopolitical act of birth planning reduces the freedom of choice for the individual person, the health discourse opens up new possibilities for the individual—but within the framework set by the government. I argue that the state faced limits to its governance in shaping the behavior of the population. The limits are not limitations which were imposed upon the population; rather, as I seek to uncover, they are limits to government itself and to its ability to take invasive measures. This leads to the question: Where was governmentality unable to reach and how were these limits negotiated?

The limits of governmentality in the discourse of health examined in the following chapters differ with respect to each topic treated: nutrition, exercise, sleep, and civilization diseases. In nutrition science governmentality is able to reach quite far before it encounters resistance. The governance of experts, that is, the state, can be easily identified in the calculations made for individual persons. This governing of the population is more prescriptive than coercive. In the environment of public dining spaces governmentality extends a bit further, as actual meal plans are handed out to institutions (canteens) and individual households to supply them with optimal nutrition. The structure of canteens and the attempt to completely govern the private life of the population during the Great Leap Forward (1958–1961) historically resulted in catastrophe, where governmentality hit a wall which it was unable to navigate around: the governed structures broke down, and life returned to an almost pre-1958 state.[38] The topic of physical exercise, meanwhile, shows how this area of human activity became institutionalized and how the individual condition of bodies posed a major problem to the total control of the nation's body, as it came down to the individual person to decide when exhaustion had struck and how a physical limit was defined. The inability to govern a body completely is even more evident when talking about sleep and rest. The activity of rest was a limit to and at the same time a source of power for labor: as the state cannot look into the minds and emotions of its population, there is no way of telling how much rest was adequate for an individual. At the same time, forcing somebody to sleep when they are not tired is often futile, unless one wants to force-feed the population sleep medication. Finally, the civilization diseases pose the most obvious limits to governmentality: while the Chinese state managed to control outbreaks of epidemics, the new and modern socialist lifestyle of wealth and often sedentary activity fostered living situations which brought about new health problems that, in spite of their education attempts, the authorities were unable to prevent.

The ultimate limit to governmentality thus seems to be the very thing which health practices are intended to form: the individual human body. We need to ask how far authorities can push and control individuals without pushback or negative reactions from the population. We also need to consider the following: How far can the governing of bodies be planned and executed effectively? What mechanisms have to be instilled in the population's "mind" so that it can be governed to the most positive effect? To accomplish the task of governing the Chinese body, the governing authorities tried to penetrate the individual space by appealing to ideology and by nudging the population to make the "right choices," that is, accepted choices. Those entailed the concept of self-care for the sake of individual as well as national health.

These self-care or personal hygiene practices came into being in combination with the arrival of biomedical inventions from the outside, and they do have the air of what Foucault described as "techniques of the self," containing practices that serve as prevention and cure. They can be performed by each individual person and do not need expert supervision, which makes them independent of medical expert knowledge. Foucault calls them "health practice" or the "framework of daily life."[39] Here self-care is the tending of an individual to their own well-being according to their environment and their abilities. These techniques of the self are vaguely reminiscent of Marcel Mauss's *Techniques of the Body*, the latter indeed being much more normative than the health practices observed in the context of the PRC.[40] The notion of self-care was ingrained into the minds of the Chinese readers of self-help literature, and became an almost medical as well as political category that was bolstered by biomedical vocabulary and observations. One has to keep in mind that the individual body is not, in this context, seen as an entity that is independent in its own right. In the PRC the individual person is never seen as separate from society, but rather as a part of it. So by using the term "individual" I merely intend to point to the single body as opposed to the general population. The choices each person can make for the sake of their own health open up a decision-making space that may be interpreted as individual, but given the facts of ideological indoctrination there is no way of telling how far this freedom to choose reaches. Still, in this process the "self" is discovered when an awareness of the body is created. The body involved in physical activity becomes two things: the body of a person and a tool of labor, with the latter being maintained to guarantee the production process.

This forms a dualism that permeates the entire discussion of the body at the time. The self that was part of the discourse of exercise, nutrition, and rest gained footing and space. With the exception of the class enemy, who during the many campaigns was deprived of sleep, food, and even medical treatment,[41] the individual body was not, as I am going to show, fully subjected to political control.

The normalization of health as the default setting of the physical body, a state that has to be upheld and to which one aspires, leads to the next questions we need to ask: What is normal? And what is a normal body? Since defining health is tricky, the general understanding may be that identifying disease and illness, with its aches and pains, is much easier. Often it is assumed that a normal physical state which is tolerable and comfortable can be identified as healthy without medical insights or examination. Disease, on the other hand, becomes abnormal. Georges Canguilhem details this observation and presents an intriguing study of normality and norm, pointing to the difficulties of this category especially when talking about health. He claims that, statistically speaking, both health as well as disease are to be considered normal, seeing as they both occur frequently in populations. Health becomes normative when it is defined as the ideal condition of the body. Canguilhem points out that "the experience of the living" includes periods when one is sick due to disease. This would mean, however, that disease is not abnormal, but part of living. He argues, that "hence it is only another way of saying that continual health is a norm and that a norm does not exist. In this misconstrued sense, it is obvious that the pathological is not abnormal."[42] According to this view, then, the healthy state as well as the unhealthy state both constitute forms of normality for the body. Thus, a disease is a deviation from a state of imagined equilibrium. This in turn entails that the pathological state is nevertheless a part of life, and hence that "being healthy and being normal are not altogether equivalent since the pathological is one kind of normal."[43] Health can, thus, be considered normative, and is often deployed as a tool in order to evaluate a situation. For Canguilhem, health is "a margin of tolerance for the inconstancies of the environment."[44] Disease can therefore be understood as a reduced margin of tolerance to the environment.

Canguilhem's ideas reflect the fact that it is much easier to identify disease than health, because a seemingly healthy body may have symptoms that point to a sickness that are only measurable by specialized instruments, and not evident to unaided perception. Disease and health are both states of the human body, but in the context of modernity with its emphasis on production the healthy state is the one that is desired. Deviations from health, that is, diseases, thus are obstacles to production, and although they may be part of life they are not part of the idealized and aspirational strong body. The normative aspect of health, as Canguilhem describes it, is at the forefront of the Chinese socialist nation-building endeavor. These issues all play a role in my analysis of the discussions on health that took place in this period, and are reflected in the fact that few source materials actually emphasize a definition of health, but focus rather on the *return* to health, where the individual body is enabled to be rid of pain or to return to work after sickness.

Arthur Kleinman elaborates on this relativity of the concept of health in his study of chronic illnesses, raising the question of when a condition is considered a disorder or an illness: "By invoking the term *illness*, I mean to conjure up the innately human experience of symptoms and suffering."[45] Chinese health literature includes the personal experience of comfort or discomfort as a barometer of well-being, often marked in the sources by invoking a reference to "one's own feelings" (*an ziji de ganjue* 按自己的感觉) on the matter of exercise, rest, or well-being. While on the outside, the Chinese authorities and biomedical experts adhere to "hard" science,[46] that is, measurable and authoritative data, the personal experience of the population never truly vanishes, although there is an attempt to standardize the criteria for health for every age and labor group.

The concept of the physical body lies at the base of this discussion, being the space where all health practices are carried out and where the negotiations of power between the state and the individual take place. It is the site of production and, in the end, of health. The body possesses its own aesthetic which in the Mao era was linked to its physical ability as a malleable object that has a function in labor and revolution. Its functionality is visualized specifically in terms of the muscles, as the part of the body where labor power is located. The anatomical depiction of muscles is a rare thing in Chinese history, as Shigehisa Kuriyama has observed: before the twentieth century the beauty of muscles was not present in Chinese art, daily life, or the discourse of the body.[47] The dissection of the physical form into a muscular apparatus and a skeletal structure marks a break with the traditional view of the body as a holistic entity, and introduces new possibilities since the new understanding of muscles locates them at the center of production. Muscles were seen as small "power plants," geared toward industrial production and so directed at the generation of economic growth by pursuing the scientification of the body and its parts. A body devoid of the needed muscles could not function in an optimized production environment and had to be avoided or changed and rehabilitated by building its muscles. The body of muscles and production strength is often described as a machine, which is one route to the very simplified and sometimes shallow understanding of the complex human organism that we find in a number of discourses related to the concept of health, production, and science.[48] This new understanding of the physical was rooted in the natural sciences and in biomedicine, a scientific discipline that was raised to prominence during the Republican period and further fostered as a central part of life and government in the PRC. *Kexue* 科学, science, was no longer merely a descriptive adjective, but a normative attribute. Anything that was labeled "scientific" automatically gained credibility and value. The employment of biomedical science, its scientific structures, and its normative quality, is evident in the establishment of Chinese health practices in this period.[49]

Behind the health endeavor, the primary and quantitative concern of the Chinese socialist state was to raise productivity as a means to achieve socialism and to attain an increased standard of living. Production goals and labor organization permeated all aspects of daily life. Labor, as the physical manifestation of production, was the reason to hone one's body, to get up in the morning, and then to return to one's bed at night: quite simply, it determined all other activities. This determination to be productive in the pursuit of a higher purpose might be deemed Weberian. Max Weber indeed saw the ascetic lifestyle of the Protestants as directed toward a higher purpose, and showed that today's emphasis on discipline and productiveness in a capitalist society derives from this Protestant work ethic. Weber described a controlling disciplinary structure—the Christian religion—which permeated all of daily life and structured its every aspect. This discipline was closely linked to morality and became the basis of everyday capitalist endeavors.[50] Interestingly, a similar progression can be perceived in the Chinese socialist system, where a productive and diligent body, working for the sake of the common good, was defined as the ultimate goal by the authorities.

In striving toward a growing economy characterized by quantifiable increases in production, the process of quantification itself plays a huge role. In pursuit of a mathematical assessment of all the parts of the production process, the measuring of the body as well as of training exercises, nutrition, and resting periods were positioned at the heart of the Mao-era health practices. This entails an objectification of the body, a standardization as remarked upon by Canguilhem, that was thought to be best achieved by the use of numbers and facts as a means to govern a population. In this process the numbers become charged with additional meaning, coming to be perceived as objective and universally understood, as Theodore M. Porter, Tong Lam, and Arunabh Ghosh have shown in their respective works.

When a population is objectified, and engaged with on the basis of quantification, the governing entity exerts control over the group thus quantified.[51] The process of "social quantification" strips people of their individuality; although this can be interpreted as invasive and negative, it does not have to be so. As Porter remarks, a statistical survey of the human population may often benefit societies, especially in seeking to improve the situation of working people, the young generation, and marginalized groups.[52]

The widespread adoption of numbers as valid expressions of the facts of daily life has had a relatively short history in China, and is broadly understood to be closely linked to the contact with Western powers, as demonstrated both by Ghosh and Lam. In this context Lam understands statistics, numbers, and the resulting depiction of facts through them, as signs of a modernity that sought to standardize and to impose norms upon social reality.[53] The numerical tables and lists of nutrition values I include in this study support this assumption, showing how every part of daily life was measured and translated into quantities of units that could be calculated and planned. The strong push at the time for the scientification of China led to a trust in numerical values by the targeted audience, that is, the general population. While this quantification surge was meant primarily to improve both life and government, it is often argued that it opened the door to the totalitarian and authoritarian character of the PRC government. According to Porter "Numbers turn people into objects to be manipulated. Where power is not exercised blatantly, it acts instead secretly, insidiously."[54] A high degree of objectification of the Chinese body can be found in the numbers and statistics that were thus built up around the conception of the body. These numbers seemed unable to cover everything, however, as the frequent reference to personal conditions, individual feelings, and physical ability demonstrates. In a Western context, "Those who fail to conform [to the expected numbers] are stigmatized, and most others have internalized the values of an ever more pervasive bureaucracy of experts and calculators."[55] In the Chinese context, shortcomings are trained out of the participants depending on their abilities, or they are subjected to an especially nutritious diet to overcome malnutrition. The values and charts created by Chinese scientists were published as standards, creating norms that the individual was held to. While this standard could be adapted if the situation required it, at the same time it was upheld as the pinnacle of bodily ability and this ideal was substantiated by ideology. Numbers are thus not only a prescription for the physical form, but in this process actually *become* the body, describing it and opening it up for control. In the context of the continuing process of scientification, trust in these seemingly objective numbers was a natural consequence. The level of acceptance of science as universal truth may be gauged from the thorough discussion of nutritional values and body measurements, as well as the quantification of sleep and resting habits. It also shows itself in the thorough examination of bodies that diverge from the previously established norm, specifically in the cases of hypertension and obesity.

Physical examinations and bodily tests were a regular part of the routine in the PRC, especially in the early decades. These tests took place all over the country. A local gazetteer from Chengde, Hebei, reports, for instance, that between 1949 and the beginning of the Cultural Revolution (1966) students of the Polytechnic College of the Hebei Normal University for Nationalities (Chengde minzu shifan gaodeng zhuankexuexiao 承德民族师范高等专科学校) were examined every year. Measurements taken included height, weight, chest circumference, eyesight, examinations of the skin, and so on. After 1979, apart from every newly arriving student, the second and third years as well as the students leaving to enter the workforce were also examined. They were subjected to a complete checkup: chest, internal and external examinations, organs and skin, eyesight, lung capacity, height, weight, and so on.[56] Similar procedures are listed for hospitals or schools in the gazetteers of Ningde in Fujian, Baofeng in Henan, or Poyang in Jiangxi.[57] The thirst for such information throughout the Mao era (and beyond) shows the importance of quantification in the eyes of the state.

These grand-scale assessments of large parts of the population, intended to gain insight into their physical condition and to make sure they were well prepared for a productive life, have changed in their appearance since the Mao era. Today, such inquiries are neither strange nor atypical, and are largely outsourced to modernity's ever-present companion, technology. Nowadays, such information-gathering is made possible by the willingness of the population to enter their vital statistics into health apps on their smartphones, allowing the device to track their movement and sleep cycles, often even logging their nutrition intake, all without coercion by a concerned state yet with the same ever-present intent to optimize health and, in the end, life.

JOURNALS AND HANDBOOKS—THE TREASURE VAULT OF HEALTH PRACTICES

To achieve its goal of elucidating the discourse around the healthy body, the present book engages directly with Chinese sources, seeking to enter into a dialogue with them while at the same time highlighting the transnational dimension of health. Interestingly, these sources are often translations from foreign language publications, adapted to the needs of the local population. The resulting new corpus of health practices was a merging of different traditions and ideas. By utilizing these texts, I attempt to bridge a gap in medical historiography, wherein the engagement with Chinese sources is still insufficient.

The difficulties of engaging with Chinese sources are manifold. For one thing, they are written in Chinese, a language often not accessible to researchers. They are also somewhat difficult to come by in a time when travel is limited and archival access or interview opportunities strongly regulated. These issues impact the approach to research, and certainly show themselves in the results here presented. Accessing any text corpus always has to be done with a certain level of reflection and a critical mindset. The publications used for this study were all published by official Chinese institutions, and thus have often been claimed by commentators and onlookers to be ideologically biased. This bias presents itself in the pervasive reference to the "great achievements of the Party" in science, the pleas to adhere to a healthy lifestyle in pursuit of the common good, as well as the choice of topics to be discussed. As Sigrid Schmalzer has emphasized, however, this does not make them unusable, but they have to be handled carefully and supplemented with additional information drawn from their historical contexts so as not to simply replicate their biases. The handbooks and articles used here are thus bolstered with additional biographical information, explanations of historical context, and further articles on the various topics, so as to shed light on the issues of nutrition, exercise, and sleep from all sides and so enable insight into the health discourse of the era. This "layered analysis," as Schmalzer calls it, enables us to engage with the topic of health in socialist China through official publications, and to come up with an intriguing new understanding of what it meant to be healthy.[58]

In the 1950s, the production, dissemination, and availability of scientific knowledge were of high priority to the Chinese state in the wake of the science popularization movement (*kepu* 科普).[59] This entailed major publication efforts of Republican, Soviet, and Western scientific material, including medical texts and hygiene-related knowledge, so that it could be handed down to the population via the channels of the CCP's political network in the countryside, and also via the newly established education system. The bulk of the material used for this research is composed of 1950s–1980s handbooks on health, food, exercise, rest, medicine, and the like, as well as journal and magazine articles. Judith Farquhar describes these handbooks and short articles on health practices as "quick fixes" that supplement and replace the advice of medical personnel.[60] These "quick-fix" texts are the basis for my analysis. The handbooks used will be introduced properly in the individual chapters; for the moment, however, I want to briefly review the magazines and journals I employ, pointing out their range, their frequency, and the problems deriving from using them.

The basis for all these publication activities were the publishing houses and companies that took charge of editing, printing, and spreading the written texts. One of the main publishing houses for health and hygiene topics is the People's Medical Publishing House (Renmin weisheng chubanshe 人民卫生出版社), which mainly produced and disseminated material on health and hygiene. Founded in 1953 in Beijing, it functioned as the publishing house to the national Ministry of Health.[61] Its frequent publications throughout the 1950s, 1960s, and 1970s appear in announcements in the *Jiankangbao* 健康报 (*Health News*) at the end of many issues. The topics related to health span from Chinese Medicine to birth control. They include translations from Russian[62] and English sources, as well as the reproduction of some Qing dynasty books. Due to this publishing house's responsibilities and tasks, it had far-reaching influence on the production of knowledge and the resulting literature. It was charged with the implementation of Ministry of Health policies, the introduction of medical knowledge from the Soviet Union, and with the merging of theory and practice to improve and disseminate both. Furthermore, it had to introduce Soviet research results, publish teaching materials, and spread and improve knowledge on medicine and pharmaceuticals, while also developing medical books for experts and lay people. The link to Soviet knowledge arises from the sense of socialist brotherhood between the two nations, but is severed as soon as the Sino-Soviet partnership ends in the early 1960s. This rupture witnesses a shift from Russian sources toward American and Japanese publications, as well as favoring original research by Chinese experts. Following the incorporation of foreign-language material in the *kepu* movement, the compilation of dictionaries and thus the determination of medical terms was another of the tasks of the People's Medical Publishing House.[63] This makes it one of the main authorities in the process of publication and dissemination, and attributes it chief responsibility for the standardization of health knowledge.[64]

While more and more information was published through these official channels, the authorship of many contributions remains obscure, especially in the period of the 1950s and 1960s. Another rather striking formal characteristic of the texts from this period is the language employed, which can vary from highly academic (*Zhonghua Yixue Zazhi* 中华医学杂志, *Zhongyi Zazhi* 中医杂志) to the popularized and vernacular (*Jiankangbao*, *Dazhong Yixue* 大众医学). The material is generally repetitive in structure, employs a redundant register of words between different publications, and contains a surfeit of metaphorical expressions to engage the newly found readership. Yet despite the fact that increasingly complex and novel concepts were introduced in it, it remains fairly simple in style.

The expert journals are the more theoretical publications tailored toward scientists with a basic understanding of biomedicine. The more popular newspapers, on the other hand, range in the topics covered and are meant for a broad audience. Together with the academic journals they show how the state shaped the discourse via different kinds of publication. The *Jiangkangbao* is one of the oldest vernacular newspapers on health and hygiene in the PRC. This biweekly newspaper was published by the Ministry of Health–adjoined Jiankangbaoshe 健康报社 (Health News Publishing) to be disseminated among the broad population. From its beginning in Ruijin, Jiangxi Province in 1931, the journal was edited by the Military Medical Office until the founding of the PRC. It was the official newspaper of the Northeast Army and the

People's Government in 1949, only to become the mouthpiece of the PRC's Ministry of Health in 1950. There were phases in which the *Jiankangbao* was not published regularly, especially before the founding of the PRC and during the Cultural Revolution, when most publishing houses stopped production: publishing ceased for 13 years and was taken up again in 1979.[65] The issues contained varying numbers of articles on the topics of *jiankang* or *geren weisheng* 个人卫生 [personal health/hygiene].[66]

Another popular journal, the *Dazhong Yixue* 大众医学 (*Popular Medicine*) is, according to its website, one of the oldest magazines to popularize medical science, having begun publishing in 1948.[67] It is published in Shanghai by the *Dazhong Yixue* Editorial Committee (Dazhong Yixue bianji weiyuanhui 大众医学编辑委员会) and printed at the Shanghai Medical Publishing House (Shanghai yixue chubanshe 上海医学出版社).[68]

The magazine *Xintiyu* 新体育 (*New Sports*), founded in 1950, is called by Lu Xiaoning "the most influential and popular sports magazine in the Mao era." "This magazine published news stories about sporting events in the PRC, featured photographs of folk exercises, introduced athletics in other communist countries, and set up such columns as 'exchange of pedagogies of physical education,' 'short stories,' and 'science of exercise and physiology.'"[69] It is edited by the New Sports Magazine Publisher (Xintiyu zazhi she 新体育杂志社) in Beijing and published by the People's Sport Publishing House (Renmin tiyu chubanshe 人民体育出版社).

Another journal popularizing medical expert knowledge is the *Zhonghua Yixue Zazhi* 中华医学杂志 (*Chinese Medical Journal*), which has been published since 1915. I used this journal mainly for its expert material on civilization diseases, biomedical analyses, and case analyses of hypertension.[70] The *Zhongyi Zazhi* 中医杂志 (*Journal of Traditional Chinese Medicine*) is an additional source for information on health and health practices. First published in 1951 as an academic platform to discuss various forms of Chinese medical practices, experiences, and the like, it includes case studies for diagnostics and treatment and shares expert information.[71]

One journal that was of use to this study despite not at first glance being connected to hygiene and health was *Laodong* 劳动 (*Labor*). First published in 1950, the journal gives insight into labor-related topics, including organization, management, labor safety, progress, and innovation. The small magazine *Jiankang* 健康 (*Health*), not to be mistaken for the *Jiankangbao*, is a monthly magazine published since 1980. Whereas the *Jiankangbao* was a mouthpiece of the CCP, the *Jiankang* is a much more low-key publication that includes a lot of lifestyle pieces and short stories, and fewer news-style articles. The topics range from retirement problems and issues of the elderly to obesity-related questions, and are written for non-expert audiences.[72]

The problem with all these publications including handbooks is the rupture during the Cultural Revolution (1966–1976), when for a few years all publication activity ceased. The length of this period is not the same for each publication, but generally stretches from 1966 until 1978. This did not impact the content, as one cannot detect a change in subjects, tone, or evaluation of subjects pre– or post–Cultural Revolution. Knowledge production itself was impacted neither by the founding of the PRC in 1949 nor by the Cultural Revolution, as I show in the course of this book. This stability of content is devoid of ideological considerations. The content of health knowledge in journals as well as handbooks remains unchanged. The stability of health knowledge is also present in the recurring reprinted editions from Republican publications. Changes in the narrative only occur due to the added forewords, which often described the circumstances of the publication and its relation to the prevailing narrative of the socialist revolution.

Published by state-run publishing houses and thus under the supervision of the state and the propaganda department, the resulting material is also prone to depict ideas that have been sanctioned by the authorities. Interestingly enough, the ideological tone and influence within these sources is kept to a minimum and can be seen mainly in the prefaces or the introductory paragraphs. The overarching goal of strengthening the nation by establishing good health in the population is rarely directly expressed in the texts themselves, and instead the whole health discourse is embedded in a nationalist narrative which is restricted to the paratext.

THE ROAD SO FAR

The study of medical history in twentieth-century China has captured the attention of many scholars in past decades. The focus of their research is often the dichotomy between traditional Chinese (*zhongyi* 中医) versus Western medicine (*xiyi* 西医), their combination, or the rise of hygiene awareness and public health shaped by transnational knowledge transfer.

The New Medicine was formulated in the 1950s as a way to provide health care to a large population with little medical personnel and is ongoing until today. According to Volker Scheid, after its institutionalization, the New Medicine was intended as a conglomerate of medical know-how and practices that were supposed to aid in the growth and development of the PRC and improve the living standard of the population. More thorough scientific experimentation with Chinese Medicine was conducted in its wake to establish it as a modern scientific discipline. Through my reading of contemporary materials, I can trace Scheid's observation of this monumental attempt at reconciling two seemingly contrasting theoretical knowledge systems. Where

Scheid has his eye on the body of Chinese Medicine as a tradition, I focus on the specific role of health as a holistic concept within this discourse.[73]

So far, scholars have been fascinated with the pathologization of patients and the creation of this hybrid system. Yang Nianqun's 杨念群 "Recreating 'patients'" (*Zaizao 'bingren'* 再造 '病人') tells of the restructuring, reinvention, and negotiation that occurred between the Chinese and Western medical systems. The focus of his research is on the local administration of medicine in China and the changes of perception of medicine and disease.[74] Similarly, Hillary A. Smith looks at retrospective epidemiology[75] in the Chinese medical system, bringing together traditional concepts of diseases with the biomedical understanding of them, and focusing on how beriberi was perceived and categorized in Meiji-era Japan. Here, the center of attention is the state of sickness, its origins, and treatments.[76] Traditional medical practices in imperial and twentieth-century China were often seen in the context of *wenbing* 温病, warm diseases. This heavily influenced how pathologies were perceived and how sickness at the time was categorized. Marta Hanson connects biomedical pathologies with these Chinese medical concepts and thus follows epidemics such as leprosy and smallpox through Chinese history, providing a thorough understanding of how diseases were understood and organized in the contemporary system.[77] The contact between biomedical pathologies and traditional Chinese medical practices is the focus of Lei Hsiang-lin's *Neither Donkey nor Horse* (2014). The encounter of Chinese Medicine, first with Western medicine and then with the state, shaped and formed today's medical landscape. Lei revisits the contact with the bubonic plague, the role of missionaries, and the conviction that Chinese Medicine was nothing but superstition, to show how different actors, including diseases, have impacted the health condition of the population and to what extent. Through the exchange with Western methods and science, Chinese Medicine finally became what it is today, which in part includes its status as "state medicine."[78]

The studies of Chinese medical history have not only included policies regarding traditional medical practice, but also addressed approaches to population control that fall into the realm of biopolitics. Part of this general shift toward biopolitical approaches to the body in the PRC included the arrival of germ theory and the understanding and establishment of chemistry, which generated new ways of dealing with disease, such as vaccination. In her *Mass Vaccination: Citizens' Bodies and State Power in Modern China* (2019), Mary Brazelton observes how immunization programs in the twentieth century were utilized to fight the age-old stigma of the Sick Man of East Asia. By vaccinating the population, the Chinese authorities not only followed the medical need to fight epidemics but also established medical control over the Chinese nation.[79] The new ways to mobilize the Chinese population through mass movements were influenced by the widespread application of science to get rid of diseases that had long prevailed in China and the empire. The Patriotic Health Campaign, starting in the mid-1950s, aimed to contain the spread of diseases but also to aid in the education of the population, in disease prevention, and to promote hygienic living.[80]

While all of these studies go into detail about epidemics, power relations, and state control, the focus firmly remains on the pathological state of China. In this context there is frequent discussion of the return of the body to health, as well as the newly emerging concept of public and personal hygiene for the ultimate goal of a strong state; but what health looked like remains unclear and is not dissected further. Rogaski sets out to answer this question for treaty-port China in the very early twentieth century by looking at the restructuring of cities and the introduction of modern city planning and public health measures, but so far a study of similar concepts in the PRC has been missing. For socialist China, bigger problems have until now been in focus, mainly concerning ideological struggles. An inquiry into the day-to-day literature, including magazines, newspapers, and self-help handbooks, thus reveals a remarkable and yet neglected discourse of health practices. The present book shows how a focus on these diverse texts—and not on the health policies themselves or the mass campaigns—can present us with a picture of health as it is negotiated between state authority, experts, and the population, and how health as a concept opens the door to self-awareness and individual choices. It also considers the instances in which this negotiation breaks down, when health problems persist or change in their nature due to the inability of the state to control everybody fully.

NOTES

1. Shu Xincheng (1893–1960) was an educationalist from Xupu, Hunan. He obtained a degree from Hunan higher normal college (*Hunan gaodeng shifan xuexiao* 湖南高等师范学校) in 1917, after which he held different functions and posts, such as a teaching position at Hunan First Normal University. He was then involved in the development and revolutionizing of the Chinese education system, and in 1928 was asked to be on the editing board of *Cihai* 辞海. After 1949, he became a representative for Shanghai at the National People's Congress. Apart from *Cihai* he also published various books on education and specifically Chinese education history. See *Jiaoyu dacidian zengding hebianben xia*, 1444.

2. One of Shu's biographies lists the following titles: 《道尔顿制研究集》 (1929), 《现代教育方法》, 《近代中国留学史》 (new edition 1989), 《中国新教育概况》 (1930), 《教育通论》 (new edition 1990/2006), 《近代中国教育思想史》 (1918/1932), 《我和教育》 (1945). See *Jiaoyu dacidian zengding hebianben xia*, 1444.

3. Shu Xincheng, *Wo zenyang huifu jiankangde* 我怎样恢复健康的 (Beijing: Zhonghua shuju chubanshe, 1956), 13–14.

4. Already in the Qing period there were governance measures in place for natural disasters such as famine, as Walter Mallory and Pierre-Etienne Will have shown: Walter H. Mallory, *China—Land of Famine* (New York: American Geographical Society, 1926); Pierre-Etienne Will, *Nourish the People: The State Civilian Granary System in China, 1650–1850* (Ann Arbor: Center for Chinese Studies, 1991).

5. Rudolph Wagner, "China 'Asleep' and 'Awakening.' A Study in Conceptualizing Asymmetry and Coping with It," *Transcultural Studies* 1 (2011): 4–139. For a comprehensive discussion of all the topics associated with the stigma, see Iwo Amelung, ed., *Discourses of Weakness in Modern China: Historical Diagnoses of the "Sick Man of East Asia"* (Frankfurt: Campus Verlag, 2020).

6. See Jia-Chen Fu, *The Other Milk: Reinventing Soy in Republican China* (Seattle: University of Washington Press, 2018); Helen M. Schneider, *Keeping the Nation's House* (Vancouver: UBC Press, 2011).

7. David Luesink, William Schneider, and Daqing Zhang, eds., *China and the Globalization of Biomedicine* (Rochester, NY: University of Rochester Press, 2019); Bridie Andrews and Mary Brown Bullock, eds., *Medical Transitions in Twentieth-Century China* (Bloomington: Indiana University Press, 2014).

8. See Xinzhong Yu, "Epidemics and Public Health in Twentieth-Century China: Plague, Smallpox, and AIDS," in *Medical Transitions in Twentieth-Century China*, ed. Bridie Andrews and Mary Brown Bullock (Bloomington: Indiana University Press, 2014), 91–105; Rachel Core, "Tuberculosis Control in Shanghai: Bringing Health to the Masses, 1928–present," Andrews and Bullock, *Medical Transitions*, 126–45.

9. See Nianqun Yang 杨念群, "Disease Prevention, Social Mobilization and Spatial Politics: The Anti Germ-Warfare Incident of 1952 and the 'Patriotic Health Campaign,'" *Chinese Historical Review* 11 (2004): 155–82.

10. Friedrich Engels, "The Part Played by Labour in the Transition from Ape to Man," in *Beyond the Body Proper*, ed. Margaret Lock and Judith Farquhar (Durham: Duke University Press, 2007 [1876]).

11. On mass education and literacy campaigns, see Vilma Seeberg, *The Rhetoric and Reality of Mass Education in Mao's China* (Lewiston: E. Mellen Press, 2000); Ruth Hayhoe, *Education and Modernization: The Chinese Experience* (Oxford: Pergamon Press, 1992).

12. For the ways the CCP used coercion and mass mobilization to reach its goals in the early Maoist period, see Julia Strauss, "Morality, Coercion and State Building by Campaign in the Early PRC: Regime Consolidation and after, 1949–1956," *The China Quarterly*, no. 188 (2006): 891–912. See also Edward Friedman, Paul G. Pickowicz, and Mark Selden, *Revolution, Resistance, and Reform in Village China* (New Haven, CT: Yale University Press, 2005); Michael Dutton, *Policing Chinese Politics: A History* (Durham, NC: Duke University Press, 2005). Production and economic development were set out in five-year plans, alongside the structures and behavior patterns of daily life. The five-year plans influenced the availability and distribution of food and the development of labor, as well as the constitutions that set the legal framework for labor and vacation laws and the development of an education system

which had a major influence on the dissemination of knowledge, the implementation of physical education, and the literacy movement.

13. For economic and industrial planning, see Rui Kunze and Marc A. Matten, *Knowledge Production in Mao-Era China: Learning Science from the Masses* (Lanham, MD: Lexington Books, 2021), 167.

14. Miriam Gross, *Farewell to the God of Plague—Chairman Mao's Campaign to Deworm China* (Oakland: University of California Press, 2016).

15. Ruth Rogaski, *Hygienic Modernity: Meanings of Health and Disease in Treaty-Port China* (Berkeley: University of California Press, 2004); Hsiang-lin Lei, "Moral Community of *Weisheng*: Contesting Hygiene in Republican China," *East Asian Science, Technology and Society* 3 (2009): 475–504.

16. Rogaski, *Hygienic Modernity*.

17. Lei, "Moral Community of Weisheng."

18. The constitution was institutionally relevant to the Republic of China, which was a member until 1950, and later to the PRC, which entered as a member in 1972. See Seung-Joon Lee, "The Patriot's Scientific Diet: Nutrition Science and Dietary Reform Campaigns in China, 1910s–1950s," *Modern Asian Studies* 6, no. 49 (February 2015): 22.

19. This definition is still in use today. Constitution of the WHO (1948) (https://www.loc.gov/law/help/us-treaties/bevans/m-ust000004-0119.pdf [accessed 22 March 2020]), 119.

20. Herbert Plügge and Rolf Kohn, "Wohlbefinden und Missbefinden," *Psyche* 12, no. 1 (1959): 40: "Im Wohlbefinden *nehme* ich nichts von meiner leiblichen Verfassung *wahr*; mein Körper ist mir als „schweigendes Selbstverständnis' (passé sous silence *[Satre]* gegeben [. . .]."

21. Drew Leder, *The Absent Body* (Chicago: University of Chicago Press, 1990), 17: "[I]n thematizing a part of the body we necessarily change its phenomenological status."

22. Leder, *The Absent Body*, 15.

23. Nathan Sivin, *Traditional Medicine in Contemporary China: A Partial Translation of* Revised Outline of Chinese Medicine *(1972) with an Introductory Study on Change in Present Day and Early Medicine* (Ann Arbor: Center for Chinese Studies, University of Michigan, 1987), 95.

24. Ralph C. Croizier, *Traditional Medicine in Modern China: Science, Nationalism, and the Tensions of Cultural Change* (Cambridge: Harvard University Press, 1968), 23.

25. Daqing Zhang, "Changing Patterns of Diseases and Longevity: The Evolution of Health in Twentieth-Century Beijing," in Andrews and Bullock, *Medical Transitions*, 32–50.

26. Core, "Tuberculosis Control in Shanghai."

27. See also Luesink, Schneider, and Zhang, *China and the Globalization of Biomedicine*.

28. See Xun Zhou, *The People's Health: Health Intervention and Delivery in Mao's China, 1949–1983* (Montreal: McGill-Queen's University Press, 2020); Gross, *Farewell to the God of Plague*.

29. Achim Landwehr, *Historische Diskursanalyse* (Frankfurt: Campus Verlag, 2018), 96.

30. Given that Chinese Medicine is known as TCM, it would seem logical to use this term, but the term itself was only invented in the 1980s. I will mainly use the term "Chinese Medicine" to describe those practices that are part of the medical system developed from folk medicine and traditional medical practices, based, for example, on the *Huangdi Neijing*. Nevertheless, it is not a suitable term. "Chinese Medicine" could also signify "medicine in China" and "medicine from China," both of which can and do also contain biomedicine. To make the differentiation easier, I stick with the term "biomedicine" for medical practices connected to what is also termed "Western medicine," although the "West" need not be its origin, and I use the term "Chinese Medicine" for any practice that is ascribed to the traditional medical system originating in traditional medical texts and folk medicine.

31. See Peter Burke, *What is the History of Knowledge?* (Cambridge: Polity Press, 2016).

32. William Sewell, "A Theory of Structure: Duality, Agency, and Transformation," *American Journal of Sociology* 98, no. 1 (July 1992).

33. See Pierre Bourdieu, Patrick Champagne, Julien Duval, Franck Poupeau, Marie-Christine Rivière, and Peter Collier, *Habitus and Field: General Sociology, Volume 2; Lectures at the Collège de France (1982–1983)*, (Cambridge: Polity Press, 2020).

34. Sewell, "A Theory of Structure."

35. Michel Foucault, *Die Sorge um sich* (*Sexualität und Wahrheit 3*) [*History of Sexuality*] (Frankfurt: Suhrkamp Verlag, 2012), 180.

36. Susan Greenhalgh and Edwin A. Winckler, *Governing China's Population: From Leninist to Neoliberal Biopolitics* (Stanford: Stanford University Press, 2005), 27.

37. Michel Foucault, *Analytik der Macht* (Frankfurt: Suhrkamp, 2005), 148–74.

38. See Frank Dikötter, *Mao's Great Famine: The History of China's Most Devastating Catastrophe, 1958–1962* (New York: Walker & Co., 2010); Kimberly E. Manning and Felix Wemheuer, *Eating Bitterness: New Perspectives on China's Great Leap Forward and Famine* (Vancouver: UBC Press, 2011); and Jisheng Yang, *Grabstein—Mùbei: Eine Dokumentation der großen chinesischen Hungerkatastrophe 1958–1962* (Frankfurt am Main: Fischer Verlag, 2012).

39. Foucault, *Die Sorge um sich*, 135.

40. See Marcel Mauss, "Techniques of the body," *Economy and Society* 2 (1973).

41. See for example the case of Liu Shaoqi: Lowell Dittmer, "Death and Transfiguration: Liu Shaoqi's Rehabilitation and Contemporary Chinese Politics," *The Journal of Asian Studies* 40 (1981), 459–460.

42. Georges Canguilhem, *The Normal and the Pathological* (New York: Zone Books, 1989), 137, 138.

43. Canguilhem, 196.

44. Canguilhem, 197.

45. Arthur Kleinman, *The Illness Narratives: Suffering, Healing, and the Human Condition* (New York: Basic Books, 1988), 3.

46. Kleinman, 9.

47. See Shigehisa Kuriyama, *The Expressiveness of the Body and the Divergence of Greek and Chinese Medicine* (New York: Zone Books, 2002), 111: Kuriyama argues that "historically, the vision of muscularity was in fact the exception. Interest in individual muscles and indeed the very notion of muscles—as distinct from flesh, tendons, and sinews—developed uniquely in medical traditions rooted in ancient Greece. Elsewhere, as in China, 'ignorance' of musculature was the rule[.]" See also for example Ko Cho and Kyoko Iriye Selden, *The Search for the Beautiful Woman: A Cultural History of Japanese and Chinese Beauty* (Lanham: Rowman & Littlefield, 2012).

48. Anson Rabinbach, *The Human Motor: Energy, Fatigue, and the Origins of Modernity* (Berkeley: University of California Press, 1992).

49. Rui Kunze and Marc A. Matten, *Knowledge Production in Mao-Era China: Learning Science from the Masses* (Lanham, MD: Lexington Books, 2021).

50. Max Weber, "Die protestantische Ethik und der Geist des Kapitalismus," *Archiv für Sozialwissenschaften und Sozialpolitik* 21, no. 1 (1904).

51. Arunabh Ghosh, *Making it Count* (Princeton: Princeton University Press, 2020).

52. Theodore M. Porter, *Trust in Numbers: The Pursuit of Objectivity in Science and Public Life* (Princeton: Princeton University Press, 1995), 77.

53. Tong Lam, *A Passion for Facts* (Berkeley: University of California Press, 2011), 1–18. Lam emphasizes the ambivalent position of social surveys in his work when he stresses that they are a tool born from the semi-colonial period of China. At the same time, they served as a way to emancipate China from its imperial past.

54. Porter, *Trust in Numbers*, 77.

55. Porter, 77–78.

56. Liu Mingxian 刘明显 and Qian Shuxin 钱树信, eds., "Shiyebian—disizhang tiyu junxun weisheng 事业篇-第四章体育 军训 卫生," in *Chengde minzu shifan gaodeng zhuankexuexiao zhi* 承德民族师范高等专科学校志 (Hebei sheng Chengde shi: Jiaoyu kexue chubanshe, 1994), 129.

57. Lin Pinxuan 林品轩, ed., "Diliubian yiliao shiye—disanzhang yizhengguanli 第六篇 医疗事业-第三章 医政管理," in *Ningde diqu yiyao weisheng zhi* 宁德地区医药卫生志 (Fujian sheng Ningde shi: Fujian renmin chubanshe, 2005), 147; Yang Liugong 杨留功, Wang Shunxing 王顺兴 and Dong Guofan 董国范, eds., "Diqizhang tiyuweisheng—disanjie weisheng 第七章 体育卫生-第二节 卫生," in *Baifeng xian diyi gaoji zhongxue xiaozhi* 宝丰县第一高级中学校志 (Henan sheng Pingdingshan shi baofeng xian: Zhongzhou guji chubanshe, 2000), 122–23; Kang Li康黎 and Cheng Guanqun 程关群, eds., "Disanzhang shehui yiwu huodong 第十三章 社会医务活动," in *Poyang xian renmin yiyuan zhi* 鄱阳县人民医院志 (1933–2008) (Jiangxi sheng: Jiangxi renmin chubanshe, 2009), 215–16.

58. Sigrid Schmalzer, "Beyond Bias: Critical Analysis and Layered Reading of Mao-Era Sources," in *Positions: Asia Critique* 29, no. 4 (November 2021): 759–81.

59. Kunze and Matten, *Learning Science from the Masses*.

60. Judith Farquhar and Qizheng Zhang, *Ten Thousand Things: Nurturing Life in Contemporary Beijing* (New York: Zone Books, 2012), 132.

61. Weishengbu bangongshi ting, ed., *Weishengbu lishi kaoji 1949–1996 nian* 卫生部历史考记1949–1996年 (Beijing: Renmin weisheng chubanshe, 2013), 184.

The People's Medical Publishing House was the result of merging the military-adjoined Huadong yiwu shenghuoshe 华东医务生活社 and the Dongbei yixue tushu chubanshe 东北医学图书出版社 into one; it is still in existence today and now is one of the main publishing houses for medical knowledge according to their website. See http://www.pmph.com.

62. The authors of several sources from the 1950s were Russian or at least from the Soviet Union. Their names were almost all transcribed into Chinese. At times the original Cyrillic version of the authors' names would also be added, but quite often it was not. This left to the researcher the task of finding out who was the author. In the bibliography and footnotes I still provide the original Chinese version, as there may be transcription errors either on my side or in the Chinese originals.

63. Weishengbu bangongshi ting, *Weishengbu lishi kaoji*, 184.

64. The other authority on spreading health knowledge is the health propaganda department of the Ministry of Health.

65. Weishengbu bangongshi ting, *Weishengbu lishi kaoji*, 182

66. For a more thorough discussion of the pre-PRC development of the *Jiankangbao*, see Fu Qisheng 傅柒生 and Li Zhengang 李贞刚, eds., *Hongse jiyi* 红色记忆 (Red Memories) (Beijing: Jiefangjun chubanshe, 2011), 132–35.

67. See the *Dazhong Yixue* website, http://www.popumed.com/about (accessed March 26, 2020).

68. The publishing house and editorial board changed in the 1970s; at that time the journal was published by the Shanghai Scientific and Technical publishers (Shanghai kexue jishu chubanshe 上海科学技术出版社).

69. Xiaoning Lu, "Promote Physical Culture and Sport, Improve the People's Constitution," in *Words and Their Stories—Essays on the Language of Chinese Revolution*, ed. Ban Wang (Leiden: Brill, 2011), 179.

70. The *Zhonghua Yixue Zazhi* was published by the People's Medical Publishing House Renmin weisheng chubanshe 人民卫生出版社 in Beijing, one of the leading publishers in health literature.

71. The *Zhongyi Zazhi* was published in Beijing by the *Zhongyi Zazhi* she 中医杂志社.

72. The *Jiankang* was published by the Jiankang zazhi she 健康杂志社 in Beijing.

73. See Volker Scheid, *Chinese Medicine in Contemporary China: Plurality and Synthesis* (Durham: Duke University Press, 2002). See also Kim Taylor, *Chinese Medicine in Early Communist China, 1945–63: A Medicine of Revolution* (London: Routledge, 2011).

74. See Jisheng Yang, *Grabstein—Mùbei: Eine Dokumentation der großen chinesischen Hungerkatastrophe 1958–1962* (Frankfurt am Main: Fischer Verlag, 2012).

75. For a thorough discussion of the concept of retrospective epidemiology, see Randall Packard, "The Fielding H. Garrison Lecture: 'Break Bone' Fever in Philadelphia, 1780; Reflections on the History of Disease," *Bulletin of the History of Medicine* 90, no. 2 (Summer 2016).

76. See Hillary A. Smith, *Forgotten Disease: Illness Transformed in Chinese Medicine* (Stanford: Stanford University Press, 2017).

77. Marta Hanson, *Speaking of Epidemics in Chinese Medicine* (London: Routledge, 2011).

78. Hsiang-lin Lei, *Neither Donkey nor Horse: Medicine in the Struggle over China's Modernity* (Chicago: University of Chicago Press, 2014).

79. Mary Augusta Brazelton, *Mass Vaccinations: Citizens' Bodies and State Power in Modern China* (Ithaca, NY: Cornell University Press, 2019).

80. Gross, *Farewell to the God of Plague*.

PART I

Nutritional Government

The history of food in China has been discussed by many authors and from many different angles,[1] but the development of nutrition science and knowledge is still a very underresearched field, not only for imperial but also for post-1949 China. Joseph Needham and Gwei-Djen Lu, on the one hand, offer one of the few academic overviews on traditional nutrition history in their 1951 essay *A Contribution to the History of Chinese Dietetics*. Regarding the influence of Western nutritional science, on the other hand, the discussion has focused on the late imperial period and the beginning of the twentieth century, as Seung-Joon Lee shows in his paper "The Patriot's Scientific Diet," Mark Swislocki in his "Nutritional Governmentality," or Jia-Chen Fu in her *The Other Milk*. So far, research on nutrition science in Mao-era China is sparse and mainly focused on the Great Famine of the Great Leap Forward, as Felix Wemheuer, Frank Dikötter, and Zhou Xun have demonstrated. Part I of the present volume aims to bridge this gap by outlining the publication efforts undertaken by the Ministry of Health (*Weishengbu* 卫生部) (founded in 1950) to disseminate basic nutrition knowledge and to shape the idea of nutrition in the process of improving the nation's health.

Nutritional governmentality is the process by which a state controls, regulates, and fosters its population's nutritional status. The notion was put forward by Mark Swislocki,[2] and expresses a process that was a precursor of the biopolitical actions the PRC has been pursuing in the past five decades. Food and food issues were long-standing problems for the (imperial) Chinese governments and the population. Administration of food and its availability were the main focal points during imperial times. Pierre-Étienne Will and R. Bin Wong give a comprehensive overview of the Qing granary management in their *Nourish the People* (1991). This governance of food supply resulted in what Swislocki observed to be a relatively well-fed population despite the nineteenth- and twentieth-century Western conviction that the Chinese body was frail and no match for the foreign powers.[3]

With the intrusion of the Western powers into the Qing empire, the idea of the Sick Man of East Asia arrived on Chinese soil, and with it the Qing began to strive to strengthen the population. The introduction of modern sciences changed the educational landscape and the way knowledge was provided for the literate population.[4] Nutrition science also entered the Chinese empire at this time, and was made into a tool to overcome the physical weakness of Asia's "Sick Man," as well as a way to govern the huge nation. Swislocki puts at the forefront of his discussion the responsibility of the imperial state and later the Republic to provide the population with sufficient food. When, in the Republican era, nutritional science shifted from this quantitative view of a good diet to a qualitative assessment of food content, the academic discussion blossomed, fueled by the returning experts and the involvement with Western research, as Jia-Chen Fu and Seung Joon Lee have shown in their respective works. In Republican China, nutrition science became a means to ensure health and to strengthen nationalism. In her *The Other Milk*, Fu examines the history of the soybean's success as a national food in the form of tofu and soymilk, telling the story of Chinese nutrition science and the soybean as interwoven with the narrative of nation-building. Nutrition science was part of the modernization attempts on the way to ridding China of the stigma of the Sick Man of East Asia. Through the example of soy, Fu shows how a strong Chinese identity was created via food and nutrition.[5]

One value that had great impact on the perception of food and the body in an industrialized environment is the calorie. As Nick Cullather underlines for the nineteenth century in his *The Foreign Policy of the Calorie*, an assessment of (mal-)nutrition became possible in the context of colonialism upon the discovery of the calorie. It was utilized by the colonial powers to evaluate nutrition in the colonies as lacking, and thus to justify their further colonization.[6] Yet despite its widespread use, the calorie as a value of fuel energy for consumption and of energy expense in the human body remains an abstract idea.[7] Wilbur O. Atwater (1844–1907)[8] likened the human body to a machine and invented machinery to gauge its energy expenses through detailed measurements.[9] The calorie, however, was not the only qualitative reference point in meals: protein, fats, carbohydrates (macronutrients), vitamins, and minerals (micronutrients) also played a major role in nutritional sciences at the time. Protein especially received attention in the late nineteenth and throughout the twentieth century, depicted as the building blocks of life.[10] Gyorgy Scrinis coined the term *nutritionism* to refer to this fragmented perception of food as consisting of macro- and micronutrients.[11] Nutritionism rationalizes the intake of nutrients for the purpose of strengthening the physical form, the body. Linked to the omnipresent governance of the CCP at the time, it became a means to enhance the physical vigor of the nation, so as to finally rid China of the Sick Man stigma. An article by Wu Xian 吴宪, one of the leading nutritionists at the time, and his colleague Zhou Qiyuan 周启源, published shortly before the official announcement of the PRC, tells of the hope and expectation experts and the Chinese governments had for nutritional development. In August 1949 Wu and Zhou published a comprehensive defense of nutrition in the *Renmin Ribao* (People's Daily 人民日报). There they argue that since the second Sino-Japanese War the government had turned toward the nutritional state of the population as a means to improve the nation's strength.[12] Instead of just demanding an improvement of food availability, they tie nutrition to a larger background and draw out its connections to agriculture and farming, to the production and logistics of food. In the end they call for more research in nutrition science and the sciences linked to it, such as physiology and chemistry. Wu and Zhou also mention the need for educational material and handbooks, films, radio broadcast, and exhibitions on the subject matter.[13] In this part of the present volume, then, the processes of the publication and organization of nutrition knowledge in the 1950s and the following decades will be surveyed to show how knowledge about food, nutrients, and scientific nourishment was disseminated, the ultimate goal being to improve the health status and build strong bodies for the socialist revolution.

NOTES

1. For example, Eugene N. Anderson, *The Food of China* (New Haven: Yale University Press, 1988); Frederick J. Simoons, *Food in China: A Cultural and Historical Inquiry* (Boca Raton: CRC Press, 1991); Jun Jing, ed., *Feeding China's Little Emperors: Food, Children, and Social Change* (Stanford: Stanford University Press, 2000); Mark Swislocki, *Culinary Nostalgia: Regional Food Culture and the Urban Experience in Shanghai* (Stanford: Stanford University Press, 2009).

2. Mark Swislocki, "Nutritional Governmentality—Food and the Politics of Health in Late Imperial and Republican China," *Radical History Review*, no. 110 (Spring 2011): 9–35.

3. See Iwo Amelung, ed., *Discourses of Weakness in Modern China: Historical Diagnoses of the "Sick Man of East Asia"* (Frankfurt: Campus Verlag, 2020), and Hsiang-lin Lei, "Moral Community of *Weisheng*: Contesting Hygiene in Republican China," *East Asian Science, Technology and Society* 3 (2009): 475–504.

4. Peter G. Zarrow, *Educating China: Knowledge, Society, and Textbooks in a Modernizing World, 1902–1937* (Cambridge: Cambridge University Press, 2018); Tze-Qi Hon and Robert J. Culp, *The Politics of Historical Production in Late Qing and Republican China* (Leiden: Brill, 2007); Shu Xincheng, *Zhongguo jindai jiaoyushi ziliao* 中国近代教育史资料 (Beijing: Renmin jiaoyu chubanshe, 1981).

5. Jia-Chen Fu, *The Other Milk: Reinventing Soy in Republican China* (Seattle: University of Washington Press, 2018).

6. Nick Cullather, "The Foreign Policy of the Calorie," *American Historical Review* 112, no. 2 (April 2007): 337–64.

7. Mildred Ziegler, "The History of the Calorie in Nutrition," *Scientific Monthly* 15 (1922): 525: "Calorie as a mere word explains nothing. It is a symbol for an idea, however, which, as we have seen, has undergone changes brought about by the development of several sciences."

8. Atwater was a scientist in the late nineteenth century involved in nutrition science and the calorie discussion. See A. C. True, "Wilbur Olin Atwater, 1844–1907," *Proceedings of the Washington Academy of Sciences* 10 (1908).

9. Wilbur O. Atwater, "Food as Building Material and Fuel," in *Principles of Nutrition and Nutritive Value of Food*, ed. Wilbur O. Atwater (Washington: U.S. Government Printing Office, 1910).

10. Atwater, "Food as Building Material and Fuel"; Kenneth J. Carpenter, "The History of Enthusiasm for Protein," *Journal of Nutrition* 116, no. 7 (July 1986); Urban Jonsson, "The Rise and Fall of Paradigms in World Food and Nutrition Policy (Commentary)," *World Nutrition* 1, no. 3 (June 2010).

11. Gyorgy Scrinis, "On the Ideology of Nutritionism," in *Contemporary Transitions*, ed. Jeffrey M. Pilcher, vol. 4 of *Food History: Critical and Primary Sources* (London: Bloomsbury, 2015).

12. "*Wo guo renmin tizhisu ruo, yuanyin guran henduo, yingyang buliang shi yige zhuyao yuanyin, zheshi buneng fourende* 我国人民体质素弱，原因固然很多，营养不良是一个主要原因，这是不能否认的。" See Wu Xian and Zhou Qiyuan, "Ruhe gaijin renmin yingyang 如何改进人民营养," *Renmin ribao* (August 30, 1949).

13. Wu Xian and Zhou Qiyuan, "Ruhe gaijin renmin yingyang 如何改进人民营养," *Renmin ribao* (August 30, 1949).

Chapter 1

Shapes of Nutrition

The forging of a connection between food and health was part of the twentieth century's modernization processes. Many health practices regarding proper food are based in nutrition science, a branch of science that explains the chemical properties and functions of food. The development of nutrition science in the PRC resulted in an understanding of food as the entity needed for a well-functioning body. Here, I first introduce the institutional background so as to guide the reader's structural understanding, before detailing two case studies on the topics of vitamin C and protein, these being examples of the institutionalization of knowledge production.[1]

Amid all its economic and political upheavals, Mao-era China did care about the quality of food and the health of the nation, and the distribution of knowledge on nutrition science in the 1950s shows this. Nutrition was understood as one part of the health and prevention work undertaken by the PRC. This kind of prevention work not only included food sanitation, but also the dissemination of nutrition knowledge, including daily intake requirements with regard to macro- and micronutrients. The adaptation of a sufficiently nutritious diet catering to the body's needs was advocated by the government and professionals alike.

Already in Republican times there existed strategies for dealing with hygiene and nutrition that were meant to improve the health of the Chinese in an increasingly globalized world. Seoung-Joon Lee discusses the "Patriot's Diet" and the prominent advertising of wheat consumption and coarse rice in the first half of the twentieth century as a reaction to two main issues: the stigma of the Sick Man of East Asia and malnutrition, for example, beriberi. Nutritional work was done to not only cure the population, but also in turn to strengthen the nation.[2]

Nutritional governmentality, being an aspect of China's imperial administration but also of her modernization, can be defined as "a state's use of nutritional knowledge to conceptualize its political objectives and manage the health of its population."[3] The introduction of nutritional ideas into the late Qing's system of governance brought about changes in the understanding of hunger and malnutrition in China at the turn of the century. When comparing the different narratives of famines and their prevention, the "scarcity-to-plenty-model"—which is perpetuated by the modern historical narrative—does not stand up to scientific scrutiny. Although the modern reading of the past denies this, the Qing's famine management system was in fact working quite well until the nineteenth century, as Swislocki has shown. The governmental institutions of the late imperial as well as the Republican era (1912–1949) were engaged in successful nutritional policies, heavily influencing nutrition research, production, and supply.[4]

Basic nutrition concepts and theories were tested first in war situations out of necessity, when soldiers had to be rationed preemptively and central planning of resources was part and parcel of military strategy. The wars at the end of the nineteenth and during the twentieth century impacted the way food was handled and rationed on a global scale.[5] In the first half of the twentieth century, Republican China developed a rationing system for the sake of the military. Born from this background of rationing, food research was deepened in order to better supply sufficient nutrition to the Chinese troops and the population more generally. New food processing methods—such as rice milling—were introduced as a way to boost these rations.[6] After the Chinese civil war and the founding of the PRC, nutrition science continued and was used explicitly by the Communist government as a means to improve and control the population's health, so as to guard it against harm resulting from low-quality or insufficient food. In other words, nutritional governmentality was increasingly concerned with the quality of the diet and less with the mere availability of calories. This chapter argues that Mao-era nutrition information for professionals and laypeople was meant (a) to build an awareness of the body and its functions and (b) to establish the correct scientific nutrition in order to strengthen the overall health of the population and so ensure production.

In the quest for perfect nourishment, food lost its original form. Food, as the object of scientific research, became the sum of its nutritional parts.[7] This changed the perception of it from a whole entity to a structure made up of parts with certain functions. The scientific methods of building a healthy diet with all the important nutrients at the body's disposal became the focus of nutrition science. Food became fuel for body functions, a predictable part of daily life, both for the individual as well as for the state that was planning for food acquisition and production. In the spirit of mass mobilization in the early decades of the Mao era, people were mobilized on a grassroots level to make increased efforts toward health. By mobilizing and educating the population in this way, much was intended to be achieved with little monetary input, as intended by the second five-year plan.[8]

The information about a scientifically "good" diet and its correlation with health was advertised by various means. Apart from mouth-to-mouth propaganda, textual and visual media were the primary channels of disseminating knowledge. This chapter reconstructs the route of textual knowledge by looking at publications and at the histories of the institutions involved. The published knowledge is the result of an interplay between the actors and the structures involved in the publication process. The structures are the institutions established by the state, while the actors are the participating experts, the institutions (once again, but now conceived of as agents) that are involved in knowledge production and dissemination, as well as the party-state and the population.

When the PRC was founded, Republican knowledge and research successes were incorporated and supplemented with foreign sources to complete its knowledge base. In the early 1950s, knowledge on healthy living and food was mostly imported from the West and the Soviet Union. Especially during the period in which the paradigm of "learning from the Soviet Union" was declared by Mao Zedong,[9] Russian publications were translated in order to form a basic canon of foreign knowledge.[10] Printed knowledge was, however, not the only source of scientific input for the PRC: knowledge was also transmitted through Soviet experts sent to China to participate in the socialist development, including in the establishment of China's health system. Soviet experts taught at Chinese universities and contributed to the PRC's science education.[11]

Despite this external input, which was both personal and theoretical, from the 1950s to the 1970s nutrition studies and food administration remained a relatively small part of the Ministry of Health, whereas there was a huge increase in health care work and a buildup of the hygiene infrastructure in a way that was unprecedented.[12] Nevertheless, a significant number of publications on nutrition can be found, especially in the 1950s, to such an extent that even during the disastrous Great Leap Forward, discussions on healthy food can be found in newspapers like the Ministry of Health–adjoined *Jiankangbao*.

THE MINISTRY OF HEALTH AS THE DRIVING FORCE

The actors and structures involved in the process of production of health knowledge were manifold, and were interlinked both with each other as well as with political institutions. The expert infrastructure was put in place primarily to generate and spread health knowledge. Since nutrition knowledge is also a part of this, it too was communicated through these channels. Before the founding of the PRC, public medical and hygiene work—which included food sanitation and rationing—of the Guomindang (GMD) and the Chinese

Communist Party (CCP) was mainly concentrated on the military sector and urban centers, as the Second Sino-Japanese War (1937–1945) and the Civil War (1927–1949) produced many wounded and sick patients and the infrastructure needed to care for them was only available in cities.

A first step in establishing an infrastructure for the spreading of health knowledge was the assembly of doctors from all over the country to provide for the growing demand for medical personnel in the first half of the twentieth century.[13] To accommodate the newly emerging medical schools and professionals, the military published materials in order to furnish a basis for learning. At the end of the 1940s, according to the *History of Healthcare and Hygiene in China* (*Zhongguo weisheng baojian shi* 中国卫生保健史, 1993), 776,220 titles on medical topics had been published, and in addition 126,750 volumes of magazines and 2,400 volumes of pictorial material had been supplied.[14] These huge amounts of publications indicate a need for theoretical material covering many aspects of hygiene and health. The interest of these materials concerns the recurring theme of prevention work, for example, the prevention of epidemics which tended to infect crowded military camps and flourished in places with low hygienic standards.[15] Medical personnel not only took care of diseases and the minor ailments (blisters, swellings) that occurred during warfare and the Long March, but also made sure that the terrain on which the companies rested was clean, while securing clean drinking water and sufficient edible food.[16]

A centralized and governmentally-led health system as a basis for knowledge dissemination became possible when a stable state emerged from the conflicts between nationalists and communists. Thus, upon the declaration of the PRC in 1949, the responsibility for providing for the population's health, especially for the workers and peasants who formed the basis of the new state's production cycle, fell to the new leaders. At first the Ministry of Health focused mainly on the fight against communicable diseases, so that such threats would no longer impact the population. Large-scale prevention work was thus the main focus at the time,[17] yet this makes the handbooks and articles dedicated to improving people's individual health through diet even more intriguing. I argue that those publications fall into the category of prevention work, though on a much smaller scale, as they sought to improve on health situations to build a strong body and immune system and thus avoid diseases.

The 1950s food hygiene work of the Ministry of Health was coordinated by the Health Care Office (Baojianchu 保健处), part of the Public Health Bureau (Gonggong weishengju 公共卫生局),[18] and strongly influenced by the paradigm of "learning from the Soviet Union."[19] The Health Care Office was concerned with nutrient problems in the population and their resolution.[20] To avoid wrong processing of food, and the poisoning of food by germs, in

1953 the state introduced food hygiene examinations, as well as nationwide nutrition inspections in different parts of China in 1959 and later in 1982. These nutrition inspections tried to evaluate the quality of the Chinese diet. They tested not only nutritional standards but also correlated diet to the population's physical state.[21] The fact that examinations like these took place illustrates the increasing awareness of the importance of the people's diet.[22]

Another subdepartment of the Ministry of Health involved in the distribution of nutrition knowledge was the Hygiene Propaganda Department (Weisheng xuanchuan chu 卫生宣传处), in existence between 1951 and 1961. It was responsible for health propaganda in the cities as well as in the countryside and factories. This bureau produced education material and also conducted education in schools. In order to guarantee the unity and high standard of publications on hygiene and health, the propaganda department introduced a review process for all submitted works.[23] The influence of this administrative system nevertheless waned over time, especially in the struggles with the Red Guards, as well during the 1960s and 1970s when most hygiene responsibilities of state organizations were handed down to grassroot levels. This loss of central state control culminated in a stop to the knowledge dissemination conducted by publishing houses and at schools, which directly translated into publication gaps.

Nutrition advice was not limited to publications for professionals in the health care system, but also included newspaper and magazine articles that were meant for everyday use and the education of the broad population. The temporal focus here lies on the early PRC period. The nutritional knowledge published in text form is mostly comprised of biomedical knowledge that was acquired through translations and from foreign sources. It also stems from the direct exchange between Chinese and foreign experts, especially the Soviet experts[24] who were responsible for the spreading of information at schools and through the health care system. It was then published in papers such as the *Jiankangbao* or the *Dazhong Yixue*.

The dissemination of nutrition knowledge mainly seems to have followed the top-down hierarchy of the socialist state, as the idea of nutritional governmentality would suggest. The knowledge published by the Ministry of Health shows the personal and institutional continuity in the knowledge production process: most of the Chinese nutrition experts received their training in pre-PRC times, and this knowledge thus continued to circulate, as some of the handbooks published in the 1950s are reedited prints from the late 1940s or earlier—such as the book by Shu Xincheng on regaining health.[25] The year 1949 cannot be understood as a major rupture in the development of nutrition science, nor in the context of general hygiene, despite the "victory" of Maoism in the ideological struggles of the 1940s.

THE CASE OF VITAMIN C

Commonly known for its beneficial attributes against scurvy as well as its benefits to the immune system, vitamin C, ascorbic acid, was identified as a vital part of the daily diet. Adequate supply—especially during the winter months—was mandatory for solid health. Its promotion was part of most health handbooks with a section on nutrients.[26]

Vitamin C, mostly called *weishengsu C* 维生素C or *weishengsu bing* 维生素丙, is generally declared to be one of the most important vitamins. Some publications also point to its other names such as *weitaming C* 维他命C, *mianju suan* 免疽酸, and *kanghuaixue suan* 抗坏血酸 (ascorbic acid): by introducing all these descriptions and linking them to the term in most widespread use, *weishengsu C*, the expression is standardized for the audience. Vitamin C is a concept that did not have any equivalents in Chinese medical theory until the introduction of Western medical knowledge. As a piece of new knowledge, it was explained as simply as possible. Most chapters on vitamins are structured similarly and use the same register to make understanding easier. They first describe the chemical compound, then the symptoms of a deficiency—illustrating the need for said vitamin—and in the end the sources of the vitamin.

The knowledge of vitamins in food and of their usefulness for a healthy body was meant to help the individual avoid deficiencies. To illustrate vitamin C's importance, in his 1950s article Wang Xunyi 王巽义 explains the deficiency—scurvy—by giving insight into its symptoms. Scurvy is sometimes described as sailors' disease, given that historically sailors often suffered from this deficiency at sea due to the absence of fresh vegetables.[27] Wang mentions the chemical reason why a lack of vitamin C is so disadvantageous. According to him, vitamin C is necessary for maintaining the binding connections between cells: these bonds break up when the body lacks vitamin C, which causes bruising and bleeding, resulting in scurvy symptoms.[28] Bleeding gums, a weak immune system, and fatigue are only a few of the obvious signs of this disease, against which Shu warns.[29] Since a weakened immune system is easy prey for bacteria and viruses and a breeding ground for infectious diseases, and since fatigue influences work performance and cognitive functioning, avoiding vitamin C deficiency was rather important to the author. It is interesting that Wang Xunyi (in 1950) and Weng Deli 翁德立 (in 1960) opt to invoke a largely Western maritime observation and transfer it into Chinese. It might have been more familiar for the average Chinese reader to refer to the lack of fresh produce in the winter months, as not only were sailors prone to scurvy but also the northern population, which had little access to fresh produce during the cold season. Especially during the winter months, with little vitamin C available, many people succumbed to scurvy symptoms.

While there is extensive discussion about its deficiency, the positive effects of vitamin C on the body are not mentioned as frequently, but Huang Chengguo 黄承国, author of the *Concise Nutrition Science* (*Jianming yingyang xue* 简明营养学) (1950), lists a few: a bolstered immune system, improved digestion of plant matter, and an improvement in energy burning can be expected by people who ingest enough vitamin C.[30] In Shu Xincheng's 1956 publication, vitamin C is praised as a compound that increases appetite, helps with teeth development, protects the circulatory system, and improves the immune system.[31] The small 1956 booklet *Diet and Health* (*Yinshi yu jiankang* 饮食与健康) by Dubuque and translated by Huang Zhenhua 黄振华and Zhang Yujian 张与健—originally in Russian—emphasizes the need to supply oneself with fresh produce to avoid scurvy. It suggests raising garden vegetables and collecting wild herbs. Vegetables suggested for growing include greens, green onions, fennel, and carrots to enhance the nutrition value of the diet.[32]

The problem with vitamin C is its water solubility and instability. Water that is used for cooking and then discarded can diminish a dish's vitamin content. Furthermore, vitamin C's strong adverse reaction to alkali and oxygen, especially in combination with copper utensils as well as heat, destroys its structure. Since the body cannot produce it, vitamin C has to be ingested directly to meet the required amount. Many of the examined texts give a range of processing suggestions to ensure a proper intake. The translation of a Russian handbook originally written by Dubuque offers an extensive list of suggestions on how to handle vitamin C:

1. If vegetables are cooked with peel, vitamins are preserved better; they should be peeled after cooking.
2. Peeled vegetables should not be soaked in water or cooked in it, because the vitamins will leak into the water and be lost.
3. Vegetables should be put into the pot after boiling a soup and not be cooked at high temperatures, as they lose nutritional value.
4. Vegetables should be cooked in enamel or aluminum pots, they should not be cooked in tin pots, as vitamin C is destroyed once it comes into contact with copper or iron.
5. When cooking vegetables, they have to be immersed in water, covered with a thick lid to prevent air from getting in.
6. The longer the vegetables cook on the stove, the more vitamins are destroyed.
7. The water vegetables were cooked in should not be discarded, but used, as it contains vitamins from the vegetables as well as minerals.

8. Dishes should not be set on one side to stand for too long, especially not on the stove or next to the fire as vitamins are lost there as well.
9. Alkali should not come in contact with food, because it damages vitamin C and B1.[33]

According to Liu Lin's 刘林 *Food Hygiene* (*Shipin weisheng* 食品卫生, 1957), not only is vitamin C susceptible to heat, but it also breaks down due to oxidization if food is cut up or stored for too long. According to Lin, adding sour substances to foods should help to preserve vitamin C and diminish the loss in nutrition upon processing.[34]

There is an abundance of vegetables and fruits that were deemed acceptable to satisfy the daily requirements of vitamin C. Vegetables that contain a sufficient amount of vitamin C and thus have to undergo this special preparation treatment during cooking include potatoes, cabbage, winter rape, carrots, tomatoes, Chinese yam, spinach, green onion, fennel, celery, mustard leaves, bean sprouts, chili peppers, cauliflower, radish, fresh peas, cucumber, green beans, and so forth. Fruits that are suggested to be eaten raw are citrus fruits (e.g., tangerines and lemons), berries and rose hips, persimmons, bananas, and so on.[35] As a way of preserving vitamin C in vegetables for the winter, pickling them is often mentioned, especially white cabbage. The vitamin content in pickled vegetables can be enhanced by preserving it in brine.

In case of vitamin C deficiency, most of the Mao-era publications agree that the solution is simply to increase the consumption of vitamin C–rich foods. Shu Xincheng concedes the possibility of taking vitamin pills, but also insists that this scientific invention does not really work as a long-term solution. In his eyes, the vitamins contained in foods that are eaten rate much higher than artificially produced vitamin pills.[36]

After this assessment of availability, the only question that remains to be answered is: How much vitamin C should be consumed? There are several possible ratios, depending on the age group, the work intensity, and individual situation. Dubuque recommends 50 grams of vegetables a day as a sufficient amount to cover a person's vitamin C needs. Other sources suggest between 30 and 100 milligrams of vitamin C per day, with increased amounts for pregnant and breastfeeding women.[37] According to the 1960 article by Weng Deli the daily intake for adults should be 75 milligrams. Pregnant women are advised to have 100 milligrams/day and breastfeeding women even 150 milligrams/day. Children, especially infants directly after birth, are said to need quite a lot of vitamin C: if the requirements cannot be met by mother's milk or food ingestion, supplements are recommended, 30 milligrams/day being seen as the minimum but some experts advocate a fuzzier range of 25–75 milligrams/day. At three to seven years of age 75 milligrams/day are recommended.[38] The suggestions for different workloads rank between 60 and 75 milligrams/day for light labor and the same holds true for moderate labor intensity with a slight increase for male workers.[39] For the case of heavy and very heavy labor the recommended amounts rise up to 100 milligrams per day. Generally, though the publications assigned importance to the ingestion of vitamin C, the amount that is required from the diet is not big and nor does it vary much. What this differentiated view on one nutrient shows, then, are the changing needs for different groups in the population. This will play an even bigger part in the following chapter, on meal plans and nutrition organization.

THE CASE OF PROTEIN

Contemporary Chinese materials on protein tap into the idea of protein as an important macronutrient for building strength. This idea has been the focus of worldwide discussions for quite some time, as evident in Kenneth Carpenter's article "The History of Enthusiasm for Protein." In some form this enthusiasm spans the twentieth century and even extends beyond the turn of the millennium. In his paper "The Rise and Fall of Paradigms in World Food and Nutrition Policy," Urban Jonsson describes the period between 1950 and 1974 as being marked by the influence of the "Protein deficiency paradigm."[40] This paradigm was prevalent in the Republican discussion of protein deficiency in the Chinese diet. Jia-Chen Fu introduces this discussion of protein quality and shows how sufficient access to protein sources involved considerations of the value of animal protein and soy protein. In the Republican era, animal proteins were seen as superior to plant proteins,[41] while the traditional soybean was understood to serve the body just as well as animal protein due to its chemical makeup and was reinstated as a valid protein source. The aim was to strengthen the nation, since protein was thought to have aided Western countries in ascending to their contemporary status as industrial powers.

In the spirit of continuity, it seems fitting that many of the Mao-era articles on nutrition emphasize protein as well. Still, the other macronutrients—fat and carbohydrates—are not forgotten in this discussion. Protein is not singled out, rather it is seen as part of a group of nutrients that are needed for optimal functioning of the human body. Nevertheless, proteins, as opposed to fats and carbohydrates, gain importance in one aspect: they are understood as building blocks of the human body and of life itself, and thus as necessary for growth and building a healthy population, as the nutrition scientist Zheng Ji 郑集 (1900–2010) emphasizes in a subchapter on protein in his 1952 publication *Practical Nutrition Science* (*Shiyong yingyangxue* 实用营养学).[42] Proteins are the material muscles consist of, so an increase in protein intake is sometimes equated with an increase in strength and vigor through muscle growth.

Interestingly, whereas paragraphs on vitamins focus primarily on deficiency symptoms and press for sufficient intake, paragraphs on protein do not tend to raise this issue as much.[43] One example of this is Chen Feirun 陈费润, who discusses deficiency in his *How to Manage Public Dining* (*Zenyang banhao gonggong shanshi* 怎样办好公共膳食) from 1954. Chen states that protein deficiency is accompanied by oedemas, especially in the feet and legs, and that these symptoms are easily overcome by increasing the ingestion of food and thus protein.[44] The 1950 *Dazhong Yixue* article "What's Adequate Nutrition?" (*Zenyang shi heli de yingyang?* 怎样是合理的营养) by Zhang Hongde 张鸿德, on the other hand, insists that while protein might be an important nutrient and that it is necessary to consume enough of it, too much may lead to health issues.[45] According to Shu Xincheng, excessive intake of this macronutrient could cause problems for the metabolism, as the kidneys could not process all of the protein ingested. This results in a loss of nutrients, which can cause ill-health for the body. Too little protein, on the other hand, might obstruct growth and result in low energy levels, which is exactly what nutrition science wanted to avoid.[46]

Proteins consist of amino acids, as explained by the handbooks. These different amino acids are listed by several sources, sometimes including their English translations which directly mark the information as imported foreign knowledge. The difference between essential and non-essential amino acids is specified, and the ingestion of the former is deemed mandatory, while the latter is considered optional as the body can produce them itself.[47] This leads to different preferences of food depending on the targeted amino acid content. While protein is associated with the buildup of muscles, carbohydrates and fats are responsible for the energy level, and this is due to their chemical structure. Some authors, such as Huang Chengguo or Chen Feirun, concur that it is possible to utilize protein as an energy source, albeit not as effectively as carbohydrates and fats. Since the breakdown of protein can cause some damage to the body, energy should be derived from fats and carbohydrates.[48]

The underlying question that interests most authors in this discussion is that of quality. What protein has the best quality relative to the human body? And how available is it? Amino acids can be found in plant- and animal-derived foods, and this is where the issue of quality arises. The latter is mostly seen as superior to the former, but when looking at the contemporary discussion in the PRC it becomes apparent that it is not only the quality of the amino acid itself which decides which protein is most suitable for consumption, but that environmental and economic factors also play a role. No judgment is passed on whether the population should consume more animal or more plant protein:[49] the sources only insist that animal proteins carry complete amino acid chains, whereas plant proteins do not. The need to consume complete proteins is a priority for most authors: Shu Xincheng, for example, prefers eggs, lean meats, and soy, because fish, grains, and vegetables contain only incomplete protein chains.[50] He does not insist on not consuming incomplete chains of amino acids, but for him in order to attain the full spectrum of proteins, it is necessary to consume both meat and plant foods. A 1965 *Jiankangbao* article published by the Nutrition Institute of the Chinese Academy of Medical Sciences and a 1979 article in the *Dazhong Yixue* by Yang Guangqi 杨光圻 display the same tone and vocabulary, lending credibility to the standardization argument.[51] The 1965 publication offers short and comprehensive explanations on macronutrients, minerals, and their importance. Yang's article goes further and gives a short overview of the historical development of Chinese cuisine as mainly vegetarian. This is seen as efficient in preventing cardiovascular diseases, but as lacking in sufficient sources of good protein. It thus gives rise to the modern need for careful introduction of animal proteins or soy protein. According to several authors, soy proves to be the cheapest protein alternative, before dairy, meat, or eggs: soy products such as tofu, soymilk, soy bean powder, and biscuits made from bean flour are all valid protein supplements.[52]

An approach to supplying sufficient complete amino acid chains is the combination of plant proteins in foods to create complete sets on the plate. In the *Dazhong Yixue* from December 1959, Tie Ju 铁菊 stresses that plant protein's only difference to animal protein is the way it should be consumed due to its incomplete amino acids. If plant proteins are strategically mixed during consumption to include all essential parts there should not be a problem. What Tie proposes is to manually form full sets of amino acids.[53] A later article by Wu Shunde 吴顺德 from November 1979 sees animal protein as easily digestible, and thus possessing high nutritional value as opposed to plant protein which is difficult to digest. For Wu animal protein suits the human physiology best: the problem was its availability and its high price. Wu recommends that increasing animal protein availability should be the focus of future endeavors to improve the Chinese diet. Protein levels should be adjusted to the rising living standard: plant proteins should be combined to form a complete set of amino acids so that no deficiencies arise when animal proteins are unavailable. Wu concludes that a diverse choice of foods should be made available, especially in public canteens, so that all needs are covered and no lack in protein can occur.[54]

Since it was a main building block for muscles—the power plants of the body—protein had to be ingested for not only health but for successful labor: thus the question arose of how much intake was just right. The recommended amount of daily protein intake varies between different social groups (divided according to sex, age, and work intensity), but remains approximately the same within each group over time. As with vitamin C, for the group of pregnant and breastfeeding women as well as children and infants, for example, Shu Xincheng advocates the consumption of higher dosages of protein than for the elderly.[55] He offers a thorough review of how people's daily protein intake should be assessed. To calculate daily protein consumption, he looks at the daily caloric intake: 10–15 percent of the daily calories should come from protein, 55–70 percent from carbohydrates, and 20–30 percent from fats. For a diet of about 2,400 kilocalories, this would result in 60–90 grams of protein a day.[56] In 1979, Wu Shunde suggests a daily protein requirement of 1.3 grams of protein per kilogram of body weight, which is higher than the suggestions in other publications.[57] He furthermore states that an intake below 1 gram per kilogram in the long run leads to adverse effects, such as loss of strength and weight, anemia, and oedema.[58]

The changes and increases in protein recommendations over time are not as huge as the claims regarding protein's importance might suggest.[59] Despite its prominent role in supporting labor, the actually recommended quantity of protein remains rather low. This leads to a range of different questions as to how experts arrived at the methods to calculate protein requirements and what prompted the small changes that we do observe. In the end, the calculated amount depends on the scientific consensus of how much protein was actually needed per kilogram of body weight to maintain health and function. What can be observed in this discussion, however, is the slow increase of recommended protein with an increase in labor strain: this links protein consumption to successful production and to the building of a "healthy army of workers."

The diet resulting from these explorations in nutrition science consists of building blocks that have to be combined according to the individual's needs, leading to calculable plans for breakfast, lunch, and dinner so as to provide sufficient energy and raw materials. Different authors including Shu Xincheng, Dubuque, Huang Chengguo, and Chen Meiyu offer differently structured meal plans, but all of them showcase the perception of food as a toolbox with which to optimize the body, as the following chapter will show.

Nutrition advice in Mao-era China was produced by a young organizational system, with the party-state as its head and publishing houses and medical personnel as its arms. From this system, a basic body of books and texts emerges to supply the readership with information on how to ideally nurture their bodies. The discussion at the beginning of this chapter has made clear, though, that the foundation for this system was laid during the Republican era.[60] Nutrition knowledge belongs to a common twentieth-century effort to modernize China, and some of the books we have examined are reprints from pre-PRC times combined with new research efforts, or were written by people educated pre-1949. The Mao era brought a widespread attempt to popularize this knowledge in a socialist context on a scale hitherto unseen. It exceeded the scope of the pre–Mao-era publication system, since the socialist state relied on mass mobilization and institutionalization to make a widespread dissemination of nutritional knowledge possible.

The origin of nutrition knowledge played a huge part in its dissemination, since although the personnel of the Ministry of Health were all Chinese, nutrition knowledge was imported from the West and the Soviet Union instead of using local (traditional) knowledge. All handbooks on nutrition stick resolutely to the biomedical path and do not introduce Chinese medical categories as a supplementary source.[61] The handbooks and articles on nutrition sciences primarily employ biomedical and biochemical information to construct their picture of nutrition. In it, food is no longer food but rather the sum of its parts, an accumulation of macro- and micronutrients with specific functions. Scientific methods are the key to determining what compounds are contained in different kinds of food and how much the human body needs daily to function at an optimal level. The fact that food is no longer seen as a whole, and that the focus is shifted toward its components, results in meal plans and food suggestions that can be compared to medical prescriptions: if symptom A occurs, take nutrient B, or, to receive the most benefits from your food, the meal has to contain the following nutrients. And while it seems practical to supplement nutrients with pills, most authors considered here still advocate nutrient intake via food, especially protein and vitamin C.

Against the backdrop of modernization in China, the human body is increasingly described as a machine that needs fuel.[62] The concept of nutrition substantiates this. This development in thinking about the body and its nourishment makes physical control possible, both through external forces (the state) and at the level of individuals themselves. Just as the body's needs can be measured, so can the quantities of fuel, that is, food. The realization that the body's needs can be calculated prepares the way for the question of responsibility. If a well-balanced diet can be communicated to the population by the leadership, then the responsibility lies with the knowing individual to nourish their body for optimal health and in turn for optimal production, making it a group effort to strengthen the nation. The push to be a healthy individual is delivered by the narrative of being a good socialist. In effect it leaves individuals with no choice but to opt for a healthy body. Nutrition science also allocates some responsibility to the state, since it makes state planning and building more accurate, so enabling a preliminary determination of how large the harvest needs to be to feed the nation properly in order to obtain healthy workers.

NOTES

1. An early version of this chapter has been published in the *Routledge Handbook of Food in Asia* (2019). It has since been reworked and completed with additional references and material.

2. See Seung-Joon Lee, "The Patriot's Scientific Diet: Nutrition Science and Dietary Reform Campaigns in China, 1910s–1950s," *Modern Asian Studies* 6, no. 49 (February 2015).

3. Mark Swislocki, "Nutritional Governmentality—Food and the Politics of Health in Late Imperial and Republican China," *Radical History Review*, no. 110 (Spring 2011): 12.

4. Swislocki offers a thorough examination of how hunger, that is, malnutrition, was perceived over time. The shift from focusing on the deficiency issues of the nobility in the Qing empire, to the famine issues of lower-class Chinese in the Republican era, show a remarkable change in perception as well as scientific assessment. See here also James Vernon, *Hunger—A Modern History* (London: Belknap Press, 2007).

5. See Lizzie Collingham, *The Taste of War* (London: Penguin Books, 2011).

6. Lee, "The Patriot's Scientific Diet," 4.

7. Gyorgy Scrinis called this phenomenon *nutritionism*. See Gyorgy Scrinis, "On the Ideology of Nutritionism," in *Contemporary Transitions*, ed. Jeffrey M. Pilcher, vol. 4 of *Food History: Critical and Primary Sources* (London: Bloomsbury, 2015).

8. Willy Kraus, *Wirtschaftliche Entwicklung und sozialer Wandel in der Volksrepublik China* (Berlin: Springer-Verlag, 1979), 187.

9. Thomas Bernstein and Hua-yu Li give a detailed account of all the facets of learning in their edited volume *China Learns from the Soviet Union, 1949–present* (Lanham: Lexington Books, 2010).

10. Xi Gao, "Foreign Models of Medicine in Twentieth-Century China," in *Medical Transitions in Twentieth-Century China*, ed. Bridie Andrews and Mary Brown Bullock (Bloomington: Indiana University Press, 2014), 185–202; AnElissa Lucas, "Changing Medical Models in China: Organizational Options or Obstacles?" *The China Quarterly*, no. 83 (September 1980): 471, 477.

11. This exchange did not progress without hiccups, which Shen Zhihua and Guy Alitto discuss in their 2002 article on the issues of Soviet experts in the PRC and the areas in which they helped build the young socialist nation, supplementing the account by Deborah Kaple in her 1998 article "Soviet Advisors in China in the 1950s." See Shen Zhihua and Guy Alitto, "A Historical Examination of the Issue of Soviet Experts in China: Basic Situation and Policy Changes," *Russian History* 29, no. 2 (2000): 377–400; and Deborah A. Kaple, "Soviet Advisors in China in the 1950s," in *Brothers in Arms: The Rise and Fall of the Sino-Soviet Alliance, 1945–1963*, ed. O. A. Westad (Washington, D.C.: Woodrow Wilson Center Press, 1998). Kaple (p. 121) lists 17 experts sent to the Ministry of Health. See also Shen Zhihua, *Sulian zhuanjia zai Zhongguo* 苏联专家在中国 (Beijing: Zhongguo guoji chubanshe, 2003).

12. This also manifested in the educational realm, as suggested by an article in the *Jiankangbao* about two open letters to the Ministry of Health by concerned professionals on the issue of sufficient dietetics classes for aspiring doctors and hygiene

personnel: "Yingyang gongzuozhong de wenti jidaijiejue 营养工作中的问题急待解决," *Jiankangbao* (June 18, 1957), as well as within the five-year plans, which concentrated on increasing the numbers of hospital beds and medical personnel, see Kraus, *Wirtschaftliche Entwicklung und sozialer Wandel*, 42–47, 95–96, 187–88.

13. Chen Haifeng 陈海锋, ed., *Zhongguo weisheng baojianshi* 中国卫生保健史 (Shanghai: Shanghai kexuejishu chubanshe, 1993), 26, 32. See also Lucas, "Changing Medical Models in China" and Gao, "Foreign Models of Medicine."

14. Chen Haifeng, *Zhongguo weisheng baojianshi*, 77.

15. Chen Haifeng, 43, 63.

16. Chen Haifeng, 63.

17. Miriam Gross and Kawai Fan, "Schistosomiasis," in Andrews and Bullock, *Medical Transitions in Twentieth-Century China*, 106–25.

18. The public health bureau was established in 1949 and renamed the Weisheng fangyisi 卫生防疫司 in 1953. It changed in rank and was reorganized so that the formerly subordinated health care office, established in 1954, was split from its structure and stood alone afterward. The health care office was closed down in 1964 and reopened in 1985. Weishengbu bangongshi ting, *Weishengbu lishi kaoji*, 23, 31, 36.

19. Lucas, "Changing Medical Models in China," 463.

20. Weishengbu bangongshi ting, *Weishengbu lishi kaoji*, 23.

21. Chen Haifeng, *Zhongguo weisheng baojianshi*, 129–30.

22. It should be noted that the improvements recorded in the 1980s' examination cannot solely be attributed to an improved health care system or enhanced knowledge about food, but possibly to higher living standards and increased food availability.

23. Weishengbu bangongshi ting, *Weishengbu lishi kaoji*, 27.

24. Gao, "Foreign Models of Medicine," 196.

25. Shu Xincheng, *Wo zenyang huifu jiankangde* 我怎样恢复健康的 (Beijing: Zhonghua shuju chubanshe, 1956). Another booklet that was reprinted in the early Mao era and which points to increased demand for and interest in the topic was Chen Feirun's work from 1954 on how to run a public canteen, both editions titled *Zenyang banhao gonggong shanshi* 怎样办好公共膳食 (Chen Feirun 陈费润, ed., *Zenyang banhao gonggong shanshi* 怎样办好公共膳食 (Shanghai: Zhonghua shuju chuban, 1951) and [Chen] Feirun [陈]费润, ed., *Zenyang banhao gonggong shanshi* 怎样办好公共膳食 [Beijing: Renmin weisheng chubanshe, 1954]). The latter is a revised version of the former, since when looking at the paragraph on proteins one can see that the later edition has a whole paragraph added with some additional information in form of tables and a quotation in Russian.

26. Huang Chengguo 黄承国, ed., *Jianming yingyang xue* 简明营养学 (Shanghai: Xinan yixue shushe, 1950), 9–10; [Chen] Feirun, *Zenyang banhao gonggong shanshi*, 15–16; Chen Meiyu 陈美愉, *Yingyang weisheng* 营养卫生 (Beijing: Renmin weisheng chubanshe, 1954), 76–80; Chen Shuqi 陈叔骐, *Yingyang weisheng* 营养卫生 (Beijng: Renmin weisheng chubanshe, 1954), 11–12; N. E. Dubuque (Qiubiyouke 裘毕尤克), *Yinshi yu jiankang* 饮食与健康, trans. Huang Zhenhua黄振华 and Zhang Yujian 张与健 (Shanghai: Xin zhishi chubanshe, 1956), 12–13; Liu Lin 刘林, ed., *Shipin weisheng* 食品卫生 (Beijing: Renmin weisheng chubanshe, 1957), 11–12.

27. Wang Xunyi 王巽义, "Weishengsu shi zenyang faxiande? 维生素是怎样发现的?," *Dazhong Yixue* 8 (1950): 142–45; Wang Xunyi was a biologist working at the Tongji hospital in Shanghai. He graduated in 1941 from Shanghai Tongji University Hospital, in 1947 he went to Basel, Switzerland, to study, and returned after the PRC was founded. He coedited the first edition of the *Shengli Huaxue* 生理化学 journal. (See the entry on Wang Xunyi in Wu Mengchao 吴孟超 and Wu Zaide 吴在德, *Bainian yixue Tongji ren: bainian lai woguo yixue shiye fazhan zhong de Tongji he Tongjiren* 百年医学同济人: 百年来我国医学事业发展中的同济和同济人 (Shanghai: Tongji daxue chubanshe, 2009): 第三节 生物化学和分子生物学，四，同济人业绩. See also Weng Deli 翁德立, "Kangxuebing 坏血病" *Dazhong Yixue* 2 (1960): 52.

28. Wang Xunyi 王巽义, "Weishengsu shi zenyang faxiande? 维生素是怎样发现的?" *Dazhong Yixue* 8 (1950): 142–5.

29. Dubuque, *Yinshi yu jiankang*, 12; Shu Xincheng, *Wo zenyang huifu jiankangde*, 9.

30. Huang Chengguo, *Jianming yingyang xue*, 10. Huang Chengguo is mentioned by Chen Feirun in his foreword as a colleague.

31. Shu Xincheng, *Wo zenyang huifu jiankangde*, 50.

32. Dubuque, *Yinshi yu jiankang*, 13.

33. Dubuque, 14–16.

34. Liu Lin, *Shipin weisheng*, 12.

35. The information within the materials utilized here was meant for all of China. There are no references to regional specifics and possible differences in diet between different places.

36. Shu Xincheng, *Wo zenyang huifu jiankangde*, 53. It can be observed when looking at the advertisements in newspapers that vitamin supplements became more and more common.

37. These two groups also get special attention where protein is concerned.

38. Weng Deli, "Kangxuebing 坏血病," 52.

39. Shu Xincheng, *Wo zenyang huifu jiankangde*; Qu Huiqing, *Jiating yingyang shipu*; Hou Xiangchuan 侯祥川, ed., *Yingyangxue jinzhan* 营养学进展 (Shanghai: Shanghai kexue jishu chubanshe, 1966); Zhongguo renminjiefangjun Nanjingjunqu junyi xuexiao, *Yinshi yingyang weishengxue jiangyi* 饮食营养卫生学讲义(Nanjing: Nanjing junqu junyi xuexiao, 1976); Zhongguo yixue kexueyuan weisheng yanjiusuo, ed., *Shiwu chengfen biao* 食物成分表 (Beijing: Renmin weisheng chubanshe, 1977); Chen Xuecun 陈学存, *Yingyong yingyang xue* 应用营养学 (Beijing: Renmin weisheng chubanshe, 1984).

40. Urban Jonsson, "The Rise and Fall of Paradigms in World Food and Nutrition Policy (Commentary)," *World Nutrition* 1, no. 3 (June 2010): 134–36. As far as the question of actual protein deficiency is concerned, it should be said here that a deficiency in protein only occurs when there is a severe caloric deficit, meaning that protein deficiency often is a sign of starvation.

41. The reason for this argument is the completeness of animal-protein-contained amino acids, whereas plant proteins do not contain all essential amino acids readily available.

42. Zheng Ji 郑集, *Shiyong yingyangxue* 实用营养学 (Shanghai: Huadong yiwu shenghuoshe, 1952), 15–24. Fu introduces Zheng Ji's work as a Chinese nutritionist in the first half of the twentieth century. Fu focuses on his view on the deficiencies of the Chinese diet. Zheng Ji is a well-known nutritionist in the PRC. He received his PhD from Indiana University and returned back home to China in 1934 where he held several different medical and academic positions and published extensively on nutrition science. Jia-Chen Fu, *The Other Milk: Reinventing Soy in Republican China* (Seattle: University of Washington Press, 2018). See also Zhou Mian 周棉, ed., *Zhongguo liuxuesheng dacidian* 中国留学大辞典 (Nanjing: Nanjing daxue chubanshe, 1999), 284.

43. This could be expected, given that there seems to have been an inherent fear of protein deficiency in the West in the 1950s (Jonsson, "The Rise and Fall of Paradigms," 134–36).

44. [Chen] Feirun, *Zenyang banhao gonggong shanshi*, 4–6.

45. Zhang Hongde 张鸿德, "Zenyang shi heli de yingyang? 怎样是合理的营养?" *Dazhong Yixue* 8 (1950): 118–19.

46. Shu Xincheng, *Wo zenyang huifu jiankangde*, 35.

47. Zhang Hongde, "Zenyang shi heli de yingyang? 怎样是合理的营养?" *Dazhong Yixue* 8 (1950): 118–19.

48. Huang Chengguo, *Jianming yingyang xue*, 5; [Chen] Feirun, *Zenyang banhao gonggong shanshi*, 4.

49. This contrasts with the sharp criticism of vegetarian protein sources in Fu's observations.

50. Shu Xincheng, *Wo zenyang huifu jiankangde*, 33.

51. Zhongguo yixue kexueyuan yingyang yanjiusuo, "Danbaizhi, zhifang, tang he wujiyan 蛋白质，脂肪，醣和无机盐," in *Jiankangbao* (November 6, 1965); Yang Guangqi 杨光圻, "Shanshide danbaizhi 膳食的蛋白质," *Dazhong Yixue* 1 (1979): 3.

52. See, for example, [Chen] Feirun, *Zenyang banhao gonggong shanshi*; Chen Meiyu, *Yingyang weisheng*; Shu Xincheng, *Wo zenyang huifu jiankangde*.

53. Tie Ju 铁菊, "Zhiwuxing shiwu neng gonggei renti bixu de danbaizhi ma? 植物性食物能供给人体必需的蛋白质吗?" *Dazhong yixue* 12 (1959): 452.

54. Wu Shunde 吴顺德, "*Dongwu danbaizhi yu zhiwu danbaizhi* 动物蛋白与植物蛋白," *Dazhong Yixue* 11 (1979): 23.

55. Shu Xincheng, *Wo zenyang huifu jiankangde*, 34.

56. Shu Xincheng, 67.

57. Usually, protein suggestions are 1 gram of protein per kilogram of body weight per day.

58. Wu Shunde, "*Dongwu danbaizhi yu zhiwu danbaizhi* 动物蛋白与植物蛋白," *Dazhong Yixue* 11 (1979): 23.

59. For a detailed discussion of the development of protein suggestions, see the following chapter.

60. Lee, "The Patriot's Scientific Diet," 30–2.

61. There are, nevertheless, Chinese Medicine publications that talk about dietary cures for diseases, such as the *Changjian jibing minjian yinshi liaofa* 常见疾病民间饮食疗法 from 1964 by Zheng Qiming 郑启明. See also Ruth Rogaski, *Hygienic*

Modernity: Meanings of Health and Disease in Treaty-Port China (Berkeley: University of California Press, 2004), 304–5.

62. This metaphor is not new to the Mao era; see Hsiang-lin Lei, "Moral Community of *Weisheng*: Contesting Hygiene in Republican China," *East Asian Science, Technology and Society* 3 (2009): 482.

Chapter 2

Spaces of Food

Food is a basic component of everyday life and is usually enjoyed in the form of meals. In the twentieth century these meals are the translation of nutrition knowledge into practical and applied techniques called cooking. This practical application of nutrition knowledge and the reassembly of previously fragmented foods shows how nutrition science controls what is considered food and how, in turn, food controls daily life. The discussion in this chapter turns to focus on the period from the late 1950s to the beginning of the 1960s, a time when, through the founding of public canteens, meals were granted their own space in the political system of socialist China, a space that was regulated, standardized, and structured by governmental authorities. I argue that meal plans were a way to structure the population's diet and to control bodies. The space of nutrition provision in which those plans were executed moved between home kitchens and public canteens due to the political and social impact of the Great Leap Forward. This movement, however, had no repercussions for the content of nutrition knowledge.

By looking at what was on the menu in public eating spaces, one can assess how nutrition knowledge was put into practice and what the ideal was supposed to look like. Apart from the disbalance between the imagined ideal and the reality as it was in fact carried out, this chapter looks into the way proper meal plans were formed and the plans for the preparation and serving of meals. Yet before diving into the source material on meal planning, adequate diet structures, and preparation routines, a few words are necessary on eating as a universal physiological need and a cultural practice. George M. Foster and Barbara G. Anderson go into detail about medical practices and anthropological observations on health, and venture down the road of nutrition to observe the problems that in the past arose globally due to malnutrition not only in adults but also in children. Against this background they look at the cultural construction and social definition of food.[1] Since food influences everything in daily life, it is not simply connected to a practice of eating, but also linked to authority, logistics, identity, and cultural and social relations. Foster and Anderson distinguish between food and nutriments, so as to sharpen the difference between what is seen culturally as edible and enjoyable and what is scientifically defined as nourishment. In the Chinese context this distinction is acknowledged but then forsaken, as the focus is placed distinctly on nutrient quality instead of the cultural notion of edibility. Thus, the distinction between food and nutriment gets lost.[2] For the sake of the modernizing and strengthening of society, a science-based diet and understanding of food takes center stage in China. This understanding changes the perception of food in a profound way, since food—viewed through a quality lens—stops being a meal or a dish and becomes fuel in the form of nutrients, as described previously.[3] Foster and Andersen further remark that food has to be adjusted to local and cultural preferences in order to be successfully adopted; although this may indeed be witnessed in many cases, it is not in fact paramount for the perceived success of a scientific diet.[4]

For China, the symbolic meaning of food and meals was always tightly linked to the idea of the traditional family. This connection was broken when, in the first decade of the PRC's existence, eating was moved from the privacy of the home to the public space of canteens. At the same time, knowledge of nutrition was supplied to the population to further the understanding of nutrition on the path to reaching the state's goal of strengthening the nation. Eating as a social and political activity in those public spaces was understood as a spatially uniform activity, that is, not displaying regional differences in nutrient needs across China. The uniform cooking instructions published for all parts of the large nation pay tribute to this understanding.

Guo Yuhua takes stock of China's generational eating habits and their meaning for society and politics in her 2000 article "The Generation Gap at the Table." Nutrition and eating used to be a matter for the family, and was often tied to generations coming together to share a meal. By exploring the dynamics of these different age groups today, the impact that nutrition science and consumerism have had on the Chinese population becomes tangible. The three current generations (the grandparent generation, the parents, and the children) symbolize three different knowledges of food: traditionalist, modernist, and consumerist.[5] The traditionalist knowledge corresponds to the grandparent generation who grew up during the Republican era. They experienced the founding of the PRC and the arrival of widespread anti-illiteracy and anti-superstition campaigns. They lived through the Great Famine and the Cultural Revolution and were traumatized in various ways.[6] Traditional food knowledge postulates that both *yin* and *yang* need to be maintained for food to be considered nutritious. Imbalances can be prevented or fixed by adjusting the essential parts of daily meals and the regulating the indulgence in diverse and natural foods.[7] The modernist knowledge of food, on the other hand, being the knowledge of the parent generation, is the science-based knowledge that entered China during the late nineteenth and twentieth centuries. This generation's attitude with respect to diet is strongly influenced by the scientific and nutritionist paradigm.[8] Today's parent generation is comprised of survivors of the Great Leap Forward and the Cultural Revolution, who are heavily influenced by the Mao era and its push for science. They rely heavily on scientific facts and discoveries when planning their children's meals, in order to provide better for them and lay a good foundation for their health. They were targeted directly or indirectly by Mao-era knowledge production, and in the process a generation was created that started to think about food in scientific terms.[9] The preoccupation with nutrition sciences results in a diet that came out of a surge of nutritionist publications that reflect what Gyorgy Scrinis termed *nutritionism*.[10] Consumerist knowledge of food, finally, is concerned with today's food choices, being influenced by a culture of consumerism and advertisements.[11]

The distinction between traditional and modernist knowledge is central for my discussion of nutrition science in mid-twentieth-century China, as it describes the transition from old (traditional) nutrition knowledge to the (new) scientific diet made up of macro- and micronutrients.

NUTRITIONAL GOVERNMENT AND THE GREAT FAMINE

Discussing food during the Mao era inevitably leads one to consider the institutionalization of canteens as spaces of nutrition, ideology, and politics. They have been discussed by scholars such as Dikötter, Manning and Wemheuer, Watson, and Eyferth[12] in their research on the period of the Great Leap Forward (1958–1962). Canteens are identified as a major contributor to the famine.[13]

During the PRC's attempt at rapid development of heavy industries and social restructuring toward a communist society, the effort known as the Great Leap Forward, the direct impact of canteens on the Chinese population's nutrition was heavy, albeit short-lived. Although the Great Leap's attempt at governing and controlling Chinese life was based on scientific standards, it failed miserably. The PRC government intended to create a fully controlled eating space for a combination of nutritional and ideological benefit. In order to implement this, first, private kitchens were abolished in the rural areas so as to free up labor, especially female labor power, and to bring family life into the open at the newly established canteens. The public dining halls and factory dining halls helped in restructuring daily life and the logistics of food distribution. Ideally, they would provide food for everybody: historical circumstances, however, led to a very different outcome. Contrary to the original intentions, droughts and misinformation culminated in severe emaciation and starvation.[14]

James L. Watson has examined the actual events at public canteens during their short period of existence and comes to a very sobering conclusion: 6,789 canteens were created as an ideological idea following a utopian vision, but in reality they never worked. For one thing, food quality was bad and often no food was served at all.[15]

The introduction of public canteens is tied to the establishment of the communes in the early PRC. The basic idea was to erase the family kitchen as a central place of social interaction in order to build up Communism. By founding communes and collectivizing everything, even kitchen tools and utensils, the act of cooking was taken from the homes and put into a public space: the public canteen, or as Watson calls it "the mess hall."[16] In exploring the "low cuisine," Watson makes a point of the fact that the dishes in these halls tasted vile.[17] The raison d'être of the canteens was the well-intentioned freeing of women's labor from domestic responsibilities: instead of doing household chores they could now work in the factories or in the fields and contribute productive labor to the Great Leap for economic development. The ideological usefulness of public canteens also extends to the rest of the working masses, following the Communist authorities' preoccupation "with the problem of time"—namely the fact that more work hours were needed. Eating at a canteen close to or on their worksite would free people from having to return home and prepare their meals on their own. By this means, the societal core, the family, and the home as a place to retire from labor and the outside world, was destroyed. Eating at home was collectivized and transformed into a public event during which political propaganda and other ideological education could be spread among the eaters.[18]

The (dis-)functionality of the canteen system centered on the problem with produce redistribution, alongside the collectivization of kitchens and the Maoist slogan "eat well, eat full." First, grain, vegetables, and even coal were redirected toward the canteens to ensure better availability for them. Then the slogan caused overconsumption in canteens, which led to future shortages. Additionally, the canteens did not function according to the required standards. Food was often lacking in quality and was cold or unsanitary.[19]

In *Mao's Great Famine*, Dikötter additionally mentions the unwillingness of the population to participate in eating at public canteens due to their inability to provide for individual tastes and preferences, and the fact that they often were located far from people's homes and worksites.[20] The association with a lack of everything, with poverty and with crippling hunger, still lives on in the public narrative of the Great Leap Famine. It is, however, often contradicted by the memory of a feeling of great solidarity and social connection.[21] This memory embodies the ideal that was sought after: a collective feeling among the villagers and patrons of the canteens. This ideal is, of course, overshadowed by the brutal account of reality, when at the height of the Great Famine the canteens proved useless to feed the population, and in fact mostly provided meals devoid of nutrition.[22] Other methods to provide nutrients were sought after, such as food augmentation, these methods being promoted when grain rations could no longer sustain the population. Despite the introduction of public canteens, food augmentation was frequent at the time, as famine devastated the population. The augmentation methods were based on the idea that by intensively processing food a more nutritious or at least belly-filling product would emerge. The idea of achieving more nutrition by cooking rice several times seems absurd, but it was attempted by the "advanced rice-cooking methods," double-steamed buns, or ingesting "superfoods" such as chlorella.[23] The actual nutritional plans I introduce are far from these dire attempts to achieve some feeling of satiation in the population via augmented foods.

Contrary to the claimed focus on food and its distribution in canteens, food itself was not the actual reason for introducing public canteens in the first place. Their rational above all else was the freeing of labor.[24] In *The Big Rice Pot—The Whole Story About Public Canteens in the Countryside* (*Daguofan—nongcun gonggongshitang shimo* 大锅饭—农村公共食堂始末), Luo Pinghan looks at statistics and official papers to reconstruct what transpired in the public canteens. Public canteens were not only supposed to supply the population with food and needed sustenance, but were also a way to control the population—as would be expected in a context of nutritional governmentality.[25] Public canteens could have functioned as a way to overcome malnutrition, but the most important aspects of them were the socialist practices to which they were linked, that is, the collective practices of eating, lecturing, and gathering. The expected increase in production potential by lessening household workload was a much more prominent point in favor of public canteens than the nutrition they provided for the workers.

The ideological pull to visit the canteens was the idea of eating one's fill at their tables. In the spirit of socialist construction, this political encouragement in the first months of the canteens' existence may have been a sign of prosperity, but it was strongly opposed to the notion of not wasting food advocated in the handbooks on eating.[26] Neither does it comply with the idea of exact planning, as eating uncontrollably hardly makes rationing possible. And it also does not comply with the idea of the specific amount of calories needed for production. It does, however, contribute to the point the CCP and the Chinese government were trying to make at the time: that the new era would bring more prosperity to everyone.

Instead of engaging with the tragedy of the Great Leap Forward, this chapter acknowledges the disaster but looks instead at the ideas and plans that were intended to improve the population's health during the Great Leap. The canteens were believed to be a way to solve the problem of nutrition by feeding the population in a controlled environment. In this particular case, however, idea and reality could not have been further apart.

Public Canteens

In retrospect, many of the accounts of the Great Leap Forward tell a story of hunger and disorganization, despite the attempts to create well-planned canteens. Canteens were seen as a tool to provide food for the masses without impacting production, and so to prevent hunger. They were not supposed to offer bland and restrictive foods, nor to be an unstructured institution. Originally, on paper, canteens were strictly planned out and given specific instructions to guarantee a hygienic, functional environment in which to serve nourishing foods.

A public canteen (*gonggong shitang* 公共食堂)[27] is a space constructed and run with the goal of feeding the workers of a factory or residents of a town. Public canteens were more than just ideologically charged spaces that allowed the population access to food: they were also a tool to control the flow of grain, the intake of nutrients, and a space where the CCP could demonstrate its influence on everybody's life. They imposed nutritional governmentality to the last calorie, since public canteens were places where nutrition knowledge could be enforced.

Nutrition knowledge could be handed directly to an individual for personal use in the form of books, lectures, and talks, but building a suitable cooking and consumption environment, that is, a canteen, made its immediate implementation possible. Regulations concerning the canteen set up, hygiene, and staff directions optimized canteen workflows, so that healthy food could be delivered to the guests. One tool to circulate this knowledge to staff, cadres, and the population were handbooks on managing canteens.[28] In them the readership finds nutrition information and explanations, cooking tips and advice on how to organize canteen infrastructure, including how to build one. The canteen layouts had to offer enough space for adequate storage, cooking, and cleaning facilities, as well as an area for eating. Compared to home kitchens, this was a highly specialized working area, which was explained in detail to the audience to enhance their understanding of a modern cooking institution.

An example of canteen architecture can be found in Chen Meiyu's 陈美愉1954 handbook *Nutrition Hygiene* (*Yingyang weisheng* 营养卫生) (figure 2.1). She not only included instructions on building well-aired storage facilities,[29] but also on how a kitchen had to be constructed in order to function well and to serve the masses hygienically. It had to have a large enough worksurface (No. 28, cemented working counter, Nos. 25 and 32, chopping

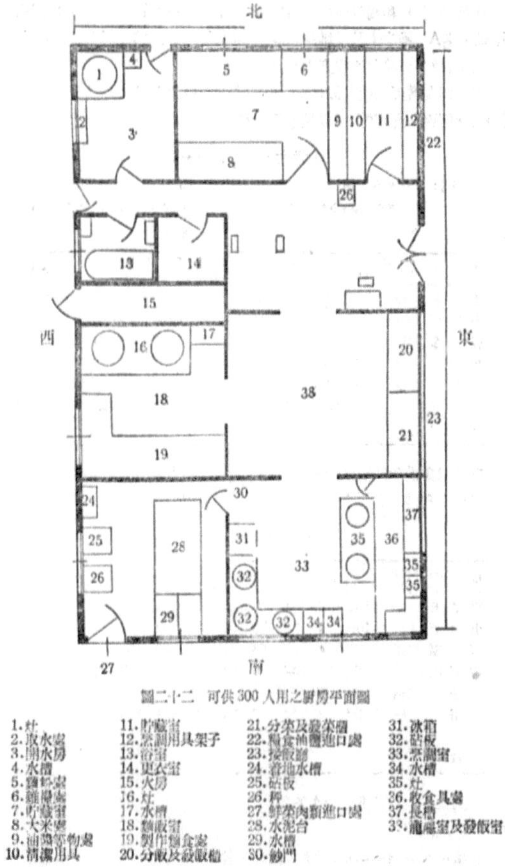

Figure 2.1. Blueprint of a canteen layout.
Source: Chen Meiyu, Yingyang weisheng, 199.

boards), building materials had to be suited for the purpose of a kitchen, there had to be a skylight for the air to leave the building, a food preparation room (No. 18, a room for the preparation of flour and rice dishes, including No. 19, a noodle-making station), a separate cooking room (No. 33) with running water and a stove (No. 35); there also had to be storage rooms (Nos. 7 and 11), an office, a bathroom (No. 13), a changing room (No. 14), and a washing room for the utensils (No. 10).[30]

The canteen administration was rationalized and bureaucratic, with structures and routines in place for purchasing, planning, and execution. Not only were separate rooms and staff assigned very specific jobs, but the procurement and production of food was also thoroughly managed. Lists of food that had to be procured were kept and updated for each purchase. In addition to this, inventory lists and calculations of the numbers of patrons and nutrient contents of daily menus had to be made by the canteen staff to provide adequate resources. Additionally, questionnaires on health status and deficiency symptoms were supplied in order to adjust the nourishment supplied, showing the need to assess the physical conditions of the populace.[31]

In the same year as Chen Meiyu's publication on nutritional hygiene was published, Chen Feirun's booklet *How to Manage Public Eating Well* (*Zenyang banhao gonggongshanshi* 怎样办好公共膳食) (1954) was reprinted.[32] Chen Feirun—as advertised by the title—touches on the issue of eating in public spaces, which includes public canteens. His focus is not only the proper management but also and especially the cleanliness and proper storage of food. He clearly warns the audience of water contamination and pests.[33] Architecturally, Chen Feirun differentiates between areas in the building such as the preparation room, the cooking room, the office, or storage. He lays out blueprints for ideal buildings and storage facilities by way of further explanation.[34] One of those is a large foldable print of a canteen for 500 people. The picture is annotated in great detail and shows all the functional rooms described by Chen Feirun and Chen Meiyu.[35]

On the topic of work done in the kitchens, Chen Feirun confirms the observations made in Chen Meiyu's text: there are thorough instructions concerning the procuring, storing, prepping, processing, and serving of food in order to guarantee the running of the kitchen, as well as hygiene standards.[36] Chen Feirun's booklet includes detailed instructions concerning the preparation process. Just as the place where meals were eaten changed fundamentally with the introduction of public canteens, so did the way food was served. There were two ways of having a meal in a public canteen: shared dishes—the more traditional way—or separate dishes—the more hygienic way, so that germs could not be passed along as easily. The sharing of food is not completely denounced by Chen Feirun, but he remarks favorably on the possibility of portioning food more correctly in the case of separate dishes for each person. This offers far better possibilities to calculate amounts, and it prevents germs from spreading.[37]

The topic of hygiene was not lost on the managers of public canteens, and appears rather often as a topos in articles in the *Jiankangbao* that report on the success of the canteens. Articles such as "Manage Public Canteens Well, Ensure Production and Construction" (Banhao gonggong shitang, baozheng shengchan jianshe 办好公共食堂，保证生产建设) (September 15, 1958), "Anguo County's Canteens' Hygiene Was Raised Remarkably" (Anguo xian shitang weisheng xianzhu tigao 安国县食堂卫生显著提高) (December 13, 1958), or "Jishan County's Public Canteens Put Nutritious Recipe Book into Effect" (Jishan xian gonggong shitang tuixing yingyang shipu 稷山县公共食堂推行营养食谱) (April 27, 1960) all link hygiene and nutrition to the canteens' success as a support for labor, despite the above-mentioned issues from which by 1959 all public dining halls were suffering.[38] These articles are not evidence of good conduct on the part of the managers or staff, but they are a vehicle to perpetuate the value of public eating, its high standards of hygiene, and the message concerning healthy and nutritious food. The articles can also be interpreted as encouragement for others to follow in opening well-run, hygienic canteens.

Planning Calories

In order to manage a public canteen efficiently, costs and menu items had to be calculated. How did the authors of public eating and nutrition handbooks figure out what a nourishing daily menu would contain? In a world that quantifies everything, the answer to this question comes from a complete measurement of the body as regards its energy needs, and the correlative quantification of foodstuffs. This is also how food becomes a tool of statecraft.[39]

In the case of public canteens, the governing aspect of the rationalization of food becomes more pronounced, as the personal choice for healthy foods is taken away from the individual peasant or worker. Instead, the daily menu orients itself along the macro- and micronutrient requirements of the different population groups (defined by age, sex, labor intensity). Depending on these parameters, each group requires different energy amounts: the heavier the workload, the more calories are supplied. The requirements are often summed up in tables containing the different target groups, their workload, and the nutriment requirements.

A proposal from the 1961 publication *Nutrition Hygiene* (*Yingyang weishengxue* 营养卫生学) illustrates this idea of adequate nutrition for each stage of life. It is very detailed and comprises a fair amount of information on age groups, labor groups and their nutrient requirements, and common ways to convey nutrition knowledge. Developed by the China Academy of Medical Sciences (Zhongguo yixue kexueyuan 中国医学科学院),[40] a detailed nutrition table shows the increase of nutrient needs with increasing age and labor intensity. While a sedentary adult male worker in this calculation receives 2,600 kilocalories a day, a heavy adult male worker gets 4,200 kilocalories. The same trend can be identified when looking at adult female sedentary workers, who are supplied with 2,300 kilocalories, but with 3,500 kilocalories for heavier physical labor. Apart from energy requirements in different work settings this table also shows the recommended protein intake, which changes only in children, pregnant, and lactating women, but remains stable in all adult groups no matter the workload. This runs counter to the understanding of an increased need for protein with increased physical stress, so as to build muscle and better withstand the demands of work.

Apart from sex and labor intensity, another defining factor for the calculation of energy and nutrient requirements was age. Meal plans were created with specific age groups in mind—babies, children, adolescents, adults, and the elderly. The plans I look at here are mostly plans for workers involved in the labor process, not for the elderly or for children. The latter two groups have different calorie needs, as children are still growing and their bodies are developing, while the elderly experience age-related changes in metabolism.[41]

Calorie suggestions all build on the premise that the body needs an adequate amount of food and nutrients to function properly. The quantities in which different kinds of foods have to be ingested is determined by the amount of calories or energy (*reliang* 热量) they contain, as well as by the nutrients they provide. The calorie is thus used to determine when somebody is defined as malnourished[42] and is a central aspect of nutrition science.[43] There are two often-used means for calculating the energy content in food: by weight and by content (calories).

The unit of the calorie is a very abstract one. It is presented to the readership as a small entity that might be difficult to pinpoint by a cook on-site, but which is essential to the calculation of a body's needs. In 1950, Huang Chengguo remarked that "the calorie unit is used very little in nutrition sciences, it is not very convenient, that is why it is increased by a thousand, thus the energy needed to heat 1 liter of water one degree is one thousand calories, which are also called kcal (kilocalories)."[44] In 1954, Chen Feirun explored the idea of calories and with it the concept of the metric weights that needed to be introduced to replace the traditional *liang* 两 and *jin* 斤-system, which often varied between different parts of China.[45] A standardization of weights makes the reproduction of recipes and nutrition advice easier and forms an understanding of quantities as a unified system. In the nutrition literature, metric weights are mostly used as measurements for cooking instead of the more precise yet less practicable calorie. Metric weights were much more practical to use while cooking, and it was also easier to bulk up food volume- and weight-wise than calorie-wise by adding water or grain husks, neither of which possess much nutritional value but do increase volume, as seen in the food augmentation methods during the Great Leap.[46] Calories are broadly applied as a value of nutrition in the context of nutrition science, that is, on nutrition charts, while recipes rely on metric weight values for ingredient measuring.

So how many calories were needed to fire up production and keep the population healthy? The physical energy needs of Chinese bodies was the topic of quite some discussion in the handbooks on nutrition science. Central to these suggestions are the calorie amounts suggested for different labor intensities and the associated micronutrient requirements. The energy amounts do not change drastically over time; rather, they even out and are quite steady.

As already observed, the different basic calorie needs are defined according to the different population groups (male and female), and then by a categorization of workers according to their workload (sedentary, light, moderate, heavy, and very heavy work). Hou Xiangchuan 侯祥川 (1899–1982) in 1966[47] and Feng Ailan 冯蔼兰 in 1985 agree with this observation and offer their own overviews.[48] Across the board, women always receive about 200–300 kilocalories less than their male counterparts in the same category of work.[49] A male moderate worker was assigned 3,000 kilocalories by most experts—except a single suggestion by Shu Xincheng, who only recommends 2,600 kilocalories.[50]

Heavy workloads were understood to require more energy, and the handbooks seem more at odds with each other's suggestions. As time passes, a significant decrease in the suggested calories can be observed, from 5,000 kilocalories in 1955 to only 3,600 kilocalories in 1985. The first suggestion came from a 1955 book on the topic of protection of health and labor ability by Lukyanov, a translation from the Soviet Union by Li Guangcheng 李广成.[51] There is no apparent justification within the materials for the decrease in calories. There is, however, another category in some handbooks called "very heavy labor" (*jizhong tililaodong* 极重体力劳动). It is possible that the two categories were combined in some of the publications. "Very heavy labor" included mining, heavy industry labor, and the like, while heavy labor included farming and physically taxing work in factories.

While from the context and the similarity in approach it seems obvious that there must be common original sources used to arrive at these numbers, unfortunately, few of the materials directly cite their sources. At the same time, uniform recommendations would be a logical consequence of our assumption that the overall policy was one of nutritional governmentality, since the state would control all publications and dictate through the Ministry of Health what kilocalorie amounts are acceptable. Behind these concise charts and the different labor categories there are different starting points employed to figure out the amount of energy needed for an individual: (1) by calculating a body's basal metabolic rate and a person's activity level,[52] or (2) by taking into account physical traits such as weight and height.

Writing in 1950, Huang Chengguo uses the term "total calorie value" (*zong reliang* 总热量) to describe the amount of calories a body needs throughout the day to not only survive but to function well. He arrives at this total value by adding the required energy for work, activities, and so on to the basic metabolic rate.[53] A similar approach is found in the 1956 Soviet translation of Dubuque.[54] Also in 1956, Shu Xincheng advocates calculating the body's basic metabolic rate by multiplying the body weight in kilograms by the 24 kilocalories per kilogram that are needed to maintain basic function, namely:

Basic metabolic rate = body weight × 24 kcal

To this Shu adds the required calories for activities and arrives at the energy expense of the body in question.[55] In a 1961 publication by the Hygiene School Research Group of the Shanghai Medicine Professional College (Shanghai yixue zhuankexuexiao weishengxue jiaoyanzu 上海医学专科学校卫生学教研组) the same method is used. It postulates that per kilogram of body weight 1 kilocalorie is burned every hour without additional activity, thus:

Basic metabolic rate = 24 × 1 kcal × body weight in kg

Additional energy expenses from activity and labor are added on top of the metabolic rate to show the actual energy need of the body.[56] The same approach is also reprinted in Du Xixian's 1980 *Dietary Nutrition Science* (*Yinshi Yingyangxue* 饮食营养学): an adult male of 60 kilograms body weight will burn 60 x 1 kilocalories per hour just to supply body functions, which amounts to 1,440 kilocalories of basic metabolic rate.[57] In 1984, Chen Xuecun calculates the energy expense of daily activities and adds 8 hours of sleep, 8 hours of work, 4–6 hours of light movement, 2 hours of walking and housework to the basic metabolic rate. He ends up with about 3,000 kilocalories for an adult male moderate worker.[58] Chen Xuecun and, in 1985, Feng Ailan suggest yet another method to calculate the energy expense of the body: by calculating the body surface.[59] This method relates weight and height and calculates the calories burned per square meter per hour. All of these technical formulae found their way into nutrition charts to display a standardized approximation of the daily physical needs of a body involved in labor at the different stages of life.[60]

Similar charts can be found in most publications on nutrition science and handbooks on nutrition hygiene, such as the 1966 publication *Nutritional Progress* (*Yingyangxue jinzhan* 营养学进展) by the nutrition scientist Hou Xiangchuan.[61] For either calories or protein there is no major difference in the nutrition recommendations between Qu's (1959/1955) and Hou's (1966) charts. A few minor differences can be identified in the suggested amounts of protein, where there is a little down-grading for the sedentary and light workload.

Hou widens the scope of the nutrition charts when he opts to include a chapter on the outcomes of a 1962 conference on nutrition. At this conference the participants mainly discussed expert nutrition knowledge, and its inclusion offers intriguing insights into what was deemed to be an issue at the time, especially concerning the actual consumption of calories. Yu Shouyang 于守洋,[62] the chapter's author, elaborates on a nutrition survey which took place in Dongbei during the 1950s and in 1960. This project was compiled by Yu Shouyang and his colleagues, who went about this research between 1949 and 1957 in North China.[63] The survey summarized the nutritional makeup of the Dongbei workers' diet, which averaged 4,329 kilocalories a day. This statistic has to be taken with a grain of salt as it is unlikely at the time of the conference in 1962 and during the period of this survey—the Great Leap had just occurred—that the actual food consumption amounted to more than 4,000 kilocalories per day. The mere fact that there was a survey, however, shows how much emphasis was actually put on the correct nutrition and food supply.

Protein

Just as calories were measured, macro- and micronutrients also underwent the same procedure. Protein, as the central building block of muscles, was essential to everyday meal planning. As a central theme of the discussion on strengthening, and despite being only one of three macronutrients, protein is put under the spotlight on the nutrition charts, where we see that only the protein needs are mentioned alongside the kilocalorie and mineral needs. Carbohydrates and fats are not depicted in the tables, but they are passively present in the kilocalorie amounts for each group.

The amounts recommended are not excessive, but the amount of protein content rises with work intensity. The reason for this increase can be traced back to the idea of muscles as power plants of the body and of protein as their building blocks. As the muscles involved in the work process need more building material in the form of amino acids to sustain the worker's strength, the body needs more protein. While a light worker is suggested to take in about 60–80 grams of protein, depending on the author, heavy and very heavy labor usually are supplied with 80–100 grams of protein per day.[64] In this comparison of different publications, it becomes obvious that protein recommendations rise only slightly, if at all.

A more practical way of recommending an adequate protein supply can be found in the 1950 work of Huang Chengguo. He suggests three different kinds of meal plans: a high-, a medium-, and a low-protein meal plan.[65] This focus on the macronutrient ratio is one way of building meals, linking nutrient levels to activity levels (higher protein meals for harder physical work). Another way to adjust the diet to the required energy expenses was to increase or decrease the number of calories, as seen with Chen Meiyu in 1954 and later Chen Xuecun 陈学存 (in 1984) or Feng Ailan (in 1985).[66]

Charts like this are an easy way to cover all the important nutrient information. However, they do not explain how this is applied to the real-life issues of cooking. Taken by themselves, the quantifying aspect of the nutrients is interesting as it aids in the planning of the population's nutrition. In order to make a meal out of these nutrient values, the handbooks on public eating additionally give concise instructions for cooking and quantifying foods and their nutrient content.

MEAL PLANS AND FOOD

How were those nutrients taken in by the population? And how was nutrition knowledge applied to daily eating practices? Generally, nutrients are depicted as isolated parts of food as part of an attitude of scientific reductionism. They are not put into context, that is, there is no mention of how much rice, vegetables, or meat had to be consumed to achieve the required nutrients in daily food intake. How, in the end, were these calories and nutrients converted back into actual foods?

Since nutrients are not in fact isolated parts in food, meal plans provide examples of what to eat and how to structure daily food intake accordingly. They are either handed out as menu sets for canteens and hospitals, or put into the dietary guidelines for home cooks. The plans are the practical link between what was suggested as basic nutrition needs and what these suggestions could look like on a plate.

Improving the Nation's Diet

Meal plans published in different handbooks suggest the daily incorporation of certain foods to achieve maximal nutritional benefits; for example, Chen Meiyu's 1954 *Nutrition Hygiene*, a handbook on anything related to nutrition and eating practices, offers the following ideal meal plan:

1) a pound of soy milk, 4 *liang*[67] tofu (if it is possible to replace soy with dairy at least half a pound)
2) half an egg, if no other dairy or meat is available, stock up to one whole egg but no more than two (will decay in intestines). For people over 40: 1 egg max.
3) 4–8 *liang* fresh vegetables
4) 4–8 *liang* fruit
5) 1–4 *liang* fish, meat
6) 1–3 pounds (*jin*) of grains or potatoes
7) fat: depending on work and weight fluctuation: use vegetable oil rather than animal fats.

Chen Meiyu measures the food—and thus the nutrients—via weight, which can be measured easily. She still uses the traditional measurements in her instructions, as they were possibly more familiar to the readership albeit less scientifically accurate. The caloric weight of Chen's meal planning lies with the grain portion of the meal plan. The plan mainly consists of whole foods (nonprocessed), and there are no processed snacks or sweets or any kind of refined sugar included.[68] She does not, however, leave her readers simply with this vague list. Instead, she offers a more in-depth look at specific meal plans in which she shows how to build a sufficient diet with accessible ingredients. She demonstrates this by talking the reader through a meal plan's setup.

Some of her examples of meal plans, such as the one above, are deficient in some ways. Thus, she offers ways to improve them. Pointing to its deficiencies (indicated in the chart by V), Chen proposes to improve this plan—here consisting only of polished rice and cabbage (see figure 2.2)—by adding some tofu and lean pork, as seen in figure 2.3, to counter the considerable lack of protein (*danbaizhi* 蛋白质), calcium (*gai* 钙), vitamin A (*weishengsu A* 维生素 A), B1 (*liu'ansu* 硫胺素), and B2 (*hehuangsu* 核黄素) in the first plan.[69]

The resulting plan then is only deficient in vitamin A and B2. This is evened out by adding an egg on top of the rice, cabbage, tofu, and pork, only leaving a deficiency in vitamin B2, according to Chen's explanation.[70] She then gives two more exemplary meal plan suggestions, both of which are much more varied and offer more sources of the required nutrients. By first building up a simple meal plan from a basic diet of rice and cabbage, Chen manages to explain slowly to the reader how simple additions can complete the required nutrient profile.

食譜一：是米1.0斤，小白菜0.5斤，油2兩

食物	通俗量	克	每人克	熱量	蛋白質	鈣	鐵	維生素A	硫胺素	核黃素	菸酸	維生素C
標準米	1市斤	500	500	1,765	40.0	200	7.5	0	0.70	0.20	16.0	0
小白菜	半斤	250	250	33	2.7	213	3.0	2,000	0.07	0.20	1.5	89
油	二兩	62	62	558	—	—	—	—	—	—	—	—
合計		812	812	2,356	42.7	413	8.5	2,000	0.77	0.20	17.5	89÷2=45
缺點					V	V		V	V	V		
高標準				2,600	60	800	12	5,000	1.8	2.0	1.8	75
低標準				2,600	60	600	8	3,500	1.2	1.5	1.2	52

Figure 2.2. Simple meal plan.

Source: Chen Meiyu, Yingyang weisheng, 198.

食譜二：　一日兩餐

早餐：標準米飯三碗　　　　　　　晚餐：標準米飯三碗
小白菜（5兩）炒肉絲（62克）　　　豆腐（2兩）燒小白菜（5兩）
油一兩　　　　　　　　　　　　　油一兩

食物	份量	總克	每人克	熱	蛋白質	鈣	鐵	維生素A	維生素B_1	維生素B_2	菸酸	維生素C
標準米	一斤		500	1,765	40.0	200	7.5	0	0.70	0 20	16.0	0
小白菜	十兩		310	40	3.4	266	3.7	2,552	0.09	0.24	1.80	112
豆腐	二兩		62	45	5.7	68	2.2		0.03	0.02	0.12	
瘦猪肉	二兩		62	309	10.4	7	0.2		0.32	0.07	2.60	
油	二兩		62	558	—	—	—	—	—	—	—	
合計			996	2,717	59.5	541	13.6	2,551	1.14	0.53	20.52	112÷2=61
∨=缺欠								∨		∨		

第二個食譜和低標準比較，祇有兩個缺欠，就是維生素A和核黃素不足。現在在食譜二上加上一個鷄蛋，且看結果如何？

食譜三：（即食譜二加上一個鷄蛋）

食物	份量	總克	每人克	熱	蛋白質	鈣	鐵	維生素A	維生素B_1	維生素B_2	菸酸	維生素C
標準米	一斤		500	1,765	40.0	200	7.5	0	0.70	0.20	16.0	0
小白菜	十兩		310	40	3.4	266	3.7	2,552	0.09	0.24	1.8	112
豆腐	二兩		62	45	5.7	68	2.2		0.03	0.02	0.12	
瘦猪肉	二兩		62	309	10.4	7	0.2		0.32	0.07	2.60	
油	二兩		62	558	—	—	—	—	—	—	—	—
蛋	一個		50	82	7.4	27	1.3	720	0.08	0.16	0.05	
				2,979	67.0	568	14.9	3,270	1.22	0.69	20.57	61
∨缺欠										∨		

Figure 2.3. Adjusted meal plans.
Source: Chen Meiyu, Yingyang weisheng, 200.

Individual Meal Plans

Chen Meiyu's general plan for any worker is made more specific in the publication *General Knowledge on the Adjustment of Nutrition* (*Yingyang tiaoji jiben changshi* 营养调剂基本常识) by the Livelihood and Welfare Office of the CCP Committee of Henan Province Committee Secretariat (Zhonggong Henan sheng wei shijichu shenghuo fuli bangongshi 中共河南省委书记处生活福利办公室) in 1959.

The meal plan for a heavy workload is first divided into main dishes and additional dishes (figure 2.4). The first are grain-based foods, such as noodles, rice, millet, corn, taro, and so on. The latter contain vegetables, beans, oil, and so forth. Additionally, the second caption reads: "Calorie distribution of the

重体力劳动每人每天食譜

类别		名称	數量	含量			
				蛋白質（公分）	脂肪（公分）	醣（公分）	热量（千卡）
主食	粮食	面粉、大米、小米、玉米、高粱等	11兩	33.02	9.18	247.68	1,236.264
	紅芋		2斤7兩	28.04	2.44	353.51	1,586.95
付食	瓜茄类	南瓜、多瓜、茄子、黄瓜等	半斤	2.25	0.30	5	32.495
	豆类	黄豆（可制成豆腐、豆汁、豆芽吃）	3兩	35.76	17.12	23.26	399.198
	植物油	芝麻、花生、黄豆等油	2錢7分	0	8.33	0	77.469
	蔬菜	白菜、紅白蘿卜、韮菜、芹菜、藕等	1斤	9	1.1	38	202.93
合計				108.07	38.47	667.45	3,536.346

說明：（1）蔬菜所含的上述营养成分及热量虽然不多，但其他鉄、鈣、維生素等較多，在調剂中应保持一定比例。
（2）上述营养素热量占总热量比例：蛋白質占13%左右，脂肪占1%左右，醣占77%左右。

Figure 2.4. Meal plan for a heavy workload.
Source: Zhongguo Henan sheng weishuji shenghuofuli bangongshi, Yingyang tiaoji jiben changshi, 6.

一般体力劳动每人每天食譜

类别		名称	數量	蛋白質（公分）	脂肪（公分）	醣（公分）	热量（千卡）
主堂	粮食	面粉、大米、玉米、小米等	10兩	30.05	8.36	225.36	1,129.929
	紅芋		1斤4兩	14.38	1.25	181.25	803.708
付食	蔬菜	白菜、韮菜、芹菜、紅白蘿卜、葱、藕等	1斤	9	1.1	38	202.93
	瓜茄类	多瓜、南瓜、茄子等	半斤	2.35	0.3	5	32.495
	豆类	黄豆（可制成豆汁、豆腐等吃）	2兩	22.5	11.4	15.5	261.82
	植物油	芝麻、花生、黄豆等油	2錢7分	0	8.33	0	77.469
合計				78.28	30.74	465.11	2,503.51

說明：各营养素热量占总热量比例：
蛋白質占12.2%，脂肪占11.5%，醣占76.3%

Figure 2.5. Meal plan for a normal workload.
Source: Zhonggong Henan sheng weishuji shenghuofuli bangongshi, Yingyang tiaoji jiben changshi, 7.

above-described nutrition should be around 13% of the calories deriving from protein, around 1%[[71]] deriving from fat, around 77% from carbohydrates." This puts the emphasis in the energy supply on the grains in the diet. This diet plan solely relies on plant-based nutrients and does not contain animal protein as part of the daily diet of a heavy worker.

The second meal plan introduced from this 1959 publication is a plan for a normal workload (figure 2.5). It differs from the heavy workload example in the number of total calories. Whereas the heavy worker in the end consumed 3,536 kilocalories, the normal worker only had to ingest 2,503 kilocalories. This reduction happens due to the lower volumes of the prescribed foods. The percentages remain roughly the same: the meal plan of a light worker in this version consisted of 12.2 percent protein calories, 11.5 percent fat calories, and 76.3 percent carbohydrate calories.[72]

Meals are part not only of a worker's life but of the military as well. In 1975, a book from the 1960s was republished by the health department of the Fujian army logistics department (Fuzhou budui houqinbu weishengbu 福州部队后勤部卫生部), called the *Textbook of the Military Health Worker* (*Minbing weishengyuan keben* 民兵卫生员课本).[73] It covers a vast array of health and hygiene topics that were deemed important for peasants and liberation army soldiers. As this booklet was intended for the southern part of China, it specifies health advice for this area's climate, terrain, and so on. Apart from medical emergency information on poisoning, CPR, and anatomy, the *Textbook* also includes a short chapter on eating and drinking. This knowledge is geared toward the needs of the PLA on the road. It offers some insight into the food that should be consumed in the South's hot climate (vitamin-rich foods to compensate for the maneuvers of the army and their nutrient expense) and how it should be prepared. The booklet emphasizes the need to consume adequate amounts of vegetables such as melons and squashes or nightshades in the hot months. If that was not an option, the booklet recommends consuming enough leafy greens. Close to the seaside, fresh seafood and fish are recommended for their protein and calcium content. As spring, summer, and autumn can prove rather hot, proper preparation and storage of foods are necessary to avoid spoilage.[74]

Whereas the previously examined meal and nutrition plans focus on a perfect diet to enhance a person's physical condition, these tips are more like practical reminders of what to pay attention to under the circumstances of the Cultural Revolution, the era in which the booklet was published. Nevertheless, this textbook makes clear use of the nutrition knowledge of earlier publications when it advises the readers to pay attention to sufficient vitamin and mineral intake, and when it refers to seafood and fish as sources of protein and calcium. While the environment of this booklet's readership differs greatly from the governed environment of the public canteens, the idea of nourishment and its importance can be seen as being transferred to this new space.

POST-MAO FOOD OR, WHERE DO YOU GET YOUR PROTEIN FROM?

After the Cultural Revolution another way of relating nutrition information emerges: lists of the nutrient contents in certain foods. In the 1977 *Foodstuff Composition Table* (*Shiwu chengfenbiao* 食物成分表) published by the Hygiene Research Department of the China Academy of Medical Sciences (Zhongguo yixue kexueyuan weisheng yanjiusuo 中国医学科学院卫生研究所), there are no explicit meal plans offered. Instead, the book consists of lists of foods and their ascribed nutrients, as well as their places of origin. This can be used as (a) a guideline when figuring out a meal's nutrition value and also as (b) a guide for putting a meal together. By supplying a nutrition table, the *Foodstuff Composition Table* puts the nutrients within foods from the food lists into context.[75] The foods—fragmented on these tables into their different parts—had to be added up into daily dishes to fulfil the energy and nutrient requirements of the individual by the person or staff cooking the actual meal. This approach is useful for any nutrition value analysis, as the foreword in the book states, but is much more abstract than a simple plan or food suggestion, as it presumes that the person planning a thought-through diet has already acquired some kind of nutrition knowledge.

The 1980s discussion of nutrition was focused more on the quality of food than on the quantity of energy. The issue of protein is taken up once more in 1980, when Du Xixian 杜希贤 in his *Dietary Nutrition Science* (*Yinshi yingyangxue* 饮食营养学) suggests a good mixture of foods to achieve an adequate amino acid supply for the body, especially regarding the essential amino acids. By combining certain amino acids present in certain foods, he creates the basis for meal planning. The rules of amino acid combination inform his whole process of meal planning. Du recommends a well-balanced mixture of meat and vegetables as well as the incorporation of noodles made from corn and bean starch, grain bases, and certain vegetables, or at least a mixture of processed and coarse grains to achieve his nutrition goal.[76] This combination method is also adopted by Feng Ailan (1985), who elaborates on the combination of legumes and grains to complete the plant-based amino acids and to supply the body with sufficient B-vitamins and minerals.[77] The mixing of different kinds of foods, thus, is not only necessary for ample protein supply, but also—as Chen Meiyu had already shown in her 1954 corrections of meal plans—crucial to vitamin and mineral supply.

In 1984, Chen Xuecun uses similar charts and tables as in the 1977 *Foodstuff Composition Table*. In appendix 4 of his book *Applied Nutrition Science* (*Yingyong yingyangxue* 应用营养学) he offers lists of foods and their nutrients, but he gives no specific directions toward what dishes should be made out of this produce.[78]

The promoted foods are nothing too special—no superfoods or foods especially designed to increase nourishment—but common produce found at local markets. There is, however, an emphasis on grains and plant-derived nourishment, not because the authorities had a vegetarian agenda, but because of the easy procurement of such produce. The meal plans are also marked by a lack of processed foods other than polished rice or noodles.

In all meal plans, grains are the calorie staple, vegetables are the source of vitamins and minerals, and proteins in the form of legumes, soy products, and animal products were to ensure growth and strength. There is actually an emphasis on soy within the meal plans,[79] which suggest having at least one pound of soymilk for breakfast and some added tofu in some dishes, or more often than not containing more legumes or soy products than animal proteins. This is usually justified by economic necessity.[80]

These paragraphs on nutrient requirements and content often serve as replacements for meal plans. The charts displaying meal plans make the information visual and so more easily accessible to the readership, since it appears in an ordered form as well as stripped down to its essentials. This "raw data" without interpretation embodies the scientification process underway in modern nutrition knowledge. It teaches the audience what food is in a science-oriented environment, and about the importance of these nutrients for a well-functioning body. It thus depersonalizes food, especially vis-à-vis the question of the taste and pleasure derived from eating,[81] and at the same time it establishes the possibility of state planning in the realm of food, as it becomes measurable. Thus, it allows the state to avoid famine by rationing food on scientific grounds, and aids in agricultural planning by mapping out how much is needed.

Scientific Cooking

Given that the diet of a worker had to be balanced and contain all the major nutrients needed to make his or her body function at its peak, the final step in making foods into dishes was the processing of the foods themselves. This also influenced the nourishment provided by foods and the availability of nutrients to the body. Not only was it important to cook food well, but also to store it properly to avoid spoilage, and this brings me back to the beginning of this chapter, where I looked at the makeup of public canteens. The kitchens of public canteens were the place where nutrients were turned into dishes, transforming nutritional knowledge into actual food that was to be served to the guests of the canteens. This process, too, was described and standardized in detail.

Writing in 1954, Chen Feirun defines the four most important stages of food preparation as availability, storage, price, and the calculation or estimation of what is needed. The emphasis he puts on the economical factor of food and its handling is common in the handbooks: after all, food had to be available at the place where it was needed, and it had to be affordable and possibly nonperishable. Meat and milk might be seen as nutritious, but storing them could prove quite difficult in pre-refrigerator times, and thus storage rooms were central to planning canteen meals. An especially tricky aspect of the management of public canteens was the planning of meals for a large number of people. Usually, the previous day's visitors were taken as an approximate headcount for the following day's cooking.[82]

Cookbooks such as the *Popular Menu* (*Dazhong caipu* 大众菜谱) from 1966 and reprinted in 1979, and the *China Menu* (*Zhongguo caipu* 中国菜谱) from 1975, offer meal-related information that differs from that found in health and canteen handbooks. The *Popular Menu* is actually an accumulation of recipes from around China, most recipes bearing a line on where they come from, localizing them in the PRC. Their ingredients may or may not have been available only in this region. The focus is clearly on the actual recipes instead of health and hygiene tips, and includes the processing steps like washing, peeling, cutting, and so on. There are three pages at the end summarizing what has to be remembered and attended to as far as nutrient preservation and kitchen hygiene goes, in order to not let this knowledge slip completely.[83]

The *Foodstuff Composition Table* (*Shiwu chengfenbiao* 食物成分表) from 1977 breaks down cooking instructions for certain dishes into the most basic form. It shows the different kinds of food and the possible ways to cook them, including short instructions on preparing, seasoning, and the specifics of cooking them. The procedures are published in charts which also show the micronutrient contents of the prepared dishes, similar to the kilocalorie charts implying the importance of being informed about nutritional contents. Vegetable and meat preparation, for example, list ways of cooking (stir fry, boil, deep fry, stew in clear soup, braise, or cook) and detailed food-specific instructions on condiments and cooking time. Adjoined information on the micronutrient contents both before and after heating forge a link with the knowledge of the chemical changes to which ingredients are subjected during the cooking process.

Potatoes, for example, have to be peeled first, then cut into pieces, before adding spices and water. Then they are cooked on high heat for 10 minutes, before decreasing the cooking temperature to low heat and simmering them for 20 more minutes. Pork, on the other hand, can be shredded into small pieces and fried with oil for 1.5 to 2.5 minutes, before it is spiced with soy sauce. This method allows for 87 percent of B1 to be kept. In another variation the pork can be cut into pieces before it is cooked in clear broth on a high heat with salt for about 30 minutes, whereby the B1 level will fall to a mere 53 percent. Knowing about the chemical changes in the end product can theoretically prevent the destruction of or deficiencies in a certain nutrient.[84]

The cooking instructions generate a picture of "pick and choose" instead of strict prescriptions. By using the information given in the theoretical chapters and pairing it with the much more explicit knowledge provided on the actual foods, a suitable diet can be built up by everyone. The cooking instructions enable the individual to (re)produce this diet every day. The cooking instructions given to public canteen staff and the ones in the later handbooks do differ slightly in their level of detail, however, with the instructions for canteen staff being more general than the instructions in cookbooks.

This discussion has illustrated the way nutrition science was put into practice in the form of meal plans and cooking instructions that were distributed among the staff of public canteens and the Chinese population more generally. It shows the way theoretical knowledge was incorporated into printed media that were distributed among target groups, mainly canteen staff and the interested population. It further shows how the workers' bodies were quantified and calculated to better suit the PRC's planned economy.

Meal plans were the realization of theoretical knowledge, or at least the attempt to put it into practice. These plans appear in different environments over time and show a remarkable consistency in content despite the turmoil in the period between 1949 and 1978. The major nutrient groups all remain important, but their representation in terms of food ranges from that of an actual meal plan designed to be realized in environments such as the public canteens of the Great Leap Forward, to the lists of foods and cooking instructions of the post–Cultural Revolution era. In other words, despite the shifts in agency, nutrition knowledge itself remained unchanged.

In this context, food is not only a tool to create health by supplying sufficient nutrients to guarantee physical function and productivity, but also a way to assert control and to regulate daily life. Meal plans make a daily structure possible by dividing the day into breakfast, lunch, and dinner time. They also mark the transition from traditional thinking about food to modern thinking, that is, food as an amalgamation of the necessary nutrients to fuel the human motor. In this, they become a way to regulate and control the bodies of the population by making food intake a question of measurement. Meal plans are the juncture between the theoretical and practical application of nutrition science in daily life. Thus, a standardization of a formerly private activity is undertaken, which is supposed to result in making the act of eating far more amenable to the processes of state planning, and also to link it more or less directly with the control of the nation's strength.

As they appear on paper, meal plans and nutrition science are not affected by the dire need resulting from the Great Famine at the end of the 1950s. Instead, they continue to propagate a utopian version of ideal nutrition without broaching the political and social issues of the time. While articles on the issue of supplementation or food replacements took a more realistic turn,[85] the handbooks on nutrition science and the ideal nutrition for the population did not take notice of this disastrous event. In the discussion of the utopian version of nutrition, or the scientifically ideal type of nutrition for the body, considerations of labor were the biggest driving force. Food was a tool for health, and the result of creating healthy and strong bodies would be increased production. Proper food was a way to avoid malnutrition, which would lead in turn to a lower level of health. The kind of diet that was agreed upon to support the labor force points toward what today is called a whole-food diet with few processed foods. Instead, there is an emphasis on the high-carbohydrate and relatively low-fat proportions of this diet. This does not only derive from a stance on the value of nutrition, but is also a question of practicability and economic availability.

As in the building of nutrition science, the Chinese government and the CCP exercised central control by using nutrition science to create an ideal diet that fostered the socialist cause. By putting a healthy body on the socialist agenda—since only a healthy body could triumph on the path to Communism—adhering to a controlled and scientifically sanctioned diet plan became the task of a good comrade and communist. The promotion of these well-thought-through plans can be categorized as another part of the biopolitical agenda of the Chinese authorities.

NOTES

1. George McClelland Foster and Barbara G. Anderson, *Medical Anthropology* (New York: John Wiley & Sons, 1978), 265.
2. Foster and Anderson, *Medical Anthropology*, 263–79.
3. This argument can also be found in Wilbur O. Atwater's research.
4. Foster and Anderson, *Medical Anthropology*, 278: "It is clear that for those who are interested in improving nutritional levels of malnourished people, the clinical analysis of dietary deficiencies is just the first step. Unless the nutritional educator also knows the social functions of food, its symbolic meanings, and the beliefs associated with it, little progress can be made."
5. Interviews were conducted in 1994.

6. Guo Yuhua, "The Generation Gap at the Table," in *Feeding China's Little Emperors: Food, Children, and Social Change*, ed. Jing Jun (Stanford: Stanford University Press, 2000), 97–98.

7. Guo Yuhua, 99.

8. Guo Yuhua, 100.

9. Guo Yuhua, 100–101.

10. Gyorgy Scrinis, "On the Ideology of Nutritionism," in *Contemporary Transitions*, ed. Jeffrey M. Pilcher, vol. 4 of *Food History: Critical and Primary Sources* (London: Bloomsbury, 2015). Scrinis defines nutritionism as a "nutritionally reductive approach to food": "This focus on nutrients has come to dominate, to undermine, and to replace other ways of engaging with food and of contextualizing the relationship between food and the body" (p. 405). He argues that the notion of nutrients, and of food as fragmented into them, is perpetuated by the food and agricultural industry and at times exploited. The idea that nutrients can be (a) connected to certain foods and (b) linked to bodily functions and health deviations is very ambiguous in his eyes: "Nutritionism creates ambiguous tendencies toward a disempowered, confused, and dependent individual on the one hand, and an active, empowered, and critically informed individual on the other. It creates the conditions for nutrition confusion, a dependence on scientific expertise, a susceptibility to food marketing claims, and a general anxiety about 'what to eat'" (p. 416).

11. Guo, "The Generation Gap at the Table," 103.

12. See, for example, Frank Dikötter, *Mao's Great Famine: The History of China's Most Devastating Catastrophe, 1958–1962* (New York: Walker & Co., 2010); Kimberly E. Mannings and Felix Wemheuer, eds., *Eating Bitterness: New Perspectives on China's Great Leap Forward and Famine* (Vancouver: UBC Press, 2011); James L. Watson, "Feeding the Revolution: Public Mess Halls and Coercive Commensality in Maoist China," in *The Handbook of Food and Anthropology*, edited by Jakob Klein and James L. Watson, 308–22 (London: Bloomsbury Academic, 2016); Jacob Eyferth, "Women's Work and the Politics of Homespun in Socialist China, 1949–1980," *International Review of Social History* 57, no. 3 (December 2012); Jacob Eyferth, "Less for More: Rural Women's Overwork and Underconsumption in Mao's China," *Clio. Women, Gender, History*, no. 41 (2015).

13. Contributing factors of canteens were for example the "eating one's fill" slogan, when food was freely given and sometimes wasted. See Jacob Eyferth, *Eating Rice from Bamboo Roots* (Cambridge: Harvard University Press, 2009).

14. Numbers of victims have never been verified, but Dikötter and Yang have tried to estimate the number of deaths: Yang points to about 3 million victims of famine in Henan alone (Yang, *Grabstein—Mùbei*, 130–8). Dikötter on the other hand sums up various published statistics and derives figures of 36–38 million victims (Dikötter, *Mao's Great Famine*, 324).

Rationing and experiments with how little a body needed to survive in connection with nutrition sciences first came into existence during times of war, as Collingham has shown in *Taste of War* (2011), her comprehensive history of hunger during wartime and the impact wartime planning had on the following generations. As war has a profound impact on people's health (destruction of land, mental and physiological disorders, injuries or famine), this is no surprise. War and its aftermath, as well as the class struggle omnipresent in socialist rhetoric, were also impacting the newly founded PRC and her population's health in the middle of the twentieth century.

15. Watson, "Feeding the Revolution," 310.

16. Watson, 308–9. Watson calls the public mess hall campaign "the collectivization of eating."

17. Watson, 310.

18. Watson, 310–1, 315. See also Yang, *Grabstein—Mùbei*, 424, 427.

19. Watson, "Feeding the Revolution," 314. See also Dikötter, *Mao's Great Famine*, 54–55, 195–96.

20. Dikötter, *Mao's Great Famine*, 53–54: "Except for the most deprived villagers, most people did not like the canteens, if only because sprawling collectives run on a shoestring could hardly cater to individual whims, tastes and diets, some people had to walk for kilometres to reach the collective facilities."

21. Ellen Oxfeld, *Bitter and Sweet: Food, Meaning, and Modernity in Rural China* (Oakland: University of California Press, 2017), 75.

22. Yang, *Grabstein—Mùbei*, 432.

23. Hua Gao, "Food Augmentation Methods and Food Substitutes during the Great Famine," in *Eating Bitterness: New Perspectives on China's Great Leap Forward and Famine*, ed. Kimberly E. Mannings and Felix Wemheuer (Vancouver: UBC Press, 2011), 171–72, 184.

24. Luo Pinghan, *"Daguofan": Nongcun gonggong shitang shimo* "大锅饭": 农村公共食堂始末 (Nanming: Sichuan renmin chubanshe, 2015), 8.

25. Luo Pinghan, 105–37.

26. See Eyferth, *Eating Rice from Bamboo Roots*, 140. See also Chen Shuqi 陈叔骐, *Yingyang weisheng* 营养卫生 (Beijng: Renmin weisheng chubanshe, 1954), 20, on taking care that food was stored properly so it was not wasted and spoilt before consumption.

27. *Gonggong shitang* 公共食堂 has been translated in various ways: public canteens, public dining halls, public mess halls, and so on. This book uses the expression "public canteens."

28. See Chen Meiyu 陈美愉, *Yingyang weisheng* 营养卫生 (Beijing: Renmin weisheng chubanshe, 1954); and [Chen] Feirun [陈]费润, ed., *Zenyang banhao gonggong shanshi* 怎样办好公共膳食 (Beijing: Renmin weisheng chubanshe, 1954); but also Jiankangbao articles on *gonggong shitang* or *gongshe shitang*.

29. Chen Meiyu, *Yingyang weisheng*, 187.

30. Chen Meiyu, 190–95.

31. Chen Meiyu, 196–98. More inventory and nutrient lists are provided at ibid., 204–7. On the topic of health check lists, see ibid., 207–8 (for health checklist), 208–10 (for symptom and deficiency correlation list); Chen Xuecun 陈学存, *Yingyong yingyang xue* 应用营养学 (Beijing: Renmin weisheng chubanshe, 1984), 280 (chart for examination), 281 (for symptoms and deficiency correlation); Feng Ailan 冯蔼兰, *Gonggong yingyang* 公共营养 (Beijing: Qinggongye chubanshe, 1985), 201f. (for symptoms and deficiency correlation).

32. An earlier version was published in 1951 by the Zhonghua Shuju Chubanshe in the *Jiankang shenghuo congshu* 健康生活丛书. The 1954 version was published by the *Renmin Weisheng Chubanshe* and was revised slightly.

33. [Chen] Feirun, *Zenyang banhao gonggong shanshi*, 63–64.

34. [Chen] Feirun, 64–65

35. [Chen] Feirun, 66f.

36. [Chen] Feirun, 74–91.

37. [Chen] Feirun, 21. For further methods from the Republican Period to avoid germs spreading, see Lei Hsiang-lin, "卫生，身体史，与身分认同：以民国时期的肺结核与卫生餐台为例," in *Jiankang yu shehui* 健康与社会, ed. Zhu Pingyi (Taibei: Lianjing chubangongsi, 2013).

38. "Manage Public Canteens Well, Ensure Production and Construction" (Banhao gonggong shitang, baozheng shengchan jianyi办好公共食堂，保证生产建设), *Jiankangbao* (October 15, 1958); "Anguo County's Canteens' Hygiene Was Raised Remarkably" (Anguo xian shitang weisheng xianzhu tigao 安国县食堂卫生显著提高), *Jiankangbao* (December 13, 1958); "Jishan County's Public Canteens Put Nutritious Recipe Book into Effect" (Jishan xian gonggong shitang tuixing yingyang shipu 稷山县公共食堂推行营养食谱), *Jiankangbao* (April 27, 1960).

39. Nick Cullather, "The Foreign Policy of the Calorie," *American Historical Review* 112, no. 2 (April 2007): 338.

40. The China Academy for Medical Sciences was founded in 1950 by the Ministry of Health and received its current name in 1956. It is affiliated with different hospitals, among them the Peking Union Hospital. It houses several different research facilities for medical issues.

41. Zhongguo yixue kexueyuan weisheng yanjiusuo, ed., *Shiwu chengfen biao* 食物成分表 (Beijing: Renmin weisheng chubanshe, 1977), 371–72.

42. See WHO report on the Energy Requirements of Adults: http://www.fao.org/3/a-y5686e.pdf (accessed November 10, 2017).

43. The calorie was discovered and named by Wilbur O. Atwater and his colleagues: see Cullather, "The Foreign Policy of the Calorie," and Atwater, "Food as Building Material and Fuel."

44. Huang Chengguo 黄承国, ed., *Jianming yingyang xue* 简明营养学 (Shanghai: Xinan yixue shushe, 1950), 12: ("[. . .] 但是卡之单位量极少用于营养学，不甚方便，古特增加千倍，即一千豪（立+毛）之水加热上升摄氏一度之热量坏为营养之卡，又称之为大卡路里[. . .]").

45. [Chen] Feirun, *Zenyang banhao gonggong shanshi*, 18.

46. In a personal discussion Felix Wemheuer remarked upon the same issue when dealing with public canteens: only the food weight is ever given, not the number of calories attributed to them. This may be for different reasons such as the possibility to enhance volume and weight by adding sand or water for bulk. This would not correlate with an increase in calories.

47. Hou Xiangchuan 侯祥川, ed., *Yingyangxue jinzhan* 营养学进展 (Shanghai: Shanghai kexue jishu chubanshe, 1966), 87–88. For more information on Hou Xiangchuan and his influence in nutrition science during the Republican period, see Fu's discussion of soy milk (Jia-Chen Fu, *The Other Milk: Reinventing Soy in Republican*

China [Seattle: University of Washington Press, 2018]). Together with Zheng Ji, Hou was involved in the establishment of nutrition science in the Republican era and beyond. Hou held a PhD from the New York University medical college, which he received in 1924. See *Zhongguo kexuejia cidian, Xiandai disi fence* (1984), 343.

48. Feng Ailan, *Gonggong yingyang*, 74.

Feng categorizes labor as follows:

Sedentary labor: desk and office workers

Light labor: shop owners, teachers, lab workers

Moderate labor: students and their daily activities, drivers, electrical engineering, craftsmen

Heavy labor: nonmechanized peasant work, steel work, dancing or sports

Very heavy labor: loading work, lumbering, mining.

49. This gender difference also includes pregnancy and lactation times when women are suggested to add more calories but also more protein into their diet to take perfect care of their offspring.

50. Shu Xincheng, *Wo zenyang huifu jiankangde* 我怎样恢复健康的 (Beijing: Zhonghua shuju chubanshe, 1956).

51. Lukyanov, *Jiankang yu laodong nengli de baohu* 健康与劳动能力的保护, trans. Li Guangcheng 李广成 (Beijing: Renmin weisheng chubanshe, 1955).

52. Chen Xuecun, *Yingyong yingyang xue*, 2. Chen Xuecun is the author of works on nutrition science, for example the "Yingyang diaocha shouce 营养调查手册" (1987).

53. Huang Chengguo, *Jianming yingyang xue*, 11–12.

54. Dubuque, *Yinshi yu jiankang*, 32.

55. Shu Xincheng, *Wo zenyang huifu jiankangde*, 65.

56. Shanghai yixue zhuankexuexiao weishengxue jiaoyanzu, ed., *Yingyang weisheng xue* 营养卫生学 (Beijing: Renmin weisheng chubanshe, 1961), 18.

57. Du Xixian 杜希贤, *Yinshi yingyangxue* 饮食营养学 (Jinan: Shandong kexue jishu chubanshe, 1980), 21.

58. Chen Xuecun, *Yingyong yingyang xue*, 5. See also Feng Ailan, *Gonggong yingyang*, 73.

59. Chen Xuecun, *Yingyong yingyang xue*, 3; Feng Ailan, *Gonggong yingyang*, 12. Another change in calorie and energy perception and calculation was the realization that environment and climate also played a role in the body's energy expenses.

60. Qu Huiqing 区慧清, *Jiating yingyang shipu* 家庭营养食谱 (Beijing: Kexue puji chubanshe, 1959), 8. This particular table derived from a 1955 food composition table of the Nutrition Department of the Central Hygiene Research Institute and is a reprint of this earlier version.

61. Hou Xiangchuan, *Yingyangxue jinzhan*, 99.

62. Yu Shouyang was part of the editorial board of the two volumes on modern medicine of the *Zhongguo dabaikequanshu* 中国大百科全书 (1995).

63. Hou Xiangchuan, *Yingyangxue jinzhan*, 152.

64. [Chen] Feirun, *Zenyang banhao gonggong shanshi*; Shu Xincheng, *Wo zenyang huifu jiankangde*; Qu Huiqing, *Jiating yingyang shipu*; Zhongguo yixue kexueyuan weisheng yanjiusuo, *Shiwu chengfen biao*; Chen Xuecun, *Yingyong yingyang xue*.

65. Huang Chengguo, *Jianming yingyang xue*, 23–26.

66. Energy needs depend also on the activities an individual engages in during the day. For an exact calculation, some authors offer charts that assign kilocalories expense to daily activities such as cleaning, walking, or sleeping; see Chen Meiyu 陈美愉, *Yingyang weisheng* 营养卫生 (Beijing: Renmin weisheng chubanshe, 1954), 11–12; Chen Xuecun, *Yingyong yingyang xue*, 5–7; Feng Ailan, *Gonggong yingyang*, 13.

67. The weight unit used by Chen is still the traditional weights and not the metric units of grams and kilograms, or other volume units. These old units were not yet unified at the time and thus not as exact as the meal plans using standardized metric system weights.

68. Chen Meiyu, *Yingyang weisheng*, 160. Chen Meiyu generally gives the traditional weight units in her text, while in the tables the more accurate metric and caloric units are used.

69. Chen Meiyu, *Yingyang weisheng*, 200.

70. Chen Meiyu, 200.

71. Here a possible printing error occurred, since the sum of 13, 77, and 1 is 91, whereas this calculation should sum to 100 percent. As the following table claims to offer a similar amount of fats in the diet plan, 38.47 grams and 30.74 grams, it stands to reason that in this instance a 0 was not printed although intended.

72. A similar distribution can be found in the earlier handbook by Shu Xingcheng (1956) who postulated 65 percent carbs, 23 percent fat, 12 percent protein. With Shu the difference is his emphasis on fat-calories rather than carbohydrate calories. See Shu Xincheng, *Wo zenyang huifu jiankangde*, 67.

73. There have been various editions of this booklet, in 1960, 1967, 1969, 1970, and again in 1975, giving weight to its importance and use.

74. Fuzhou budui houqinbu weishengbu, ed., *Minbing weishengyuan keben* 民兵卫生员课本 (Beijing: Renmin weisheng chubanshe, 1975), 139.

75. Zhongguo yixue kexueyuan weisheng yanjiusuo, *Shiwu chengfen biao*, 368–69.

76. Du Xixian, *Yinshi yingyangxue*, 10.

77. Feng Ailan, *Gonggong yingyang*, 36.

78. Chen Xuecun, *Yingyong yingyang xue*, 382–95.

79. The question of whether soy is a worthy protein alternative to animal protein has been asked since the Republican period, as Jia-Chen Fu has shown in her *The Other Milk* (2018).

80. Liu Yugu 刘毓瑴, "Dadou he women de yingyang 大豆和我们的营养," *Dazhong Yixue* 8 (1950): 131–35.

81. See for example Christine Ott, *Identität geht durch den Magen* (Frankfurt: S. Fischer Verlag, 2017).

82. [Chen] Feirun, *Zenyang banhao gonggong shanshi*, 56.

83. Dazhong caipu bianxiezu bian, ed., *Dazhong caipu* 大众菜谱 (Beijing: Qinggongye chubanshe, 1979), 192–94.

84. Zhongguo yixue kexueyuan weisheng yanjiusuo, *Shiwu chengfen biao*, 364–65.

Similar instructions can be found in Shanghai yixue zhuankexuexiao weishengxue jiaoyanzu, *Yingyang weisheng xue*, or in Feng Ailan, *Gonggong yingyang*, 35–43, where not only the nutrient contents of food can be found, but also the ways to prepare them.

85. The titles of *Jiankangbao* articles range from “Eat a Lot of Nutrient-Rich Sweet Potato” (Duochi yingyang fengfu de ganshu 多吃营养丰富的甘薯) (October 8, 1958), to “Guizhou’s Hygiene Work in Public Canteens Continues to Improve” (Guizhou sheng shitang weisheng gongzuo buduan tigao 贵州省食堂卫生工作不断提高) (July 6, 1960), to “Processing Staple Grains and Nutrition” (Liangshi jiagong yu yingyang 粮食加工与营养) (March 15, 1961).

PART II

Physical Government

A healthy body, according to common scientific understanding, is not generated merely by appropriate nourishment. As an organism that is made to survive the natural elements as well as times of scarcity, the physical body needs both to be in motion and to experience regular periods of stillness. And as a part of the modernized and industrialized world, the human body not only has to survive but also work within the social and labor structures that have been emerging since the beginning of industrialization.[1] These structures were often perpetuated on the basis of political and ideological positions, which saw them as meaningful since they served the needs of the greater good, that is, the flourishing of the population at large. In this context, health practices emerge that actively promote the training and creation of fit and able bodies; and alongside the discourse of physical activity and exercise, the discourse of rest is created as well. These two polar opposites of activity and nonactivity have influenced the labor discussion ever since.

The human body had to be made compliant with the increased pressure of labor that was disconnected from the change of the seasons, and was oriented instead toward production requirements. Ultimately, the production process had to make do with human bodies that had limited energy supplies and other physical limitations such as strength, concentration, or eyesight, and it had to include downtime in order to recharge the body and build it up, so it could endure the new stresses.

In order to succeed in this endeavor, at a time when theoretical discussions centered around the correct deportment in a socialist society, the PRC started to introduce spaces for and knowledge of physical training and resting periods. An ideological discussion of Marxism and of Mao Zedong's thought can be found in some texts on physical health and fitness, but its presence is not overwhelming. Still, we need to keep in mind the ideological backstory of the time when looking at training schedules and rest regulations, since it gives them an additional layer of meaning. The practical approach to the application of popular exercise and resting strategies follows Mao Zedong's original discussion in *On Practice* (1937), which explains the relation between knowledge and practice as well as between knowing and doing. Relating to the introduction of scientific knowledge, Mao expresses his conviction that knowledge had to be generated through practice. Such an emphasis on practice is obvious in the disciplines of physical education and resting: here, the continued retelling of personal anecdotes delivers practically tested and scientifically appraised knowledge to the readership, who are then encouraged to apply it again to a real-life scenario in order to benefit from it.[2] Mao followed his 1937 piece with a short essay entitled "Where Do Correct Ideas Come From?" (1963), which shines the spotlight on objective matter and conceptual knowledge; it is this which provides the framework for the following two chapters of the present volume. Mao postulates that practically applicable knowledge and conceptual knowledge are two stages of knowledge that have to work together in order to form matter.[3]

The following two chapters thus dissect how physical education came to be an expected part of a worker's daily routine, while resting and sleeping were established as a precondition of labor success and as a solution to labor-caused exhaustion. Both of these practices belong to a functional body's daily schedule, and both discourses display the practical approach of Maoism in the implementation of (scientific) knowledge. While the initial information is generated by experts from established institutions, it is then checked against its practical applicability and possibly changed to suit the physical condition of the population or the situation in which it is utilized. Through this process, an awareness—or in Mao's words, a consciousness—about physical need is created that would serve as a measuring bar for the individual person as well as the state.

Despite the focus on practice, a theoretical awareness of the body is also necessary, both in the context of exercise as well as in the context of sleep, although these two activities serve the common goal via contrary applications. In order to perform physical exercise properly and engage the body in a positive way to achieve a strong physique, anatomical and biomedical knowledge was introduced to the readership. Similar proceedings can be found in the discussion of sleep, which as a passive activity was, nevertheless, examined thoroughly so as to provide the population with arguments for its importance and information about the proper resting procedure.

The contradictions in the socialist society created in the PRC were a major source of friction, and this was addressed in Mao's writings. These contradictions can be found in some parts of the health discourse, but they are not irreversible and are more of a circumstantial nature, as in the case of mental and manual workers.[4] Mao insists that through the integration of mental workers, that is, intellectuals, into socialism, all parts of the population will be activated to do the right thing, and the mental workers thus are assimilated to the manual workers. The general consensus of the primary sources on health practices for mental workers on the other hand does not display any judgments or correctional attempts to alter their type of work. Instead, mental as well as manual workers are considered to be parts of the population who both need physical training and rest in order to function properly. They do, however, require different approaches to resolve common problems (fatigue) deriving from different origins (physical exhaustion versus mental exhaustion). The health experts pass no moral judgment on either, and are more concerned with the practical rehabilitation after physical disease and the prevention of further deterioration.

NOTES

1. Anson Rabinbach, *The Human Motor: Energy, Fatigue, and the Origins of Modernity* (Berkeley: University of California Press, 1992).
2. Mao Zedong, "Shijianlun 实践论 [On Practice]," in *Mao Zedong xuanji* 毛泽东选集 (Beijing: Renmin chubanshe, 1968), 259–73.
3. Mao Zedong, "Where Do Correct Ideas Come From?" in *Selected Readings from the Works of Mao Tsetung* (Beijing: Foreign Language Press, 1971), 502–4.
4. Mao Zedong, "On the Correct Handling of Contradictions Among the People [1957]," in *Selected Works of Mao Tsetung* vol. 5 (1977), 384–42.

Chapter 3

Plans for the Body

As early as in his 1917 essay *A Study of Physical Education* (*Tiyu zhi yanjiu* 体育之研究), Mao Zedong had postulated the importance of physical exercise in the molding of a strong and resilient people;[1] and in 1949 Mao and his comrades-in-arms had not forgotten the importance of physical strength, not only for their continuing revolution but also for the economic development they sought. Exercise, for them, served primarily as a way to strengthen bodies in pursuit of increased production. To reach the production goals, the exercise regimen had to be adjusted individually so that it benefitted everyone, which means there was no one-size-fits-all approach to exercise.

This chapter investigates the processes of negotiation between the state and individual bodies by observing the ways fitness knowledge was communicated to the Chinese population. The discussion is based on widely distributed newspapers such as the *Jiankangbao* or the *Xintiyu*, but also the *Dazhong Yixue* and other health-inclined journals or handbooks for everyday use, as well as teaching materials for schools, universities, and medical personnel. The primary focus is put on radio calisthenics (*guangbo ticao* 广播体操) and running (*pao* 跑) to illustrate the propagation, institutionalization, and implementation of fitness knowledge. Both serve as case studies for exploring the meaning of fitness and the social construction of health.

Radio calisthenics—a form of orchestrated mass gymnastics—is a highly institutionalized and collective practice, whereas running can be considered an individualized form of activity. The investigation of these two different ways of physical training allows for the examination of collective versus individual training methods. Chinese calisthenics, in particular, has been employed as a form of mass education since the 1950s.[2] Although nowadays these practices are mainly limited to schools, they do show a long continuity. Running, on the other hand, has always been present in the fitness discourse but was never nationally institutionalized.

Previous research on sports and physical education in late Qing, Republican, and PRC times has emphasized the collective character of sport and the need to submit to the goal of strengthening the nation and not merely benefitting oneself. In the nineteenth century, the Qing government modernized and reformed the empire's army by establishing training schedules to rid itself of the negative image as the Sick Man of East Asia. Nicolas Schillinger argues that the "reforms not only transformed military culture in a complex process of cross-cultural appropriation and adaptation but also led to the epistemological reconceptualization of both the physical body and masculinity in China."[3] By incorporating foreign knowledge and including foreign experts in the process of restructuring the army and the military training, the Qing reformers completely restructured the military. Considering "the body [as] an object of governance,"[4] controlled and regulated by authorities for a greater cause, is in line with the present work's observations regarding an even broader social group, that is, working adults of both sexes.

The development of physical culture was continued during the Republican period. For this period Andrew Morris focuses on the link between the individual body as entangled in the *tiyu* (体育) discourse, and the young Chinese nation. In the Republican period *ticao* (体操) became a common physical practice among the Chinese population and was part of the integration of physical culture into daily life.[5] Following these Republican attempts to dispel the image of the Sick Man, the new socialist China developed elite athlete programs nationally and internationally, as well as exercise programs for the broad population. The so-called Labor and Defense System (*Laodong weiguo zhidu* 劳动为国制度)—a Soviet-borrowed institution—was part of this push for a more physically fit nation, as was the "sport for everyone" movement. The excitement about physical education had waned by the 1960s, but continued in lay sports, paramilitary exercises, and workplace-related activities.[6]

THE MACHINE METAPHOR AND ITS SIGNIFICANCE FOR THE PRC HEALTH DISCOURSE

Physical education and exercising are played out on the site of the body, which since the Industrial Revolution has been reinterpreted as a functional and productive part of society. In the PRC it becomes a true production tool, a part of the machinery that propels the development and progress of the nation. As part of the production mechanism in industrialized countries, the human body had been enveloped in the discussion of labor safety and labor efficacy since the dawn of factories. The development of the metaphor of the human machine, a process that had been ongoing since the beginning of the Industrial Revolution, profoundly changed the understanding of human labor and the body.[7]

Some of the first thinkers to make the body-machine comparison are René Descartes, in his *Discourse on Method* in 1637,[8] and later Julien Offray de la Mettrie, who in 1747 published *L'homme machine*.[9] The change in the nature of labor changed the way the human body could be accessed, and altered the impact which the development of science has had on it since the dawn of the age of industrialization. This is observed by Anson Rabinbach on the topic of the political decisions made in Europe and the United States on labor safety, hygiene, and physiology, which all influenced the way human life has been formed and shaped over the past two hundred years. One of the prevalent themes in the theoretical discussion surrounding these changes was the energy aspect of the human machine: for La Mettrie the human body had an innate supply of energy, like a *perpetuum mobile* which supplied the work process endlessly (though this assumption turned out to be rather optimistic).[10] The discovery of thermodynamics by Helmholtz in the middle of the nineteenth century helped scientists to begin to imagine the body's physiological work, its sources of energy, the mechanics of movement, and its stress limits.[11] The body has frequently been compared to a machine in the context of labor, which—among other things—resulted in the formation of a field called *Arbeitshygiene* in Germany. This new field included any topic connected to labor conditions, security, and improvements of the labor process. The connection between labor and the body was thereby stressed, which led to thinking about the body in terms of the social and productive relationships that directly influenced production. Given that work in the factory had become rationalized by the end of the nineteenth century, a way to rationalize the body as a means of production now heralded the dawn of a completely thought-through and transparent work process. The machine metaphor was prominently used in European and US industry until the beginning of the twentieth century. It experienced a new transformation after World War II when cybernetics began to seek ways to enhance body functions and perceptions.[12]

The human body, nevertheless, was not so easily transformable as the factory owners, business elites, and governments had envisaged. From the nineteenth-century perspective, the possibility of comparing the human body to an inanimate object underwrote certain ways of commodifying it.[13] The industrial backdrop against which these ideas were formulated was rather fertile for the scientific assessment of the body.[14] Considering the body as a machine made it predictable and replaceable, just like any part of an actual machine or factory. The body as a work tool was enfolded in a depersonalized, rationalized process, and could be influenced by adding certain kinds of fuel (nutrition) and implementing routines to keep it running smoothly (movement, hygiene, and rest).[15] Especially where manual labor was concerned, this depersonalization resulted in the fragmentation of the body into its primary usable parts, as seen in the reference to "workers as hands."[16] In this environment the individual parts get lost in the machinery of production and become part of it. These ideas can be identified in the Chinese context, especially in the Marxist context where they provide a framework for thinking about the body, as the following quote illustrates:

> 火车要烧足了煤才有劲儿, (. . .) 人也是这样(. . .)。[17]
>
> [The train needs enough coal to burn so it can be strong, [. . .] people are just like this [. . .].]

This quote by Chen Shuqi from the 1950s uses the machine metaphor to describe the body and its functions, and thus defines its task in life. In Europe the metaphor has made continual appearances in the nutrition sciences since the nineteenth century, and, as Jia-Chen Fu noted, in the 1930s it even made its way into the Chinese discussions of nutrition science.[18] The idea of comparing a human being to a machine or factory was, according to the historian Bu Liping, introduced to 1930s China by "Fritz Kahn's interpretation of man as a place of industry." This changed the traditional view of the human body from a "microcosm to the modern idea of chemical composition," thus interpreting it "as scientifically analysable and quantifiable."[19] The metaphor became part of the understanding of modernization in the Republic of China and later the People's Republic.

This mechanical understanding of physical bodies was entertained most prominently in the context of production, where the body took its place in lieu of actual machines. This idea served the political and economic goals of the PRC in more than one respect, since China—either before 1949 or after—was barely mechanized.[20] Accordingly, there has not only been a "human–machine continuum" as Tina Mai Chen has argued—the extension of the human body via tools and machines—but also the recognition of the body as machinelike in the labor process. Chen describes the "continuous remaking of individual minds and bodies as a means of social revolution" under Mao, elevated by the extension of human bodies into mechanical hybrids.[21] Mao himself recognized the human body's propensity to act as a machine in his "Talk on Sakata's Article."[22]

> The tools of cognition should comprise such things as the axe, machinery, etc. Man's cognition stems from practice. We use the axe and machinery to transform the world, and our cognition is thus deepened. Tools are extensions of human organs. The axe is an extension of our arms while the telescope is an extension of our eyes. The human body and its organs can all be extended.[23]

This physical change would then lead to social change and result in improvements for production and society.[24] While physical enhancement so as to foster production was one way to effect change, I argue that the body in its entirety was seen as a machine: it was a tool and a machine in the production process, although it still had needs of which the state was aware. While machines and bodies can, according to Chen's discussion, be molded, they were considered not only malleable but also as in need of a certain degree of care and maintenance in order to boost body function. Physical exercise not only formed the body, but was also therapeutic for it.

The (Healthy) Body

Anatomical knowledge had a part in the Qing and Chinese strengthening movement and medical discourse,[25] as authors such as Schillinger, Luesink, and Heinrich have shown.[26] Anatomy is used to describe bodily functions as well as medical conditions to the population. The "new" vocabulary and bodily understanding was communicated unceasingly both to the military recruits and to the population involved in the mass movements. Medical knowledge was introduced by missionaries, and through Western as well as Japanese influence.[27] By engaging the target groups according to foreign-tested practices, the Qing as well as the Republic of China aimed to emulate the Western success in warfare. These practices included German gymnastics and physical exercises, and military medical know-how often taught with the help of foreign experts.[28]

In the socialist Chinese context, the body is communicated to the population by the popular media and through education in an effort to overcome the phenomenon that Leder has termed "the absent body" (1990). Making the population aware of the body is a central concern of articles in the *Xintiyu*, which explain anatomical details of the body, muscle contractions, or the digestive system. The 1954 Soviet article by Kavelnikov titled "Training of the Body can Enhance Health" (Shenti xunlian neng zengjin jiankang 身体训练能增进健康) includes a thorough discussion of the physical benefits of exercising: not only is it good for respiratory function, but also for the circulatory system. The article describes in detail how the respiratory system provides oxygen, which is transported to the muscles via the blood stream and aids in generating energy.[29]

Another, later, example of the use of anatomical and organic knowledge to explain the body's function and the process of it becoming visible is a 1980 *Xintiyu* article by Wu Zhenying 武真英 titled "Do Not Run Excessively" (Buyao pao de guofen 不要跑得过分). Wu describes the symptoms of physical fatigue due to excessive training and does not neglect to mention how joints, muscles, and tendons will ache after too much exercise. The article includes both sides of the absent/present state of the body: it exemplifies how pain arises from misconduct, that is, overdoing it in training, and also how to return to a state of not feeling the affected body parts anymore.[30]

This information on making the body and its physical experience tangible is envisioned as a step to better health. These thorough descriptions of the body's mechanics and movement apparatus are a means of the health literature to assign scientific names to the parts of the human being.[31] A discourse on the healthy body thus becomes possible, while at the same time suggesting ways to influence it. The discussion of biochemical and physiological elements not only introduced new knowledge, but also constructed an awareness of the role of the healthy body in the context of labor. The health regimes that were proposed in post-1949 China were tailored to the different groups of the population, and showed a remarkable capacity to differentiate between individuals' life stages and the awareness that they may have cultivated on the way.[32]

How does the "absent" body, the machine, then figure into the body-labor discourse in the PRC? For one thing, the "absent" body had to become visible in the process of turning it into a machine. A machine can be taken apart and fully observed. The body of the Chinese person (i.e., the Chinese body, conceived of as a machine)—upon being reassembled—was then integrated into different discourses: nationalism, class struggle, modernization, production, medicine, and hygiene.[33]

Making the previously "absent" body visible was important for production as well as for military and political purposes in all modern nations in the twentieth century, and the Republic of China and the PRC were not exceptions, as revealed by *Jiankangbao* articles like "For the Fight for Health of the Laboring People" (Wei laodong renmin de jiankang douzheng 为劳动人民的健康斗争) (1956), "The Limitless Care of the Party and the Government for the People's Health" (Danghezhengfu dui renmin jiankang wuxian guanhuai党和政府对人民健康无限关怀) (1957), or "Improving the Health Standard Boosts Production" (Tigao jiankang shuiping cujin shengchan 提高健康水平促进生产) (1960).

Apart from technical and specific knowledge on strengthening exercises and training measures, a more general sense of health was also established in the population. This sensitivity had to be generated in order to discover symptoms of illness so that the body could be optimized for labor, as Miriam Gross has shown for the example of snail fever (schistosomiasis). In the case of physical education and self-care, this happened via education through handbooks. In health care publications the human body is clearly detailed so as to introduce the concept of anatomy to the readers—muscles and their functions are, after all, the basis of labor power, and the skeleton frames the human form. In these anatomical explanations the body is fragmented into different parts and structures, such as the nervous system (*shenjing xitong* 神经系统), the cardiovascular system (*xinzangxue xitong* 心脏血系统),[34] the respiratory system (*huxi xitong* 呼吸系统), digestive system (*xiaohua xitong* 消化系统), temperature (*tiwen xitong* 体温系统), urinary system (*miniao xitong* 泌尿系统), and the skeletal (*guge xitong* 骨骼系统) and muscle system (*jirou xitong* 肌肉系统).[35] By dissecting the formerly holistic conception of the Chinese microcosm body,[36] a new body is formed: the scientific body. This body is a tactile organism, it is explained by means of biomedical principles, and becomes an entity that needs to be taken care of.

A 1977 text by Wang Xuliang 王序良 titled "How to Train the Body in the Countryside—Gymnastics" (Zai nongcun zenyang duanlian shenti—jiqiao 在农村怎样锻炼身体——技巧) links anatomical knowledge with physical training practices. This report offers insight into gymnastics training in the countryside, and explains the necessity of muscles and their development in the context of exercise. It stresses the necessity for everyone to participate in exercise so as to help labor-fatigued bodies recover.[37] Apart from descriptions such as this, other texts use visual material to depict the biomedical body and thus make it visible.

Anatomical depictions display the body as a biological entity.[38] Pictures of skeletons allow readers to peer inside the body and so render the hidden visible. They are sometimes supplemented by schematic depictions of the body, which simultaneously make the living organism more corporeal and yet more abstract. Those schemes often list the bones of each body part, the individual organs, and so on.[39] Knowing about anatomy and the internal structure of the body can be considered part of personal hygiene, since it made it possible to think "scientifically" about the body.

Personal hygiene (*geren weisheng* 个人卫生) included self-care and the proper handling of the individual physical needs, akin to the Foucauldian "techniques of the self." One part of personal hygiene was the right way to exercise and to apply the physiological knowledge of biomedicine. A 1965 booklet describes personal hygiene as a practice of regularity and consistency. The regular training of the body aided in its strengthening. A regular schedule was important, as was the incorporation of morning gymnastics, these being considered a way to prepare the body for work, school, and all the activities of the day.[40]

SPORTS AND PHYSICAL CULTURE

In the Chinese context, a distinction is made between *sports* and *physical culture*: the latter belongs to the health practices here described and is part of personal hygiene. These physical education practices are meant to aid in the building of a healthy body to achieve a healthy nation; they differ, therefore, from the training drills and practices of professional athletes or athletes as such. The differentiation between athletic, professional sports and a more health-oriented version akin to the German *Körperkultur*, which Brownell termed *physical culture*, was made by experts in the Soviet Union and later in Mao-era China. Physical culture in socialist China was equivalent to the Russian *Fiskultura*.[41] It continued the practices of physical culture established in the first half of the twentieth century, as described by Morris (2004) and Schillinger (2016).

The intention to prove a nation's ability on the international platform of sports competitions was closely linked to *Fiskultura* in the Soviet Union. As John Washburn and Reet Howell discuss in two articles written twenty years apart (1956 and 1975), the Soviet Union made use of mass education in the field of sports to foster their internationally competing teams and their military potential, and to improve the population's health at the same time.[42] There was a distinct line drawn between sport, and especially competitive sport, and physical culture or education. On the one hand, in its engagement in international competitions the Soviet Union strove for better outcomes; on the other, physical education was meant to indoctrinate and train the population, especially post-1917 when the population was being prepared for fighting and production.[43]

In the spirit of learning from the Soviet Union, the PRC's sport culture repeated Soviet policies from about thirty years earlier and introduced a fitness program similar to the GOT (*Gotov k trudu i obrone* [Ready for Labor and Defense]). This program imparted physical education to the population with a reward system that gave incentives for participation.[44] Prior to its implementation, different Soviet expert groups had discussed the relative benefits of sports systems built either on a hygienist or a competitive basis. The hygienists' reasoning against competitive sport but in favor of physical education was based on seeing physical activity as a means to improve the quality of life and work, as opposed to a competitive and thus elitist system based on achievements and geared toward winning.[45]

Before the introduction of the "Ready for Labor and Defense" system in 1931, the Communist Party of the Soviet Union "defined the forms of physical education; they were to include 'physical exercise in the form of sport, games, gymnastics, public and personal hygiene in work and everyday life, the use of natural forces (sun, air, water), and correct régimes of work and relaxation.'"[46] These routines were supplemented by competitive activities monitored by experts to generate a fit and able population with an interest in sports.

"[I]nternational sports competitions [. . .] helped people imagine their identity within the Chinese nation and China within a 'world of respected modern nations,'"[47] as Shuman observes. This forged a link between professional or competitive sport and the rest of the population, who by participating via watching could engage in the formation of identity. The search for identity was further supported by the attempt to overcome the lingering Sick Man of East Asia stigma, which fostered a nationwide enthusiasm for sport. In order to achieve this, the body's endurance and health had to be improved, not only by prestige-fostering victories in sports competitions but by establishing a basic fitness level in the population. Health was thus utilized as a signpost of proper socialist conduct and became a way to encourage the larger population to engage in the building of fitness. This included personal hygiene as well as successful participation in competitions.

The Soviet training model is an exact blueprint for what was introduced in the PRC. During the 1950s, the maxim of "learning from the Soviet Union" informed Chinese physical education.[48] Soviet experts and sports delegations[49] introduced the new training methods and helped establish institutions such as the "Ready for Labor and Defense"[50] system (*Laodong yu weiguo zhidu* 劳动与卫国制度), or for short *Laoweizhi* 劳卫制, duplicating its Soviet counterpart.[51] This was introduced and implemented by sports leaders in China in the first half of the 1950s, but prior to its nationwide implementation, the organization and infrastructure for physical education had to be improved, which included a preparatory physical education program for the youth beginning on May 4, 1954.[52] In the following years, curriculums were created and competitions were held at schools to assess the students' progress. The exercise routines were also introduced into work units, and the workers therein participated in them.[53]

Schools and work units were thus involved in the Labor and Defense System, showing how far-reaching this institutionalization of sports and its participants was. The end of this system came with the crisis of the Great Leap Forward and the Sino-Soviet split. Participant numbers sunk, as did passes at the standard tests. The system was replaced by the "youth *tiyu* exercise standards" in 1964,[54] but this standard did not survive after the 1980s and is not a permanent or central part of the self-care and training practices communicated in physical education handbooks.

CASE STUDY 1: MOVING IN LINE—*TICAO* 体操

Calisthenics, or *ticao*, are part of the healthy socialist lifestyle, and gradually evolved from military gymnastics to the Mao-era collective exercise.[55] *Ticao* is a highly institutionalized practice which supposedly conferred vast health benefits if one trained regularly. Not only was it a way of controlling bodies so as to achieve a better physical state, but it was also a way to break the daily rhythm of labor and to alleviate symptoms of stress and work-related pains.

The arrival of *ticao*, or gymnastics, in China has been documented by Schillinger.[56] The first mention of *ticao* occurs at the end of the Qing dynasty, when the Qing military system was reformed. In connection with the borrowing of German and Japanese military terms, the concepts of gymnastics, body weight exercises, and exercises with apparatuses were incorporated, as was the Japanese term *taisō*, which corresponded to the English "gymnastics" or "physical exercise."[57] The gymnastics introduced to China were of Swedish (less strenuous) and German (more strenuous) origin. Schillinger translates the basic meaning of *ticao* as "physical drill" or "military gymnastics" for the late Qing and early Republican period. They were used to build the basic fitness of recruits so they were physically able to participate in military drills and all brought up to the same fitness level.[58]

Gymnastics were continued in Mao-era China as a starting point for fitness training—not only for soldiers but for the entire population. Sports for the masses was embedded in the mass mobilization of the 1950s and 1960s with the goal to create a socialist collective and revolutionary spirit.[59] The movement toward better public and personal health included the widespread introduction of several kinds of gymnastics or calisthenics *ticao*: artistic, with/without apparatus, for bodily hygiene, and so forth. Some of these kinds of *ticao* were institutionally and centrally governed physical education methods, as in the case of radio calisthenics. These mass-oriented *ticao* exercises originating in the 1950s did not require any expertise or excessive training on the part of participants, nor any sports equipment or anything more than a flat spot on the ground.[60] Individual gymnastics training was not dismissed either, in particular after gaining expertise through the participation in radio calisthenics or *ticao* classes. To be most effective, *ticao* exercises were meant to be done regularly, at least once a day, as a 1951 handbook by the Publishing Society of New Education (Xinjiaoyu shebian 新教育社编) claims. The exercises were carefully communicated in the clearest way possible so no misunderstandings or ensuing injuries could occur.[61] The movements included in any *ticao* routine, whether radio calisthenics or any form of nonprofessional gymnastics, were stretching, twisting, the loosening of joints and muscles, and strengthening moves.

A 1954 publication by Brykin stresses that *ticao* exercises were not competitive exercises and did not require frequent, vigorous training for prestigious competitions, but were seen as an important way to uphold productivity in workers by engaging them in regular orchestrated movement.[62] Brykin also encouraged the use of radio or broadcast calisthenics for these exercise breaks, as this particular form offered an easy way to communicate the forms and rhythm of the exercises and only took about ten minutes to do, fitting easily into a structured factory workday. Further exercise suggestions for daily use included the gymnastic exercises of the *Laoweizhi* or simple free gymnastic moves, also called health gymnastics (*weisheng ticao* 卫生体操).[63]

A 1957 *Xintiyu* article titled "What Benefits Do Inter-work Calisthenics Have?" (Gongjiancao jiujing you shenme haochu 工间操究竟有什么好处？), written by the sports medicine expert Qu Mianyu 曲绵域, suggests that *ticao* was easily incorporated into everyday routine. It took the form of morning exercises (*zaocao* 早操), exercise before work (*qiangong cao* 前工操), during a work break (*jiangong cao* 间工操), and exercise after work (*hougong cao* 后工操).[64]

The discussion of work and exercise highlights the fundamental difference between two groups of workers: manual workers (*tili laodongzhe* 体力劳动者) and mental workers (*naoli laodongzhe* 脑力劳动者).[65] The first are characterized by their work being physically taxing, involving a lot of bodily strength and exertion of power in order to master their tasks, and include peasants, mine workers, factory workers, and so forth. The second group worked without too much energy expenditure during their shifts, perhaps in administration, in studying, doing research in laboratories and so on, largely behind a desk and doing their main work inside their heads, thus being labeled with the befitting term "brain worker." This phenomenon was often connected to life in urban areas and the new living situations that arose in the 1950s. Articles such as the originally Russian 1951 article "Mental Workers' Exercise" (Zhili laodongzhe de tiyu 智力劳动者的体育),[66] the 1956 *Xintiyu* article "The Significance of Physical Culture for Mental Workers" (Tiyu yundong dui naoli laodongzhe de yiyi 体育运动对脑力劳动者的意义),[67] or the 1957 *Xintiyu* article "Health Methods of Intellectuals" (Zhishi fenzi de jianshen fangfa 知识分子的健身方法) by Tang Wuyuan 唐午园 all describe the sedentary mental workers' striving for more activity.[68]

The various forms of *ticao* were seen as an effective way to loosen up the daily working schedule of both worker groups. Mental workers, today often called sedentary workers, spent all day sitting down, which led to reduced blood flow, fatigue, and loss of efficacy; hence articles such as the 1957 one by Xie Bin 谢彬 on the elimination of fatigue by practicing gymnastics encouraged them to move during their breaks.[69] A year earlier, Shu Xincheng had suggested that mental workers get up during their work, take a short break, and do some stretching in front of an open window, which would get their blood flow going again.[70]

Workers with physically challenging jobs encountered different physical problems, linked to the mechanical repetition of the movements associated with their tasks, as demonstrated by a 1957 article titled "Miners' Physical Education" (Kuanggong de tiyu 矿工的体育) by Zhao Gezhuang 赵各庄 of the mining association. Zhao comments on miners' labor conditions and the strain they put on their bodies, elaborating on the exercise routines that may be performed before and after work, which allegedly alleviate physical stress. Stress may lead to an imbalance in their muscles, and the resulting tension may negatively influence the production process.[71]

While these *ticao* variants could be done alone or in groups, radio calisthenics was mostly a group activity, and could be done alongside anyone in the community: "Calisthenics [. . .] had a goal of teaching people how to cultivate their bodies as part of the socialist collective,"[72] and thus included people from all walks of life and all classes, the whole body of the nation. The Chinese radio calisthenics (*guangbo ticao* 广播体操) have been incorporated into the mass sports movements since 1951, and were part of physical culture, immersing the population into the discourse of physical exercise at the grass-root level.[73] Shuman terms them "*tiyu* for everyone," and indeed this did not just mean everyone, but also anywhere, be it at school, at work, at home, or in other public spaces where bodily fitness could now gain footing.

Chinese radio calisthenics have their origin in Japan and were heavily influenced by the German military system. Returnees from Japanese universities were employed in the process of creating this fitness regimen for the nation. One of these returnees was Yu Lishuang 于丽爽. She recounts the specifics of *guangbo ticao*'s creation, when in 1950 Yang Lie 杨烈—a former exchange student in Japan and secretary of the Preparatory National Sports Committee (*Tizong shouweihui* 体总筹委会)—wrote a thorough report on how to improve the population's health standard.[74] In the aftermath of this evaluation, a colleague of Yang Lie, Liu Yizhen 刘以珍, was hired to create the first sequence of *guangbo ticao*.[75] Both women were involved with sports, Yang Lie being the only woman to join a delegation that visited the Soviet Union in the 1950s to investigate their sports system, while Liu Yizhen had studied Japanese calisthenics.

Both were also involved with committees of the All-China Sports Federation (Zhonghua quanguo tiyu zonghui 中华全国体育总会).[76] In Yu's text, Liu and Yang serve as specific faces of the creation of *ticao*, but all the important institutions were involved: the Ministry of Health, the Ministry of Education, the National Sports Assembly, and the All-China Federation of Trade Unions. The wide scope of the institutions shows how all-encompassing this exercise regimen was considered to be. Apart from professional experts like Liu Yizhen, foreign experts were also part of the process. Suggestions from the population on the most recent sequence were incorporated as well, as two 1954 articles from the *Renmin Ribao* and the *Xintiyu* mention.[77] This leads to the assumption that the implementation of *guangbo ticao* was not merely done in a top-down manner, but also encompassed some bottom-up knowledge transfer. These reports of course cannot be taken at face value, as it is hard to test whether actual suggestions and complaints were integrated, but they display how information exchange between the authorities and the population supposedly functioned in a heavily governed environment.[78]

The Evolution of PRC Radio Calisthenics

The synchronized radio calisthenics were introduced primarily as a form of mass mobilization, but they were not a one-time occurrence: in fact, they have persisted until today. Nine *guangbo ticao* sequences have been created and broadcast over the past 60 years. For the sake of unity, this chapter only examines the first six sequences, published between 1949 and 1986. One reason for the continuing evolution of *guangbo ticao* sequences was allegedly the physical development and improvement of the participants: the original ten movements of the first *guangbo ticao* sequence[79] were, for example, changed, supplemented, and made more difficult in the second sequence in order to keep the movements interesting and the population moving.[80] The first six sequences were made up of eight to ten different kinds of movements that were anatomically grouped:

1. Lower body movements *xiazhi yundong* 下肢运动
2. Four limbs movement *sizhi yundong* 四肢运动
3. Chest movements *xiongbu yundong* 胸部运动
4. Side movements *tice yundong* 体侧运动
5. Twisting movements *zhuanti yundong* 转体运动
6. Front and back movements *fubei yundong* 腹背运动
7. Balancing movements *pingjun yundong* 平均运动
8. Jumping *tiaoyue yundong* 跳跃运动
9. Aligning movements *zhengli yundong* 整理运动
10. Breathing *huxi yundong* 呼吸运动.[81]

The last two types of movements were abandoned with the second sequence introduced in 1954, as they were part of the other eight movements anyway.[82] They were supposed to cover all anatomical parts of the body and were thus valued as a beneficial way to activate and engage the body in soothing movements. This breaking down of exercises according to body parts demonstrates the inclusion of biomedical and anatomical knowledge of the body, and also shows the connections made between body parts and movements, as well as their meaning for the physical constitution.

In recounting the inception of radio calisthenics, Yu Lishuang included in her report a description of the *guangbo ticao* training structure, similar to those handed out with the published picture sequences of each practice sequence. According to her, the first two movements (movements for the lower body and four limbs) were supposed to be a warm-up for the whole exercise, whereas the following six movements were the centerpiece of this short training sequence, and the last two (ordering movements and breathing exercises) could be interpreted as what nowadays is called the cooldown portion.[83] This structure has not changed over the years and was accompanied by music. The scope of these exercise patterns exceeds the daily radio calisthenics activity, since (*guangbo*) *ticao* is often proposed as a warm-up for the actual training.

The purpose of *guangbo ticao* was to improve the workers' state, helping them by taking part in this kind of exercise to feel less exhausted (*pilao* 疲劳), to improve the health of the body, to train the body to become stronger, and to replenish energy levels drained during labor.[84] And this in turn aimed at the overarching goal of increasing productivity (so that five-year-plan goals could be reached) and supporting national defense.[85]

The first sequence was introduced in 1951 as a way to encourage the population to do exercises so that they would be comfortable and strong enough to partake in other physical (including military) activities, as a *Renmin Ribao* article from 1951 explains.[86] The second sequence, first published in 1954 in both the *Renmin Ribao* and the *Xintiyu*, was set up for more vigorous training, as were all those that followed. The movements were supposed to be deeper and more complex, designed to train the whole body, but this time a more scientific vocabulary was used in the explanation of the sequence's usefulness.

> [The second sequence] contains upper limb movements, lower limb movements, full body movements, side movements, front and back movements, balancing movements and [again] full body movements, because of this as long as one practices consistently for a long time, one can develop muscles, enhance lung capacity, boost the cardiovascular system, eliminating growing decline or deformations occurring in body functions due to not exercising for a long while, thus improving metabolic function, and strengthening the ability to resist the onslaught of disease.
>
> [它包括了上肢运动、下肢运动、全身运动、体侧运动、腹背运动、平均运动和全身运动，因此，只要长期坚持锻炼，就可以使肌肉发达，肺活量增加，促进血液循环，消除身体机能某些部位因长期得不到锻炼而引起的衰退或畸形发展的现象，从而增进新陈代谢作用，增强抵抗疾病侵袭的能力。][87]

The reference to biomedical and anatomical concepts such as muscles, the cardiovascular system, and the metabolism underline the scientific framework through which the benefits of these exercises were conceived.[88]

In the third sequence, from 1957, the exercises are said to be partly derived from martial arts, thus borrowing a traditional style and embedding *ticao* in the more familiar tradition of Chinese defense practices.[89] A 1957 article from the *Xintiyu* titled "The Third Radio Calisthenics Sequence Is Promulgated" (Di san tao guangboticao gongbule 第三套广播体操公布了) connects weight loss and curing ailments to the practice of radio calisthenics. This short article, by Wu Jiangping 吴江平 and Jiang Youzhen 蒋佑桢, reports that a number of people from different work environments (the Party School [Zhonggong zhongyang gaoji dangxiao 中共中央高级党校], a textile plant in Zhejiang [Zhejiang sheng Jiaxing Minfeng zaozhichang gongbu 浙江省嘉兴民丰造纸厂公布], the Tiantan Research Institute in Beijing [Beijing Tiantan shengwu zhipin yanjiusuo 北京天坛生物制品研究所], and a telecommunications plant in Changchun [Changchun youdian qicai chang 长春邮电器材厂]) had been monitored while regularly participating in the third sequence: attendance rates had ranged between 80 and 90 percent, and most participants lost weight or experienced other positive side effects in the process. Among the participants of the Party School and the textile plant, while some people gained a little weight while participating, some lost up to 6 kilograms. The article lists 13 fat people (*pangzi* 胖子)[90] who managed to lose weight, while 29 reported increased appetite and 41 participants had better sleep. In the last two work environments, the research institute and the telecommunications plant, it was observed that diseases declined and that the basic training led to overall health improvements for the participants. It was also stressed that this third sequence was designed specifically for the needs of people spending their days in a very sedentary way, such as students and office workers.[91] This article thus describes a study of very controlled environments, such as schools, factories, and other institutions, where observations like this were possible. Since being out of shape was a problem mainly among urban sedentary workers who had to deal with seated employment, this emphasis is not misplaced: their engagement in regular physical exercise was seen as an improvement to their labor situation.

The *ticao* routines were reportedly eagerly received by the working population, as different accounts in the *Xintiyu* suggest. A 1962 report on a Shanxi textile mill by Fang Fu 方芾 mentions that the introduction of regular exercise between shifts was a cause for joy among the workers. Levels of exercise participation and of morale were observed over a period of four years (1958–61), with the conclusion that all the shift workers were very satisfied with their small routines. *Ticao* was welcomed because it alleviated the pain and exhaustion caused by the daily work posture, and helped people to relax after a work day or to prepare for the next one.[92]

The fourth sequence, from 1963, introduced nine movements for the whole body that were deemed original and new. They were also—apparently for the first and only time—disseminated in four different languages, Chinese, Mongolian, Tibetan, and Uyghur, thus including the three minorities in the discourse during a time when standard Chinese was not spoken by the entire population. In a short commentary (*duanping* 短评) in the *Renmin Ribao* from April 1963 titled "Everybody Is Doing Radio Calisthenics" (Dajia dou laizuo guangbo ticao 大家都来做广播体操) radio calisthenics were declared a cultural recreational activity (*wenhua yule huodong* 文化娱乐活动).[93] The introduction of the fifth sequence in 1971 mainly follows the rhetoric of strengthening.[94]

A positive review of the inclusion of *ticao* into the daily work schedule was published in a 1973 piece by the Party Branch Revolutionary Committee of Department Stores in Nantong. In this case, employees of a department store were studied just after the fifth sequence had been introduced. It was seen as a health activity, but also as a revolutionary act and a social activity, as all employees would assemble outside to join in this active break, which was also a lesson in correct performance, as comparisons would be made between the participants and corrections offered. Again, just as with the 1962 report, heavy emphasis was put on the regularity of participation for optimal benefit.[95]

The sixth addendum to the *guangbo ticao* tradition, from 1981, emphasizes that its movements were supposed to be more elegant (*dongzuo youmei* 动作优美), vigorous and powerful (*gangjian youli* 刚健有力), coordinated according to music (*yinyue dongting* 音乐动听), to have a big energy expenditure (*yundongliang jiaoda* 运动量较大), and were—as opposed to the fifth sequence—both more scientific (*gengyou kexuexing* 更有科学性) and more artistic (*yishuxing* 艺术性).[96] When the sixth sequence was published the connection between physical activity and relaxation was emphasized. This sequence introduced the idea of balance between work and resting time (*laoyi jiehe* 劳逸结合), an idea that can be subsumed under today's buzzword "work-life balance." From this point forward *ticao* was considered a traditional manner of physical activity in China.

From the feedback in these articles, the significance of radio calisthenics becomes apparent. To enhance its reach and institutionalization, radio calisthenics was employed in governed environments such as schools, factories, and urban areas, where workers and students were guided through the exercises for the good of the nation and the work force, according to the overall maxim of doing one's own body good. Despite the good intentions, however, this is not in fact how it played out. According to the articles elaborating on the publication of the second *guangbo ticao* sequence in 1954, participation by the population had dropped after two years of always doing the same first sequence of movements. One reason for this decline in enthusiasm was identified as a lack of education for workers and students on the subject.[97] According to a 1954 *Renmin Ribao* article, people were unsure about the physiological and ideological meaning of this kind of exercise, and were simply bored by the unchanging repertoire of ten movements: in addition, their bodies had supposedly adapted to the exercises and were now able to handle a more challenging practice.[98] This last issue was addressed by gradually increasing the sequences: only by passing the lower sequences was one safe to do the more difficult and challenging ones.

Alongside calisthenics, collective sports such as basketball[99] or track and field training[100] were recommended as suitable for after-work activities, as they take up more time, are harder to get proficient at, and often require a set number of participants. That does not of course mean that they are not eligible as exercises to be pursued, but they were much harder to schedule.

CASE STUDY 2: RUNNING FOR HEALTH

Running, as one of the hard-to-schedule activities, was introduced as an additional and easy way to train the body. Fitness experts considered it a method to improve endurance and engage the cardiovascular system. Although running (*pao* 跑 or *paobu* 跑步) was less institutionalized than radio calisthenics, standards still existed that had been defined by experts. Especially after the 1960s, newspapers, magazines, and handbooks mostly advertised running as a non-competitive activity—yet the media also included news on highly professionalized athletic teams that participated in national and international competitions. This linking of the lay to the professional way of running reinforced the ideal of personal health and national strength.

The broad population was measured against certain standard level tests of the *Laoweizhi*, which took place at schools and *danweis*, and "encouraged everyone to become a competitive athlete on a level appropriate to their age and ability."[101] The standard of the *Laoweizhi* system can be seen as one of the few means to evaluate running exercise.

In this standard, different expectations for the different participants were laid out. It differentiates between male and female participants, and between four different age groups, which for men were adolescents (16–17 years), young adults (18–30 years), middle-aged (31–40), and elderly; the age groups for women are significantly shorter, and women over 36 years of age are already considered part of the elderly group. The differences between the two sexes manifest elsewhere too, as longer running distances are defined for men (1,500 meters) as opposed to the much shorter distances for women (800 meters).

The second level of the *Laoweizhi* expects more from its participants. Since they were already trained, and thus in better shape than the first-level participants, the long-distance run here is 3,000 meters and is only assigned to male participants, while females still only ran 100 meters and 800 meters.

For both sexes the times for these runs had to be shorter, that is, they had to run the distances faster. The abilities of males and females are defined by this standard via working out how far and how fast a person is expected to run.

Unlike *guangbo ticao*, running and walking were not firmly institutionalized, and remained more of a leisure (*xiuxi* 休息) activity that was suggested to everyone. There were no nation-wide training schedules for running,[102] and it was more like an addition to daily life. It was organized individually, sometimes in the form of running groups that would form in factories, as the back cover from a 1959 January issue of the *Xintiyu* illustrates.[103] Running and walking both require very little equipment: even special running shoes are not mandatory, which made it accessible to a larger part of the population.[104] Furthermore, running and walking both build on a natural way of movement that does not include any complicated and learned forms. As a social activity it supposedly offers time with colleagues, friends, or other members of the same community, but can also be—and sometimes should be—practiced alone, as a 1979 translation from Japanese stresses.[105]

Knowledge of Running

The idea that running improves health was imported to China via popular American fitness books that had been translated in the Republican era.[106] In the 1950s, Soviet sources additionally became available and complemented the already existing canon.

One example is the 1930 publication *Individual and Mass Athletics*, written by S. C. Staley and published in Shanghai translated as *Geren yu tuanti zhi jingzhi yundong* 个人与团体之竞技运动 by Wang Yicheng 王毅诚 and Jin Feijun 金非均. Soviet sources include the *Soviet Exercise Teaching Materials* (*Sulian tiyu jiaocai* 苏联体育教材) originally published in 1949 by Cherevkov and translated by Qiu Biao 仇标 in 1952. This contains forty pages of insight into methods of running and walking.[107] More Soviet articles on running were translated into Chinese in the *Xintiyu* during the 1950s, but this exchange stops at the time of the Sino-Soviet split. This shows how the circulation of knowledge was susceptible to political and ideological shifts.

The 1955 publication *Sport and Health* (*Tiyu yu jiankang* 体育与健康) by Chen Su 陈苏 reaffirms the Soviet ideas and emphasizes that track and field abilities (i.e., running) are the basis for most sports. Chen describes running as muscle-building, strengthening of the organs, and additionally as a mental exercise.[108] The *Soviet Exercise Teaching Materials* and *Sport and Health* both show how running was not only taught via publications and the Labor and Defense System's program, but was also utilized by teachers during physical education (PE) classes. School education, including PE, was one pillar of the nationwide dissemination of fitness knowledge.

By consuming translations of international books on the topic, the Chinese population took part in the international fitness trends outside of state institutions. In the 1970s, for example, *The Complete Book of Running* by James F. Fixx was published in the United States and by 1980 had been translated into Chinese by the Xinhua chubanshe under the title *Paobu* 跑步 (Running). The colloquial style of this volume reappears in the Chinese translation, intertwining anecdotal evidence by the author with biomedical knowledge.[109]

Despite the fact that the discourse of running was communicated similarly to the case of *ticao*, running remained an individual practice, as is suggested by the relative absence of reports on "in-between-work runs" whereas "in-between-work gymnastics" (*gong/kejiancao* 工/课间操) was practiced between classes or in order to break up the working day.[110] This points to running (and walking) as being an individual activity, yet it was still part of the discussion of health. The articles frequently remind the readership that successful and efficient training needed more time than the ten minutes allotted to said breaks. The frequent reference to running as a beneficial part of daily training can be seen as a gentle nudge in the "right" direction of health and fitness. Here, authors and authorities only assume the role of informant, not of enforcer as in the case of radio calisthenics.

Like everything in the fitness and health discourse, running was divided into different varieties. These were introduced in the "running-tips-literature" so that the readership could get a decent grasp of what sprinting, moderate, and long-distance running, or relay racing really meant. A *Xintiyu* article from 1977 titled "Running" (Pao 跑) sums up the different techniques for improving individual performance, and shows how difficult it would have been to incorporate running as an interwork break, as it proposed to start with 10–15 minute runs in order to gain some endurance, which would have ruled out runs of more than about 3 kilometers. It defines 500 meters to 3 kilometers as middle-distance and 3–10 kilometers as long-distance running. The aspiring runner first had to train at low intensity and gradually add more and more distance, until they were able to make 3–5 kilometer runs.[111] Given how long it took to do proper running training, it had to be moved from work time into one's spare time.

Toward the end of the 1970s, long-distance running (sometimes even marathons) emerges as a frequent subject of discussion, such as in the article "Q&A on Hygiene Knowledge in Long-distance Running" (Changpao duanlian weisheng zhishi wenda 长跑锻炼卫生知识问答), which answers questions on breathing techniques, exhaustion, or the cooldown after a run.[112] In the 1980s, a special category was introduced in the *Xintiyu*: *Changpao aihaozhe* 长跑爱好者 (long-distance running enthusiasts). This establishes a platform for people to come for advice alongside the recurring information on short-distance running, jogging, and walking, including Q&A sections.[113]

The Science of Running and Walking

The establishment of a framework for correct form was meant to aid aspiring runners in their performance. Different training methods are introduced by different contemporary authors. An anecdotal example is the story of Ma Yutao 马玉涛 who wanted to establish a fitness routine including running and walking to benefit her daily life. Ma—a singer born in 1936—decided on running as a way to train her lungs for singing, and to improve her immune system and her stamina. Stories such as her "Running Slowly is also a Set of Skills" (Manpao ye shi yixiang jiben gong 慢跑也是一项基本功) show how routines were incorporated into daily lives: Ma Yutao did not run a marathon, but she made use of basic running techniques to enhance other parts of her life.[114]

It has to be noted that in this context running and walking, both part of fitness training, differ greatly from the European "walk" or "stroll." While the English "taking a walk/stroll" and the German "einen Spaziergang machen" are often used as direct translations of the Chinese terms *sanbu* 散步 and *zou* 走, they are not the activities suggested as a fitness regimen. "Taking a walk" in this particular case is a means to an end and contrasts with "strolling along," an activity that is connected to the immersion into nature, a purposeless activity that is engaged in by those who can spare the time.[115] Instead, *sanbu* here is seen as part of a healthy lifestyle benefitting the body, as well as a mode of travel.

As a step up from walking, running was considered the next level of cardio intensity. Running tips and "how-to"s usually offer all the information needed to succeed: training frequency, intensity, speed, and distance as well as body posture. Most experts (authors, doctors, etc.) considered it important that potential trainees did not start their training unprepared. In their eyes, intensity should be built up slowly: pace and time were increased depending on the individual's progress so as not to lead to exhaustion (*pilao*). The following paragraphs offer an overview of how the discussion of proper training played out.

Returning to 1956 and Shu Xincheng, we can see that he recommended that people walk as part of their daily regimen.[116] Walking could be done to and from work, he argued, but should also be incorporated after every meal to aid digestion, thus greatly benefiting the whole body. These short walking breaks during work and after lunch did not even have to be long; Shu insists that three to five minutes are enough.[117] He stresses that exercise as a whole—including running and walking—should increase in intensity according to individual progress, so as not to overly exhaust the cardiovascular system, since that may negatively influence muscle and heart activities.[118] He also emphasizes the need to adjust training individually to each person's ability and local conditions, with a wide variety of exercises that supposedly benefitted different people.[119]

Following Shu Xincheng's example, Chen Zhonghuang 陈中煌 also stressed the positive influence of cardio activity on the metabolism, the cardiovascular system, and the muscles themselves in his 1959 *Xintiyu* article "Methods to Improve Speed and Endurance in Long-distance Running" (Tigao changpao sudu he naili de fangfa 提高长跑速度和耐力的方法).[120] Chen reports that more and more workers and students like to go for a quick run of 1,000 or 2,000 meters in their breaks, and that they consider this "comfortable" (*shufu* 舒服). Due to this enthusiasm, he introduces some training schemes to inform his readers of the possible ways in which they might improve their running. He insists that training needs to be frequent to build up endurance, and that one must have determination and make high demands on oneself. With this mindset, Chen suggests that runners slowly add more and more distance to the length covered by running, again taking it out of the scope of interwork time. He recommends, for example, jumping, running for intervals with knees to elbows, or running with quick small steps. In the end, Chen suggests a week's training plan:

Monday: run for 60 min.

1. 3 km runners: 1) 8 x 100 m; 2) 2 x 1200 m
2. 5 km runners: 1) 8 x 100 m; 2) 2 x 1600 m
3. 10 km runners: 1) 8 x 100 m; 2) 2 x 2000 m

Additionally: weight exercises.

Tuesday: run for 60 min with varying speed.

1. 3 km runners: 1) 5 x 200 m; 2) 10 x 400 m; 5 x 200 m
2. 5 km runners and 10 km runners run the 400 m intervals 5 and 10 times more than the 3 km runners

Additionally: far and high jump training

Wednesday: light exercises

Thursday: same schedule as Monday but: run the 100 m interval only five times and the 1200–2000 m interval three times.

Friday: same schedule as Tuesday, but run the 400 m intervals in two sets with 5, 6, or 7 repetitions, according to distance group.

Weekend: go cross-country running, play basketball, or something else.[121]

While Chen introduces a rather technical training plan, in his 1959 *Xintiyu* article "How to Run" (Yinggai zenyang pao 应该怎样跑) Song Linhai 宋麟海 suggests a combination of walking as a base and then running as the next step in the quest for endurance, building up the ability to run further or with more vigor and improved stamina. He advises beginners to train by alternately running and walking, and to gradually increase the distance that is being run, in the end replacing walking with running completely.[122]

In the 1965 booklet *Practical Sports Medicine* (*Shiyong yundong yixue* 实用运动医学), Qu Mianyu 曲绵域, Gao Yunqiu 高云秋,[123] Pu Junzong 浦钧宗,[124] and Chen Jidi 陈吉棣[125] affirmed these methods of gradually increasing the intensity of one's exercise, but also stressed that consistency and regularity as well as changing external stimuli (hot/cold weather, water) were all key to a successful exercise regimen. Not exercising was considered a sure way to suffer from colds, angina, or pneumonia. The publication stresses three important principles with regard to exercising:

1. Proper order and gradual advance: gradual increase in intensity, and the best way to start training was in the warmer seasons.
2. Frequency: training needed to be frequent, no matter which season; if a break or a stop to training occurred, the results would suffer.
3. Changes in stimulation intensity: training in different seasons is important as different skill sets can only be trained in different seasons; resistance to cold can only be trained in cold winter weather while resistance to heat can only be trained during summer.[126]

These tips focus on external stimuli that may influence training, but they also emphasize how these external factors will additionally train and strengthen the body.

In 1973, Wang Fuxing 王福兴 and Cui Yunhai 崔云海 published an article titled "How to Practice Long-distance Running" (Zenyang lian changpao 怎样练长跑). They insist once more that running training had to be adjusted to individual abilities to avoid complications. If a person was fit and healthy there was no problem pushing them, but if they got out of breath easily softer methods were recommended. By gradually increasing the training intensity, one's abilities were adjusted and, in the end, perfected. For optimal (long-distance) running training Wang and Cui suggest an alternation between running and walking, as well as running frequently, sprinting a set distance, and cross-country running.[127]

A year later, in 1976, the book *Sport and Health* (*Tiyu yu jiankang* 体育与健康) answered questions on running, stating that to avoid injuries due to fatigue and weakness, proper nutrition and hydration prior to and after the run were important.[128] This book uses a question-and-answer scheme as its format, where specific questions are answered one by one as if the reader were asking them directly of the experts. This is how the reader learns to take his or her pulse to arrange a suitable training schedule for running, which is a method that is considered very scientific by the authors.[129]

The 1979 booklet *Life Lies in Movement* (*Shengming zaiyu yundong* 生命在于运动) is a collection of essays on exercising and running translated from English, Russian, and Japanese. One essay titled "Running for Health" (Weile jiankang er paobu 为了健康而跑步), first published in the Soviet Tajik magazine *Paper of the Tajik Communist Party* (*Tajike gongchandangren bao* 塔吉克共产党人报), not only offers advice for running, but first defines health according to Pavlov,[130] namely that health is a state of balance of the organism and the environment.[131] The essay argues that if people want to become strong, they need to run, as running was said to be the activity of primitive men which made them sturdy and brave on their daily hunt for food and clothing. The article stresses, though, that not everybody needed to become a marathon runner; instead it recommends moderate running routines for the readers' benefit. It strongly advocates walking every day (sometimes 10 km a day), for example, by commuting to work on foot.[132] The short essay also advises readers to gradually increase training intensity and frequency.[133]

A year later, in 1980, Zhuo Dahong 卓大宏[134] published "A Healthy Method of Walking" (Sanbu jiankang fa 散步健康法). In it, Zhuo points to a history of taking walks, discussing important historical figures such as Lenin's preference for taking walks, thus situating this form of activity in a longer—yet not Chinese—tradition.[135] This reference to authoritative figures gives more credibility and power to the act of walking. Accordingly, walking was seen as especially good for people who were not very fit, such as the elderly, people with chronic heart diseases, and overweight people. As a method to strengthen the metabolism, Zhuo even went so far as to claim that walking before and after meals would postpone the onset of diabetes. One additional mentioned benefit was the calming effect of walking. As exercise, walking would warm up the muscles and help the whole body relax, so that the walking individual would most certainly feel better.[136] In his discussion, the physical activity of walking is thus clearly considered to be a curative method or a way to increase basic fitness and to prevent chronic diseases.[137] It operates as a non-pharmaceutical cure for people who are feeling unwell and are not considered healthy. By curing their unwell state with movement, medical expenses could be avoided, while also avoiding the logistical demands required by hospitals, medical care, and so on.

In 1980, Wei Mingyan 魏铭炎 published *Health, Happiness, Longevity* (健康· 愉快· 长寿) in which he introduced ways to achieve the three things in the title. He includes a chapter titled "Life Lies in Running" (Shenming zaiyu Paobu 生命在于跑步), exploring the health benefits as well as the international history of running. He goes as far as to claim that in the 1970s there was a "running fever" (*paobure* 跑步热) in several nations (namely the United States, Japan, West Germany, and elsewhere) leading to a widespread surge in running activities and interest in this kind of sport.[138] He sums up the history of marathons and professional running to elaborate on the developing discipline and explores the reasons for its popularity. Apart from being an instrument of leisure, Wei stresses, running can also be seen as a widely utilized hygienic method for mental and physical health, or even as a means to treat asthma—although, if overdone, running can also do more harm than good, especially in regard to people older than 35. The author thus recommends a full-body checkup before starting training.[139]

All these accounts show very similar training methods. The general advice is to start slowly and increase intensity gradually. The articles mostly stress the strengthening aspect of running, both physically and mentally, and mention the importance of daily training, even if that simply means to incorporate walks to and from work. The curative aspect is another distinctive feature of these texts. The simple acts of walking and running are seen as a way to cure certain diseases, and are also elevated into a preventive method in line with the calls for prevention over treatment. This last aspect of the discourse on running becomes more and more pronounced with time.

The Individual Experience

As with any other health tips, information on running is disseminated via anecdotes, these being short personal stories by the authors about their personal journey and their opinions on the subject. In the Mao and post-Mao era there is no opposition between anecdotes and scientific evidence, consistent with the communist epistemological perspective on the link between practice and theory: anecdotes were used to confer value upon and explain the theory in the eyes of the readers. Anecdotes, which were published in politically engaged journals and magazines, are thus an illustrating example of propaganda and personal coercion, while scientific journals and magazines display the academic side of the discussion.

In 1959, for example, Zhu Qingbo 朱清波 recounts that he experienced an amazing change in his health status after taking up a basic fitness routine of running 3 to 5 kilometers a day. He was even able to score well in the standard *Laoweizhi* tests, and realized his concentration had improved, which in the end showed in his work and productivity.[140] A 1973 article by Tan Yibin 谭义斌 compares the author's physical state from before 1949 with his state after the introduction of health practices, and ends with the reassuring notion that his ill-health all but disappeared thanks to the incorporation of daily exercise.[141]

The recollections of individual training experiences are a tool to demonstrate the practical application of training tips and advice or even regulations. They are a vehicle to convince the readers to join the exercising part of the population. And they also illuminate an aspect of this discussion that would otherwise be hard to perceive: the individual decision to engage in exercise. This exercise, as already mentioned, could have been any exercise that corresponded to the scientific standard. The benefits of cardio training such as walking and running were not considered unique in contrast to any other form of physical training: the aims of all forms of training were muscle build up, increased overall strength, and weight loss, as well as the overcoming of fatigue and replenishing energy. They all led to the same goal: more strength and an improved immune system, and hence more productive work, fewer sick days, and better endurance in production. Running as well as radio calisthenics or other forms of gymnastics were used in the name of production and medicine, combined with therapy for physical impairment (fatigue, overweight, weakness, bad posture) and prevention.[142] As radio calisthenics was a collectively organized activity held in a controlled environment, the individual participant, of course, did not have to invest as much preparation time in it as opposed to a training schedule for running. The internal feedback in the case of *guangbo ticao* nevertheless remained important to determine the boundaries of safe activity, and given that most participants offered positive feedback, these seem not to have been breached. In 1954, according to Zhang Ruohong's report, Zhu Chenglin 朱成林, for example, managed to cure his ailments by attending these orchestrated exercises, at least according to his own recollection. He suffered from the aftereffects of his working situation and had to be convinced that calisthenics might help him, but the urging of doctors and the propaganda prevailed and, in the end, he succeeded in regaining health with the aid of radio calisthenics.[143]

Running had to be dosed carefully, though, depending on individual requirements and abilities, as a 1977 article by Cui Yunhai 崔云海 on long-distance running and shift work shows. Cui declares that working the nightshift meant increased stress on the body as this went against the natural rhythm of sleep. Work shifts were unavoidable in a nation that was expanding its industrial sector as fast as the PRC had planned, especially during the Great Leap Forward. Instead of molding the daily routines to the requirements of the workers, physical activity was adjusted to the needs of the industry and to the needs of the bodies in it. This meant that intensive running paired with nightly work was not recommended, due to the risk of exhaustion. Instead, readers were encouraged to adapt their training schedule so as to avoid fatigue and the feeling of being exhausted during their shifts. In Cui's article the personal feeling about exercise and its merits was put into focus. The parameters for training had to be set with respect to an individual's mental and emotional condition.[144]

We have at this point to acknowledge two different things: first, that the standards for running and its benefits were set by an authority (the state or experts) who offered suggestions and determined the targets that should be reached or aspired to; but, second, the targets and practices also needed to be checked against the participants' individual feelings and their emotional or energetic state. If the individual suffered from fatigue and a lack of energy, no amount of running would cure that, since running is an intense and stimulating form of exercise that would not calm the body and the mind sufficiently for it to get a decent break. For instance, in 1977 Dong Tian'en 董天恩 published a short article in the *Xintiyu*'s Q&A section on long-distance running. The article was on training for long-distance running at night, and comes to the conclusion that running as a form of exercise may be positive for the body, but was not a good form of training to engage in after work or before sleep, when the individual should actually engage in exercises to wind down. A light walk might do better than an intensive run as a means to provide relaxation and better sleep, wrote Dong.[145] During running the individual experience is an important benchmark as it provides clues to the physical condition. In the same year, in his "How Does One Examine Whether the Exercise Intensity of Long-Distance Running is Suitable?" (Zenyang guancha changpao de yundongliang shifouheshi? 怎样观察长跑的运动量是否合适？), Dong postulated individual feeling and pulse as two ways of monitoring whether the run's intensity was adequate for the individual. This introduces an objectively measurable constant that is also individually defined.[146] He allows some scope for personal feeling to decide how much is too much within a space otherwise governed by authorities. This is used to avoid exhaustion in the population and opens up the possibility of choice for the individual body: to run or not to run.[147]

As Shuman argued, "*tiyu* served to mold ideal socialist subjects [. . .]."[148] The two case studies—radio calisthenics and running—have shed light on two different—though combinable—ways of governing a person's health and fitness, both of which were a means to introduce body knowledge to the population. Radio calisthenics was an institutionalized practice, while running depended on an individualized training plan. Exercises were not mandatory for everybody in the population at the same degree of intensity, but were adjusted to the individual situation according to sex, age, and workload.

The state—as the main authority—could go as far as spreading this knowledge and implementing activities at work or at school, but that is where its influence stopped, and where the need for individual feedback on personal comfort came into play. The "self," as the entity giving this feedback, was the last control mechanism that the state could not penetrate, even while it tried to implement exercise programs such as the *Laoweizhi* or radio calisthenics as ways to raise the quality of bodies, to control and regulate them. Despite its efforts, the state could not dictate whether a person felt discomfort or not. Short of employing excessively coercive methods to mold the larger part of the population, the state had to accept the barrier of individual bodily conditions and the sensations attached to them. This acceptance of the individual person's feelings concerning their well-being can be seen in the words of caution not to overdo one's exercise and to respect bodily boundaries. This caution was especially important for fitness and physical activity, as each person had a different basic bodily precondition. If this was not taken into account, injuries might occur, leading to losses in production and income where workers were unable to do their daily chores. A basic understanding of one's own body and its limits thus was indispensable for smooth economic production in the eyes of the state.

At the same time, exercise was seen as a way to engage the body and strengthen it for the sake of production. The resulting strong body was part of a nation that was growing ever stronger—or at least so the authorities hoped. By utilizing physical education for the purpose of production, exercise was institutionalized and filled with ideology, situated as an essential part of a truly socialist way of life.

NOTES

1. Mao Zedong, "A Study of Physical Education (Tiyu zhi yanjiu 体育之研究)," *Xin Qingnian* (April 1917).

2. Nine sequences had been published by 2011.

3. Nicolas Schillinger, *The Body and Military Masculinity in Late Qing and Early Republican China: The Art of Governing Soldiers* (New York: Lexington Books, 2016), 3.

4. Schillinger, 320.

5. Andrew D. Morris, *Marrow of the Nation: A History of Sport and Physical Culture in Republican China* (Berkeley: University of California Press, 2004), 18.

6. Amanda Shuman, "The Politics of Socialist Athletics in the People's Republic of China, 1949–1966" (PhD diss., University of California, 2014), ix. See also Susan

Brownell, *Training the Body for China: Sports in the Moral Order of the People's Republic* (Chicago: University of Chicago Press, 1995), 28.

7. Rabinbach, *The Human Motor*; Drew Leder, *The Absent Body* (Chicago: University of Chicago Press, 1990); Drew Leder, *The Body in Medical Thought and Practice* (Dordrecht: Kluwer Academic Publishers, 1992); Drew Leder, *The Distressed Body: Rethinking Illness, Imprisonment, and Healing* (Chicago: University of Chicago Press, 2016); Ben Carrington and Ian McDonald, *Marxism, Cultural Studies, and Sport* (New York: Routledge, 2009); Alfons Labisch, *Homo hygienicus: Gesundheit und Medizin in der Neuzeit* (Frankfurt am Main: Campus Verlag, 1992).

8. See René Descartes, *Discourse on Method*, trans. John Veitch, 2008, https://www.gutenberg.org/files/59/59-h/59-h.htm (accessed March 19, 2020).

9. Labisch, *Homo Hygienicus*, 107.

10. Rabinbach, *The Human Motor*, 51.

11. See for example Rabinbach, *The Human Motor*, 65.

12. Lesley A. Sharp, "The Commodification of the Body and its Parts," *Annual Review of Anthropology* 29 (2000): 287–328.

13. Sharp, 290.

14. See Rabinbach, *The Human Motor*; Nick Cullather, "The Foreign Policy of the Calorie," *American Historical Review* 112, no. 2 (April 2007): 337–64.

15. Leder, *The Absent Body*, 21: "The mechanist world-view allows the crucial shift from passive contemplation to the active manipulation which characterizes the modern age."

16. Leder, 293.

17. Chen Shuqi 陈叔骐, *Yingyang weisheng* 营养卫生 (Beijng: Renmin weisheng chubanshe, 1954), 3. Quotes like this are not widespread, but the vocabulary used in connection to the body and its utilization in physical education and training remains very technical, for example, energy *reliang* 热量.

18. Jia-Chen Fu, *The Other Milk: Reinventing Soy in Republican China* (Seattle: University of Washington Press, 2018), 9.

19. Liping Bu, "Anti-Malaria Campaigns and the Socialist Reconstruction of China, 1950–80," *East Asian History* 39 (2014): 122f.

20. The comparison of the human body to a machine or a tool does not stop with nutritional science, physiology, or production. It is also utilized in the revolutionary rhetoric to describe it as a machinery in which the participants are just screws and cogs. In order to succeed, and for the greater good of the nation, the participation of everyone was important. See Xie Yueming 谢月明, "Zai shanqu duanlian sixiang ganqing 在山区锻炼思想感情," *Renmin Ribao* (June 21, 1965). The article elaborates on intellectuals' experiences in the *xiaxiang* 下乡 movements in the beginning of the Cultural Revolution (and even before) and their involvement in the revolutionary machinery.

21. Tina Mai Chen, "The Human-Machine Continuum in Maoism: The Intersection of Soviet Socialist Realism, Japanese Theoretical Physics, and Chinese Revolutionary Theory," *Cultural Critique* 80 (Winter 2012): 155.

22. Sakata Shouichi (1911–1970) was a Japanese physicist who was interested in Marxist philosophy and revered by Mao Zedong. See Edward Friedman, Paul G.

Pickowicz, and Mark Selden, *Revolution, Resistance, and Reform in Village China* (New Haven, CT: Yale University Press, 2005).

23. Mao, "Guanyu bantian wenzhang de tanhua," translation quoted according to Tina Mai Chen, "The Human-Machine Continuum in Maoism," 158. The original reads: "认识工具当中要包括镬头、机器等等。人的认识来源于实践。我们用镬头、机器等等改造世界，我们的认识就深入了。工具是人器官的延长。镬头就是手臂的延长，望远镜是眼睛的延长，身体、五官都可以延长。"

In a discussion of Sakata Shouichi's work, Mao Zedong noted the machine-likeness of thc human being and its excellent ability to invent tools to help it strive. In this quotation he sums up the ability of humans to extend their bodies with tools, an ability that he does not extend to animals.

24. Chen, "The Human-Machine Continuum in Maoism," 158.

25. For a thorough discussion of the introduction of anatomy studies in the Republican era, see David Luesink, "Anatomy and the Reconfiguration of Life and Death in Republican China," *Journal of Asian Studies* 76, no. 4 (November 2017): 1009–34. Luesink stresses for the 1930s that "*Tiyu* specialists like Wan Weicun argued that knowledge of basic physiology and anatomy for physical education was essential for all educators, athletes, and trainers" (p. 1017). This shows that the connection between theoretical knowledge of anatomy and movement had already been introduced to the Chinese population before the founding of the PRC.

26. Schillinger, *The Body and Military Masculinity*; Luesink, "Anatomy and the Reconfiguration of Life and Death"; Larissa Heinrich, *The Afterlife of Images: Translating the Pathological Body Between China and the West* (Durham, NC: Duke University Press, 2008).

27. Luesink, "Anatomy and the Reconfiguration of Life and Death." See also Bridie Andrews and Mary Brown Bullock, eds., *Medical Transitions in Twentieth-Century China* (Bloomington: Indiana University Press, 2014), and He Lydia Liu, *Translingual Practice: Literature, National Culture, and Translated Modernity—China, 1900–1937* (Stanford: Stanford University Press, 1999).

28. Schillinger, *The Body and Military Masculinity*, 52.

29. Kavelnikov (Keliesituonikefu 可列斯托尼科夫), "Shenti xunlian neng zengjin jiankang 身体训练能增进健康," trans. Liang Ziqin 梁子勤, *Xintiyu* 3 (1954): 23–24.

30. Wu Zhenying 武真英, "Buyao pao de guofen 不要跑得过分," *Xintiyu* 12 (1980): 31. In this short article, Wu also reminds the readers to listen to their own body to avoid training too much and so harming it.

31. The discussion only centers around health, not beauty *mei* 美. The question of aesthetics is not raised in this context. In fact, the contexts of bodily aesthetics and of health do not greatly intersect; beauty might be a result of health, but during the first three PRC decades it is not seen as a requirement.

32. The categories to distinguish bodies mentioned here were age, school, work, or pregnancy, which are all different environments that need different attention to the body.

33. Brownell, *Training the Body for China*, 58.

34. This is also sometimes called "circulatory system" *xunhuan xitong* 循环系统, see Fuzhou budui houqinbu weishengbu, ed., *Minbing weishengyuan keben* 民兵卫生员课本 (Beijing: Renmin weisheng chubanshe, 1975), 22.

35. Tiyu yu jiankang bianxie xiaozu, *Tiyu yu jiankang—yundong shengli weisheng changshi* (Beijing: Renmin tiyu chubanshe, 1976).

36. For discussions of the microcosm body, see Angela Zito and Tani E. Barlow, eds., *Body, Subject, and Power in China* (Chicago: University of Chicago Press, 1994), and Thomas P. Kasulis, Roger T. Aimes, and Wimal Dissanayake, *Self as Body in Asian Theory and Practice* (Albany: State University of New York, 1993).

37. Wang Xuliang 王序良, "Zai nongcun zenyang duanlian shenti—jiqiao 在农村怎样锻炼身体——技巧," *Xintiyu* 1 (1977): 55–56. Wang Xuliang, born in 1937, was a gymnast and an athlete. In 1960, Wang graduated from Shenyang Sport University. He is a member of several national gymnastics associations (*Ticao dacidian*, 体操大辞典 [Beijing: Renmin tiyu chubanshe, 1999], 658).

38. These visual materials on the skeleton, muscles, and sinews have been in use since the Republican period, see Luesink, "Anatomy and the Reconfiguration of Life and Death."

39. Hebei shifan daxue tiyuxi bian, eds., *Shengli weisheng* 生理卫生 (Beijing: Renmin tiyu chubanshe, 1978), 10.

40. Qu Mianyu 曲绵域, Gao Yunqiu 高云秋, Pu Junzong 浦钧宗, and Chen Jidi 陈吉棣, *Shiyong yundong yixue* 实用运动医学 (Beijing: Beijing daxue yixue chubanshe, 1965), 193–95. This material was originally considered a *neibu faxing* 内部发行, an internal release for the direct use of cadres and government members. The leading author Qu Mianyu, born in 1924, was an expert in sports medicine. He held a research position and a professorship at the medical school of Peking University. (See *Yundong jiepouxue, yundingyixue dacidian*, 运动解剖学、运动医学大辞典 [Beijing: Renmin tiyu chubanshe, 2000], 484.)

41. See Mike O'Mahony, *Sport in the USSR—Physical Culture—Visible Culture* (London: Reaktion Books, 2006).

42. John N. Washburn, "Sport as a Soviet Tool," *Foreign Affairs* 34, no. 3 (April 1956): 490; Reet Howell, "The USSR: Sport and Politics Intertwined," *Comparative Education* 11, no. 2 (1975): 137.

43. Howell, "The USSR: Sport and Politics Intertwined," 138.

44. Nina S. Levent, *Healthy Spirit in a Healthy Body: Representations of the Sports Body in Soviet Art of the 1920s and 1930s* (New York: P. Lang, 2004), 39.

45. James Riordan, *Sport in Soviet Society: Development of Sport and Physical Education in Russia and the USSR* (New York: Cambridge University Press, 1977), 95–101.

46. Riordan, 108.

47. Amanda Shuman, "Elite Competitive Sport in the People's Republic of China 1958–1966: The Games of the New Emerging Forces (GANEFO)," *Journal of Sport History* 40, no. 2 (2013): 261.

48. Brownell, *Training the Body for China*, 19.

49. Shuman, "Politics of Socialist Athletics," viii, 61.

50. The *Laoweizhi* was a fitness standard that institutionalized physical education and physical hygiene. It thus influenced everyday life on a very basic level. Different standards and norms were formulated in this system and were used to test the population on their fitness status.

51. Shuman, "Politics of Socialist Athletics," viii, 93–111.

52. Shuman, 119–20, 122.

53. Shuman, 127–34.

54. Shuman, 146–47.

55. For a short discussion of the origin of the words *ticao* or *yundong*, see Morris, *Marrow of the Nation*, 6.

56. Schillinger, *The Body and Military Masculinity*.

57. Schillinger, 50.

58. Schillinger, 51.

59. See Shuman, "Politics of Socialist Athletics"; Brownell, *Training the Body for China*.

60. See, for example, Shu Xincheng, *Wo zenyang huifu jiankangde* 我怎样恢复健康的 (Beijing: Zhonghua shuju chubanshe, 1956), 113–16; Wu Bangwei 吴邦伟, *Tiyu lilun jiben zhishi* 体育理论基本知识 (Beijing: Renmin tiyu chubanshe, 1957), 80–81; "Cankao xiaoxi" bianjibu, *Shengming zaiyu yundong* 生命在于运动 (Taiyuan: Shanxi renmin chubanshe, 1979).

61. Xinjiaoyu shebian, *Xintiyu de lilun he shixian* 新体育的理论和实践 (Shanghai: Huadong renmin chubanshe, 1951).

62. A. T. Brykin (Bu Leijin 布雷金), *Ticao. Shang ji* 体操. 上集, trans. Fang Bin 方瑸, Li Guozhen 李国珍, and Liang Ziqing梁子勤 (Beijing: Renmin tiyu chubanshe, 1954), 17: "Production calisthenics *shengchan ticao* 生产体操."

63. Brykin, *Ticao*, 10.

64. Qu Mianyu, "Gongjiancao jiujing you shenme haochu? 工间操究竟有什么好处？" *Xintiyu* 8 (1957): 16.

65. For a discussion of manual versus mental workers, see Joel Andreas, *Rise of the Red Engineers: The Cultural Revolution and the Origins of China's New Class* (California: Stanford University Press, 2009), 162.

66. Just as with nutrition requirements, different workloads require different exercises and movements. See, for example, the admonition that sedentary, mental workers, also described as intellectuals, had to specifically attend to their exercise routines: A. Kolabrev (A. Kelabuliefu 恩•柯拉布列夫), "Zhili laodong zhe de tiyu 智力劳动者的体育," trans. Gao Feng, *Xintiyu* 17 (1951): 13. For Kolabrev exercise is part of a resting strategy for mental workers. For them it was important to get up regularly and get fresh air. As exercise suggestions, they should do gymnastics every day for 15–25 minutes, walk (a natural, beneficial way of exercising), and incorporate calisthenics, games, and movement into daily routines.

67. Bertschnikov, "Tiyu huodong dui naoli laodongzhe de yiyi 体育活动对脑力劳动者的意义," trans. Li Haiping 李海萍, *Xintiyu* 21 (1956): 32–33: Bertschnikov suggested that as mental work was exhausting, breaks were needed by those engaging in it. After work they should go for a walk, swim, do exercises or physically taxing work, or participate in cultural entertainment. These activities were good breaks from

mental work and helped to relax the worker and improve brain function, according to the author. His daily recommendation for mental workers was to do 15–20 minutes of hygiene calisthenics (radio calisthenics) every day in the morning, while at night they should frequently take walks for 30–60 minutes.

68. Tang Wuyuan 唐午园, "Zhishi fenzi de jianshen fangfa 知识分子的健身方法," *Xintiyu* 13 (1957): 22–24.

69. Xie Bin 谢彬, "Zuocao neng xiaochu pilao 做操能消除疲劳," *Xintiyu* 9 (1957): 20. The article specifically discusses the engineer Cheng Mingsheng's 程明升 experiences with exercise and exhaustion. Cheng Mingsheng was the assistant to the director of the department for electrical industry (*dianli gongyebu buzhang zhuli* 电力工业部部长助理).

70. Shu Xincheng, *Wo zenyang huifu jiankangde*, 116–17.

71. Zhao Gezhuang, "Kuanggong de tiyu 矿工的体育," *Xintiyu* 19 (1957): 20–21. A much later article which sums up the same benefits of exercising and calisthenics for peasants is the 1977 article by Wang Xuliang, "Zai nongcun zenyang duanlian shenti——jiqiao 在农村怎样锻炼身体——技巧," *Xintiyu* 1 (1977): 55–56.

72. Shuman, "Politics of Socialist Athletics," 74.

73. Shuman, 72–73.

74. Yu Lishuang 于丽爽, "Guangbo ticao, bange shiji de quanmin jianshen jiyi 广播体操，半个世纪的全民健身记忆," in *Lishi de beijing* 历史的背景, ed. Beijing ribao jishi caixiezu (Beijing: Jiefangjun wenyi chubanshe, 2009), 231.

75. Yu Lishuang, "Guangbo ticao, bange shiji de quanmin jianshen jiyi," 234–36.

76. The All-China Sports Federation was founded in 1949 and met regularly from 1952 onward. It was involved in spreading physical education to the grassroot levels and in the planning of national and international sporting events. See *Zhonghua renmin gongheguoshi cidian*, ed. 朱建华 and 郭彬蔚 (Guilin 吉林文史出版社, 1989), 305.

77. Zhongyang tiyu duanlian weiyuanhui guangbo ticao xiaozu, "Di'er tao guangbo ticao gongbu le 第二套广播体操公布了," *Xintiyu* 8 (1954): 20: "Before the creation of the second sequence, the suggestions of the masses on the first sequence were collected. According to these suggestions a number of principles for the second sequence were researched established . . . " [在第二套广播体操编製以前，搜集了羣众对第一 套广播体操的意见，根据这些意见，研究和提出了第二套广播体操编製的几个原则 [. . .]].

"Zhongyang tiyu yundong weiyuanhui he guangbo sheye ju deng danwei yi bianzhi chu de er tao guangbo ticao 中央体育运动委员会和广播事业局等单位 已编制出第二套广播体操," *Renmin Ribao* (July 27, 1954): "they took up the people's suggestions, revised them a few times . . . " [吸收了广大群众的意见，多次进行修改].

78. A similar, though much more profound, exchange between scientists, the state, and the population would take place in agriculture during the Mao era; see Sigrid Schmalzer, *Red Revolution, Green Revolution* (Chicago: University of Chicago Press, 2016), 100–28.

79. Zhonghua quanguo tiyu zonghui choubei weiyuanhui guangbo ticao yanjiu xiaozu, "Dajia dou lai zuo guangbo ticao 大家都来做广播体操," *Renmin Ribao*

(November 25, 1951); and "Guangbo ticao tujie 广播体操图解," *Renmin Ribao* (November 25, 1951).

80. Over the years the movements were repeated in various forms. Some were changed and became just a little more complicated by deepening stretches or adding arm movements.

81. Yu Lishuang, *Guangbo ticao, bange shiji de quanmin jianshen jiyi*, 236. These descriptions and names concur with the ones on the form sheets published in the *Renmin Ribao* and the *Xintiyu*.

82. Yu Lishuang, 242.

83. Yu Lishuang, 242; Zhonghua quanguo tiyu zonghui choubei weiyuanhui guangbo ticao yanjiu xiaozu, "Dajia dou lai zuo guangbo ticao 大家都来做广播体操," *Renmin Ribao* (November 25, 1951).

84. This breakdown can be found at the beginning of each introduction of a new sequence. This introduction puts radio calisthenics in the PRC into context and each time displays the development it has undergone.

85. "Dali puji guangbo ticao 大力普及广播体操," *Xintiyu* 12 (1951): 6.

86. "Tui guangbo ticao yundong fazhan renmin tiyu shiye! 推广播体操运动发展人民体育事业!" *Renmin Ribao* (November 25, 1951).

87. "Jinyibu kaizhan guangbo ticao yundong (duanping) 进一步开展广播体操运动（短评）," *Renmin Ribao* (July 29, 1954).

88. Zhongyang tiyu duanlian weiyuanhui guangbo ticao xiaozu, "Di'er tao guangbo ticao gongbu le 第二套广播体操公布了," *Xintiyu* 8 (1954): 20. "Zhongyang tiyu yundong weiyuanhui he guangbo sheye ju deng danwei yi bianzhi chu de er tao guangbo ticao 中央体育运动委员会和广播事业局等单位　已编制出第二套广播体操," *Renmin Ribao* (July 27, 1954).

89. Li Menghua 李梦华, "Dajia lai zuo de san tao guangbo ticao 大家来做第三套广播体操," *Renmin Ribao* (October 7, 1957). Li Menghua was born in 1922, and since 1954 has been working for the National Sports Committee, holding various positions in Chinese sports committees and organization groups. He headed the Olympic planning committee for the 2008 Olympics in China. (See *Zhongguo tiyu baike quanshu* 中国体育百科全书 (Beijing: Renmin tiyu chubanshe), 128.)

90. The article does not mention where the overweight came from. It does not clarify whether the workers had sedentary or physically taxing jobs.

91. Wu Jiangping 吴江平and Jiang Youzhen 蒋佑桢, "Disantao guangbo ticao gongbule 第三套广播体操公布了," *Xintiyu* 19 (1957): 34.

Wu Jiangping, born in 1914, was a member of the National Sports Committee and of the China Wushu Association. He researches and practices Wushu and Qigon. (See *Zhongguo wushu renming cidian* 中国武术人名辞典 [Beijing: Renmin tiyu chubanshe, 1993], 319.)

92. Fang Fei 方芾, "Xin jiang fangzhi guang tiyu huodong sanji 新绛纺织广体育活动散记," *Xintiyu* 2 (1962): 5–7.

93. "Dajia dou lai zuo guangbo ticao大家都来做广播体操," *Renmin Ribao* (April 18, 1963).

94. "Guanyu zai quanguo shexing xin guangbo ticao de tongzhi 关于在全国试行新广播体操的通知," *Renmin Ribao* (September 1, 1971).

95. Nantongshi baihuo shangdian dangzhibu, geweihui, “Women shi zenyang jianchi guangbo ticao 我们是怎样坚持广播体操,” *Xintiyu* 11 (1973): 26–28.

For another anecdote on the curative properties of *ticao*, see Zhang Ruohuang 张若煌, “Guangbo ticao gei Zhu Chenglin le jiankang 广播体操给朱成林了健康,” *Xintiyu* 8 (1954): 37.

96. “Jiji tuixing di liu tao guangbo ticao 积极推行第六套广播体操,” *Renmin Ribao* (September 1, 1981).

97. It is safe to say that it was not meant as practical but as ideological education.

98. “Jinyibu kaizhan guangbo ticao yundong (duanping) 进一步开展广播体操运动（短评）,” *Renmin Ribao* (July 29, 1954).

99. Ma Yuehan 马约翰, “He qingnian tan tiyu duanlian 和青年谈体育锻炼,” *Xintiyu* 1 (1957): 4–6.

100. Lukyanov, *Jiankang yu laodong nengli de baohu*, 93; Tiyu yu jiankang bianxie xiaozu, *Tiyu yu jiankang—yundong shengli weisheng changshi*, 362ff.; Imamura Yoshio, Kinbara Isamu, Ishiko Toshihiro, and Kuroda Yoshio, eds., *Riben zhongxue baojian tiyu* 日本中学保健体育, trans. Wang Deshen 王德深 (Beijing: Wenhua jiaoyu chubanshe, 1982), 17.

101. Shuman, “Politics of Socialist Athletics,” 13, 15. These “sports programs in the Mao years also aimed to build a corps of elite athletes who could represent the Chinese socialist nation in international competition.” Of course, running (short-, middle-, and long-distance running) was considered a competitive sport that could be trained for and excelled in, but basic running training was also incorporated into daily health regimen for the broad populace.

102. In this case, the institutionalization took the form of offering basic tips on running, such as in Yang Shoubo 杨守博, “Tantan bai gongchi saipao de wenti 谈谈百公尺赛跑的问题,” *Xintiyu* 56 (1955): 29.

103. See Gao Ming 高明, “Beipiao meikuang gong changpao dui jianchi dongji duanlian 北票煤矿工长跑队坚持冬季锻炼,” *Xintiyu* 2 (1959). The picture shows a long-distance running group from a coal mining company in Beipiao practicing in winter.

104. The fact that sports practices had to make do with very little resources is also mentioned by Shuman (“Politics of Socialist Athletics,” 14).

105. Hikita and Oda, “Qing ni yigeren paobu 请你一个人跑步,” in *Shengming zaiyu yundong* 生命在于运动, ed. “Cankao xiaoxi” bianjibu (Taiyuan: Shanxi renmin chubanshe, 1979). Hikata and Oda strongly suggest that running alone is a good practice so as to adjust one’s running requirements to one’s own ability, and not to run with the group.

106. See Seward C. Staley, *Geren yu tuanti zhi jingzhi yundong* 个人与团体之竞技运动, trans. Wang Yicheng 王毅诚 and Jin Feijun 金非均 (Shanghai: Shanghai renwen yinshuguan, 1930).

107. M. Cherevkov (Qiliefukefu 契列甫柯夫), *Sulian tiyu jiaocai* 苏联体育教材, trans. Qiu Biao 仇标 (Shanghai: Beixin shuju, 1952).

108. Chen Su 陈苏, *Tiyu yu jiankang* 体育与健康 (Nanchang: Jiangxi renmin chubanshe, 1955), 15–16.

109. Another example is Laurence E. Morehouse and Leonard Gross, *Total Fitness in 30 Minutes a Week* (Granada: St. Albans, 1977), which was introduced by a 1980 article in the *Xintiyu* (Liao Xin 廖心, "Yu jianshen yundong yu richang shenghuo 寓健身运动于日常生活," *Xintiyu* 3 (1980): 40) and as part of the 1979 publication *Shengming zaiyu yundong* 生命在于运动 by the "Cankao xiaoxi" bianjibu, that lists the "14 myths of fitness."

110. *Guangbo ticao* routines kept on coming, but no more Labor and Defense System norms.

111. Yuan Dan 袁旦, "Pao (Zai nongcun zenyang duanlian shenti) 跑(在农村怎样锻炼身体?)," *Xintiyu* 4 (1977): 34–36.

112. Beijing tiyuxueyuan tiyuweisheng jiaoyanshi, "Changpao duanlian weisheng zhishi wenda 长跑锻炼卫生知识问答," *Xintiyu* 11 (1977): 41. Other Q&A sections were, for example, Dong Tian'en, "Changpao wenda: Wanshang lianxi changpao heshi bu heshi 长跑问答: 晚上练习长跑合适不合适?," *Xintiyu* 1 (1977): 62–63.

113. Yu Weili 余维立, "Lian changpao hou duanpao chengji hui xiajiang ma? 练长跑后短跑成绩会下降吗?" *Xintiyu* 9 (1977): 60. Ma Yutao 马玉涛, "Manpao yeshi yi xiang jibengong 慢跑也是一项基本功," *Xintiyu* 2 (1980): 27. Zhuo Dahong 卓大宏, "Sanbu jiankangfa 散步健康法," *Xintiyu* 5 (1980): 36–37. Deng Shuxun 邓树勋, "Changpao aihao zhe: 'Yong duanpao li kuai pao daiti mansu changpao haobuhao?' 长跑爱好者: '用短跑离快跑代替慢速长跑好不好?,'" *Xintiyu* 11 (1980): 32–33.

114. Ma Yutao 马玉涛, "Manpao yeshi yi xiang jibengong 慢跑也是一项基本功," *Xintiyu* 2 (1980): 27.

115. For a closer look at the Chinese habits of "*spazieren*" and the history of this specific idea, see Wolfgang Kubin, "Warum und zu welchem Zweck geht ein Chinese (nicht) spazieren? Ein Versuch," in *Kopflandschaften, Landschaftsgänge: Kulturgeschichte und Poetik des Spaziergangs*, ed. Axel Gellhaus et al. (Köln: Böhlau, 2007).

116. Shu Xincheng, *Wo zenyang huifu jiankangde*, 114.

117. Shu Xincheng, 121. Another article discussing the problems of over- and underweight people confirms Shu's suggestion: Wu Zhuzhong 吴柱中, "Pan ren yu shouren de wenti 胖人与瘦人的问题," *Xintiyu* 22 (1956): 21. See also Jiang Qiyuan 姜淇远, "Fa hou weisheme bu keyi zuo julie huodong 飯後為什麼不可以做劇烈活動," *Xintiyu* 18 (1952): 40.

118. Shu Xincheng, *Wo zenyang huifu jiankangde*, 110. Shu also addressed (p. 111) the issue of people misinterpreting sore muscles as fatigue or a negative impact of sport, and stopping as soon as they experience this "pain," although it would be necessary to persevere and push through in order to attain all the benefits physical training can offer.

119. Shu Xincheng, 113. There still is a reminder of attention: *Zhuyi weisheng* 注意卫生: Exercise should not be done alone; a person should keep track of their food intake; they should take post-workout breaks.

120. Chen Zhonghuang 陈中煌, "Tigao changpao sudu he naili de fangfa 提高长跑速度和耐力的方法," *Xintiyu* 6 (1959): 26.

121. Chen Zhonghuang 陈中煌, "Tigao changpao sudu he naili de fangfa 提高长跑速度和耐力的方法," *Xintiyu* 6 (1959): 27.

122. Song Linhai 宋麟海, "Yinggai zenyang pao 应該怎样跑," *Xintiyu* 24 (1959): 27.

123. Gao Yunqiu 高云秋 (born 1930) was a professor and head of the sports medicine research institute of the Beijing Health Science University. He was on the editorial board of the *Zhongguo yundong yixue zazhi* 中国运动医学杂志 and of the *Tiyu kexue* 体育科学. (See *Yundong jiepouxue, yundingyixue dacidian*, 487.)

124. Pu Junzong 浦钧宗 (born 1934), like Gao Yunqiu, was a professor and part of the sports medicine research institute of the Beijing Health Science University. He was on the editorial board of the *Zhongguo yundong yixue zazhi* 中国运动医学杂志. Pu graduated in 1955 from Harbin Medicine and Science University. (See *Yundong jiepouxue, yundingyixue dacidian*, 491.)

125. Chen Jidi 陈吉棣 (born 1930) was the head of the nutrition and biochemistry research unit at the sports medicine research institute of the Beijing Health Science University. She was also a professor and graduated in 1959 from Beijing Health Science University. (See *Yundong jiepouxue, yundingyixue dacidian*, 402.)

126. Qu Mianyu et al., *Shiyong yundong yixue*, 193–95.

127. Wang Fuxing 王福兴 and Cui Yunhai 崔云海, "Zenyang lian changpao 怎样练长跑," *Xintiyu* 1 (1973): 30–31. According to the article, Wang Fuxing 王福兴 worked with vehicles at the Fengtai district of the Beijing railway bureau (Beijing tielu fenju Fengtai cheliangduan gong北京铁路分局丰台车辆段工); Cai Yunhai 崔云海 worked at the Beijing Erligou car manufacture plant (Beijing Erligou qiche zhizaochang gong 北京二里沟汽车制造厂工).

128. Tiyu yu jiankang bianxie xiaozu, *Tiyu yu jiankang—yundong shengli weisheng changshi*, 362–84.

129. Tiyu yu jiankang bianxie xiaozu, 376.

130. Ivan Pavlov (1849–1936) was a Soviet scientist who is famous for his physiological experiments that included behavior modifications and research on the connection between stimuli and physiological reactions. He was heralded as *the* big Soviet scientist in almost any Chinese science publication before the Sino-Soviet split.

131. "Cankao xiaoxi" bianjibu, *Shengming zaiyu yundong*, 19.

132. "Cankao xiaoxi" bianjibu, 20.

133. The essay suggests the following: Starting from twice a week, after 1–2 months the runner should run 3–4 times a week. In the beginning this should be no more than 10–20 minutes at an easy running pace, which can be increased after confirmation with a doctor. Then an increase to 45–60 minutes is considered fine. The article strongly urges readers to make this practice into a habit. See "Cankao xiaoxi" bianjibu, 21.

134. Zhuo Dahong 卓大宏 (1932–) graduated from Huanan medical school in 1955. He specializes in sports medicine and convalescent medicine. (See *Yundong jiepouxue, yundingyixue dacidian*, 489.)

135. Zhuo Dahong 卓大宏, "Sanbu jiankangfa 散步健康法," *Xintiyu* 5 (1980): 36–37.

136. Exercise methods of Zhuo Dahong: 1. normal walking, 2. fast walking, 3. set distance and time method, 4. walking with forceful upper body movement, and 5. walking and massaging the abdomen.

137. As a curative method it is suggested to cure not only weight problems, but also bad conditions of the body, such as *bazi jiao* 八字脚; see Li Liangbiao 李良标, "'Bazijiao' hui rongxiang paode sudu ma '八字脚' 会彤响跑的速度吗?," *Xintiyu* 8 (1978): 33.

138. Wei Mingyan 魏铭炎, *Jiankang. Yukuai. Changshou* 健康· 愉快· 长寿 (Guangzhou: Kexuepuji chubanshe guangzhou fenshe, 1980), 18.

139. Wei Mingyan, 23–24.

140. Zhu Qingbo 朱清波, "Paobu gei wo haochu duo 跑步給我好处多," *Xintiyu* 7 (1959): 33.

141. Tan Yibin 谭义斌, "Duanlian shenti yao zijue 锻炼身体要自觉," *Xintiyu* 11 (1973): 14–16.

142. The notion of adding exercise to a labor-intensive day as a way to prevent the deterioration of the body can be traced through some articles, specifically the following: Shen Shen 深深, "Dongji lun changpao 冬季论长跑," *Dazhong Yixue* 2 (1960): 76; Wang Xuliang, "Zai nongcun zenyang duanlian shenti——jiqiao 在农村怎样锻炼身体——技巧," *Xintiyu* 1 (1977): 55–56; Zhuo Dahong, "Yundong jiushi shengming, duanlian keyi fang bing 运动就是生命，锻炼可以防病," *Xintiyu* 11 (1977): 12–15; Pu Junzong, "Changpao duanlian weisheme neng fangzhi shenjing shuairuo 长跑锻炼为什么能防治神经衰弱?" *Xintiyu* 12 (1977): 38–39.

143. Zhang Ruohuang, "Guangbo ticao gei Zhu Chenglin le jiankang 广播体操给朱成林了健康," *Xintiyu* 8 (1954): 37.

144. Cui Yunhai 崔云海, "Sanban dao gongren shenme shijian changpao hao 三班倒工人什么时间长跑好," *Xintiyu* 12 (1977): 39.

145. Dong Tian'en, "Changpao wenda: Wanshang lianxi changpao heshi bu heshi 长跑问答: 晚上练习长跑合适不合适?" *Xintiyu* 1 (1977): 62–63.

146. Dong Tian'en, "Zenyang guancha changpao de yundongliang shifou heshi? 怎样观察长跑的运动量是否合适?" *Xintiyu* 12 (1977): 18.

147. Interestingly enough, there were no notions of overdoing it at radio calisthenics provided one went through the sequences as intended. This may be because the circumstance under which radio calisthenics happened were monitored.

148. Shuman, "Politics of Socialist Athletics," 11.

Chapter 4

Time to Rest

The notions of rest (*xiuxi* 休息) and sleep (*shuiyan* 睡眠, *shuijiao* 睡觉) are central parts of a healthy lifestyle in popular Mao-era medicine and physical health-related publications. Fatigue (*pilao* 疲劳), caused by too much stress, a lack of sleep, or as a natural by-product of labor, posed a danger to the socialist reconstruction of the nation. Accordingly, it was addressed by the state in the form of resting routines intended to prevent labor-related exhaustion.

The discussion of sleep has so far mainly been restricted to its biomedical and psychological aspects, and has been neglected in the humanities. Yet the few studies on sleep and exhaustion open up an intriguing research field that exists at the intersection of biomedicine, psychology, sociology, and labor studies. Hannah Ahlheim's *Der Traum vom Schlaf im Zwanzigsten Jahrhundert* (2018), Eluned Summers-Bremner's *Insomnia—A Cultural History* (2008), and Kenton Kroker's *The Sleep of Others* (2007), but also Rabinbach's *The Human Motor* (1992), have introduced the humanities to thinking about sleep, and here serve as a base for my considerations of the role and significance of sleep in the Mao era. By referring back to these studies, this approach does not imply that sleeping habits in Mao China were identical to those in Europe or North America; rather I want to emphasize that sleep is a universal activity that can be observed worldwide. This observation is corroborated by the fact that medical information on sleep was highly informed by research in Europe, the Soviet Union, and the United States. Chinese experts replicated such knowledge almost word by word and applied it to their social context.

Contrary to their lack of prominence in existing historical research, sleeping and resting were accepted as a central part of social and bodily hygiene in the first three decades of the PRC. This period has often been viewed as overtly inhumane, marked by the exploitation of the population for the greater aim of socialist reconstruction, as for example during the Great Leap Forward or the Cultural Revolution. Long hours of hard work reduced both the quality and quantity of sleep, which led to a loss of vigor, thus endangering productivity.

Conceptually, even though it is part of the human condition and an element of the daily routine, sleep itself is rather difficult to grasp—not only as a subject in and of itself, but also as a focus of research. Primary sources on this subject dating from the Mao era are rare, but some do exist, and these provide a good overview of the discussion. As a focus of this chapter, instead of seeking to unearth the social reality of sleep, I concentrate on how ideal ways of sleeping and resting were communicated to the populace and how they were integrated into everyday life. My focus lies on the understanding and implementation of sleep within daily life, and the establishment of basic knowledge about it. I attempt to fill the scholarly gap in the study of sleep in China by introducing the handling of sleep, and specifically rest, in the contexts of health and labor.

Observing the practical advice given to the broad population by the state, one has to ask why the party-state had to intervene with regards to sleep and rest, and why in the end it was mostly excluded from this most private human activity? The answer may well be that in the beginning of the twentieth century a different rhythm of life set in, and the population needed advice on resting as a coping strategy for surviving in an unfamiliar environment that often did not pay attention to the physical limits of human bodies. Globally, since the age of industrialization, many populations have had to adjust to the new production systems and new rhythms caused by the fragmentation and acceleration of labor. In fact, labor and production became the main reason for exhaustion in this era. Summers-Bremner adds to these observations the notion that "in order to sleep, we need to know we are tired, and if neither we nor the system we inhabit can recognize tiredness, an increase in sleep problems, coupled with an inability to locate causes, will result."[1]

The fast-paced modern work environment did not seem to leave its employees any time for rest, as observed by Deborah Kaple in *Dream of a Red Factory*.[2] She traces the influence of Stalinism on the Chinese labor system and gives insight into labor organization and the environment the factories turned into. This intense work environment was not only an integral part of the socialist systems in the Soviet Union and PRC, but had already played out in the industrialization of Europe of the eighteenth and nineteenth centuries. In the drive to make factories even more productive, the rationalization of work flows by taking apart each work step had famously been promoted by F. W. Taylor in his work on the scientific method for running a factory.[3]

When looking at the modern labor environment and the medical knowledge of sleep, even a sufficient degree of knowledge transmission would not have helped to improve the workers' situation: indeed, there could be no improvement unless room was made for the realization of sleep, not just its theoretical understanding, and unless at the same time the workers became aware of their exhausted state. Does this mean that time to rest had to be made compulsory by authorities in a top-down approach that forced people to rest and disciplined them to follow this requirement? How could such a policy work if workers themselves did not even recognize their exhaustion?

In the case of the PRC—theoretically—all this health and sleep knowledge was provided by the state to avoid the absolute exploitation of individual energy resources.[4] In the PRC, the objectives of the five-year-plan system, epidemics, and the constant push for revolution constituted additional strains on the labor force and so posed dangers to the state's development goals.[5] If labor power was thus not unlimited, and so had to be fostered and cared for, the labor force had to be taught about bodily limits.

FATIGUE, SLEEP, AND ENERGY

In China's case, exhaustion and fatigue were approached from an energy perspective, which mostly manifests physically to show the extent to which daily life, including labor, impacted an individual. While this study looks closely at the labor environment, it does not undertake an in-depth discussion of psychological issues such as neurasthenia and insomnia.[6]

The idea of calculating a body's energy was part of the European industrialization discourse on production and bodies and the ensuing modernization of life. At the time, industrial elites perceived that both the factory owners and the workers had to understand their bodies' requirements for rest so as to even out their energy balance and serve the production process. This understanding was not implicit and had to be taught.[7] In 1958, Plügge and Kohn made clear in their explorations on exhaustion that just because a person had *reached* a certain state of unease (not-well-being), this did not mean he or she could *feel* or *identify* it.[8] In this sense, workers needed to know that they would have to take a break, while the owners of factories had to be taught about the workers' need for rest in order to keep up the production process without too much collateral damage.[9]

According to Rabinbach, the phenomenon of fatigue as a symptom of overwork was discovered by the 1870s, when "fatigue [was] [. . .] identified [. . .] with the weariness produced by the work of the community."[10] In the relatively short time since its discovery, fatigue has attracted a fair amount of interest both in China and in the Western Hemisphere because of the industrialization and rationalization of work environments. Rabinbach links the Industrial Age to a change in the perception of the body, and identifies emerging areas of conflict associated with this change, such as the limited energy of the human body. In nineteenth-century France there was an increasing number of studies on the issue, and observations were made that the population, especially young people, was exceedingly fatigued.[11] A distinction between mental and physical fatigue emerged, where the former was called fatigue or neurasthenia (nervous exhaustion and pathological fatigue) while the latter was rather defined as bodily exhaustion—the precondition for fatigue—which often could be resolved by sufficient rest.[12] The fatigued state of body and mind was often seen as a "malady of civilization" because it was considered to be brought about by modernity and the fast-moving life of modern times.[13] The increasing number of discussions on fatigue, be it mental or physical, were also seen as part of modernity, a circumstance deriving from the rapidly changing environment, with which the population—especially the working population—was coping rather poorly. However, before physical exhaustion came to be considered to be part of the pathology of fatigue, a therapy of labor was actually suggested to patients with this condition. When the "malady of overpressure [in students and intellectuals] [was replaced] with the malady of impaired energy and resistance to the performance principle"[14] a change became visible in the perception of fatigue as an energy problem.

In the early 1900s fatigue was then defined as the "accumulation of fatigues which where only incompletely restored."[15] This lack of energy may even have resulted in an "aversion to work (Unlust zur Arbeit)."[16] Yet it was still often proposed to be cured by a turn to activity. Supposedly, activity could return the individual worker back to the daily structure and rhythm of labor. Some experts even assumed that regularity and an adherence to a kind of rhythm aided in counteracting fatigue: "All natural activities of the animal body appear to be dominated by the regulation of thrifty energy use."[17] Regularity is a recurring theme in the discussion of rest: there is an emphasis on regular sleeping times, regular work hours, and thus a regulated daily routine that leaves enough time for recovery—the underlying purpose of sleep—and regular breaks throughout the day.

Sleepy Bodies: Historical Perspectives

The positive outlook on rest as a way to replenish the body's energy sources and counteract exhaustion was a new phenomenon in the twentieth century. In comparison to the situation in Europe, which had prevailed from the sixteenth until the nineteenth century, the meaning attached to resting, that is, doing no purposeful action or being idle and without something to do, changed fundamentally. Doing nothing (except for sleeping) had been frowned upon in the sixteenth century especially in Protestant circles. Idleness was scorned and seen as moral weakness.[18] The state of doing nothing was not accepted as physiologically necessary for the working body: such laziness was seen as detracting from the day's achievements, as Max Weber details in his discussion of labor ideals and the ascetic lifestyle in Protestant belief.[19]

Once the rhythm of work was no longer directed by the seasons, and the processes of production and the market economy were transformed, this perception changed, leading to a rise in the need for time off. In fact, "Max Weber concluded that a victorious capitalism no longer needed the religious ascetism of the work ethic. [. . .] The traditional work ethic became the ethos of labour power."[20] Suddenly, human energy was an important currency, and with the discovery of thermodynamics a fear of the loss of this energy arose.[21] In the newly industrialized and rationalized world, workers and employers needed their strength for production in order to form a sturdy labor force, and in this labor environment time was structured by the clock. It, too, helped bring an end to the traditional seasonally influenced labor rhythm.[22]

When time is split up into production and leisure time, a different meaning is assigned to each. This is how, in the nineteenth century, leisure and breaks became an important part of everyday life, now understood as the time of day that was used to replenish the body's energy sources. Rest thus became an activity with a concrete purpose: avoiding fatigue and, by extension, ensuring a long-term healthy body.

Kenton Kroker defines the experience of sleep as the "annihilation of experience,"[23] which is what makes it so hard to grasp and focus on—unless one focuses on the dreams associated with the act of sleeping. Concentrating on something that is made up of the absence of everything, of course, poses certain problems, such as the assessment of what is happening in this state and why it may be important to the sleeping individual. While in Aristotle's time sleep was defined "as the periodic powerlessness of the organs of sensation,"[24] by the time of industrialization it was recognized as essential for a well-functioning body. The act of sleeping raised philosophical questions about whether a sleeping person was actually conscious and aware of reality. While in the seventeenth century Thomas Hobbes still wondered about how to distinguish between being asleep and awake,[25] Chinese authors of the twentieth century were rather oblivious to this issue. For them there was no problem in distinguishing a wakeful state from dreaming. If it was remarked upon at all, dreaming was considered a by-product of sleeping that could interfere with it (if it was experienced too strongly), and was not at all a precondition for healthy sleep. Historically, sleep in China had been connected to dreams, but also to rulership, which was in turn characterized by the absence of sleep since "sleep follows on success, not vice versa," as Summers-Bremner observes.[26]

Sleep in early classical Chinese literature is the subject of only sporadic attention, despite the fact that human beings spend up to one-third of their life in this state. It was most often connected to specific social settings. In the pursuit of success and achievements protagonists went to great lengths to avoid it.[27] The time spent unconscious in sleep was considered better spent on conscious matters, and if worries sometimes kept the troubled person awake these worries were seen as worth losing sleep over. If anything, falling asleep was a weakness—not unlike the European notion of disdained idleness.[28] This notion of avoidance runs counter to the thinking of twentieth-century industrialization, when the act of sleeping turns from an imperfection into a source of vitality.[29]

The awareness of sleep requirements produced coping mechanisms to accommodate this need. In the PRC, awarding sleep space in daily life was not only a matter of temporal planning but also a matter of physical space. Sleep and rest are usually practiced in the privacy of the home, but the separation of public versus private spaces of activity became porous when health became an official matter. When the focus of sleep observation turned toward the examination of the actually sleeping body, separate from the dreaming mind, sleep as a subject was opened up to the public's interest and to possible interference from the outside.[30] At the same time, the necessary discipline to stick to a resting schedule that optimizes physical and psychological stamina was expected by the PRC authorities (and, according to them, by science). This schedule was handed down to the population by the state authorities as a measure intended to structure that part of the day to which the state originally did not have any access. Government influence can be observed at university dormitories all over the PRC today, where specific hours for shutting down electricity, curfews, and limitations of running water are set. After that, all students are supposed to be in their sleeping quarters, sleeping and thus resting for the following day.

Being Fatigued in China: The Notion of Pilao

One reason for the young PRC to seek to ensure sleep and rest was to avoid the state of *pilao*—exhaustion—among workers and peasants. *Pilao* is understood as physical and mental exhaustion that is brought about by intense labor as well as the revolutionary state, which was acknowledged to drain the population's energy. Over the following pages I answer the question of how *pilao* was defined in the 1950s–1970s and how one was seen as at risk of suffering from *pilao*.[31]

Pilao arose from a lack of time to replenish one's energy. It was unavoidable in a production environment built on the human labor force, and mechanisms had to be put in place to cope with the physical repercussions of labor. At the same time the constant narrative of revolution and class struggle also required an energetic input from people's bodies in order to change the status quo of the PRC. Both class struggle and the former exploitation by what the communist propaganda called "feudalism" were additional energy drains on society. While exploitation at the hands of landlords, class enemies, and old traditions had supposedly been abolished by the communist takeover and the adherence to Marxist ideology,[32] revolution, political agitation, and shock work campaigns also resulted in *pilao* linked to the overambitious production plans in agriculture and industry.

While the burden of the past continued to influence the Chinese body and its energy levels, the more pressing problem was labor-derived exhaustion. Intense labor cycles were promoted and aspired to, so as to boost industrial production. Contrary to the cautious words that we have seen expressed on this kind of fatigue, in the 1950s shock workers and model workers in the Stakhanovite[33] movement were supposed to increase production by doing intense work cycles in a short amount of time, as the notion of shock work suggests. In the original Soviet sense, this was not the aim of shock work, since "[w]orking to exhaustion was associated not with communist zeal but with backwardness. An ideal life for Stakhanovites was someone who worked 'at the factory exactly seven hours, since Soviet power does not permit anyone to work more, who regularly goes to the cinema, visits others, engages in sports and at the same time fulfils all production tasks.'"[34] The intense concentration on work[35] was not supposed to interfere with the body's time to rest, but rather to be achieved within the normal work shifts. There were different kinds of exhaustion the workers had to be wary of, according to Rapoport in 1952. There was a perceived difference between short-term exhaustion due to work (*juandai gan* 倦怠感 [feeling worn out]) and the fatigue that built up due to the long-term maltreatment of the body.[36]

Fatigue and Its Victims

It was not only shock workers who were prone to suffer from fatigue, but in general every worker and peasant, every man and every woman, could and would suffer from exhaustion. The Chinese state distinguished between two different social groups that could succumb to it: mental workers (*naoli laodongzhe* 脑力劳动者) and physical (or manual) workers (*tili laodongzhe* 体力劳动者). This distinction is prominent in virtually any discussion of labor in the PRC. In the context of rest, however, mental workers are not mentioned with the same negative connotations as they are in other areas of Maoist discourse. Instead, there is a sense of equality ascribed to the bodies of the PRC's subjects when talking about fatigue and rest. The Communist regime indeed fought for a narrowing of this gap between manual and mental workers. Joel Andreas describes these groups as being perceived as opposites within a hierarchy which positioned the manual workers (and peasants) on top. The difference between them arose not only from the kind of work they were doing, but from the ideological status assigned to that work. While workers and peasants were rated higher in this system, experts were supposed to share their knowledge with the population to aid in education. One way to reduce the gap between the two groups was the system of reciprocal learning.[37]

To succeed in this endeavor, new ways to educate the broad population were introduced, and new schools and universities were opened. The length of training at these institutions was shortened, so that students could graduate quickly and take up productive jobs. "The aim was to make all education combine theoretical knowledge and manual skills, preparing students for occupations that would require both."[38] Intellectuals were reeducated and put in touch with peasants and manual workers in factories to give them manual work experience, in line with Mao's emphasis on practice.[39] Yet this initiative did not evolve in as smooth a manner as the government would have hoped. Mental workers, due to their very different level of education, spoke a different language from the manual workers and thus were incomprehensible to the peasants, and neither did they share class ties which would have aided in communication.[40]

Yet while this ideologically charged distinction between manual and mental labor was reproduced in the context of class struggle, and especially during the Cultural Revolution, it is only marginally important for the topic of this chapter, since both types of workers had to rest. Nor does the Taylorist distinction between manual and mental workers apply here, as it merely distinguishes between workers who only do manual work and the thinkers who conceptualize the work process, without positing a hierarchy between them. In Europe and the United States this separation between thought and manual production led to harsh criticism of Taylor's theory.[41] Yet for the purposes of the discussion of sleep, the distinction between manual and mental is merely a functional one. In the health literature on rest, neither side was the object of negative comments or preferred treatment. Both groups had similar health problems which had to be resolved to provide labor power for economic growth. The pressing concern for the health authorities was the ability to guarantee the productivity of both groups in this environment. A tension might have existed due to ideological reasons, but it did not lead to a neglect of efforts to secure the health of either group's bodies. Mental workers fell victim to *pilao* just as much as physical workers in factories or in the countryside did, though their fatigue had different origins. A mental worker who made use of their mental faculties during their workdays eventually burned out mentally. Additionally—and as most authors and autobiographical texts never tire of mentioning—the unnatural working environment of being seated all day caused their bodily condition to deteriorate. Apart from physical weakness they also suffered from low energy levels and bad sleep. This called for a quick solution, thus health literature included pleas for regular and purposeful breaks during work.[42]

For mental workers, a purposeful break did not need to include a nap or lying down of any kind, but could include movement and exercising, as the 1954 story of Zhu Chenglin 朱成林 tells. According to the story's author, Zhang Ruohong 张若煌, Zhu was a worker in a Zhejiang textile mill who was transferred from a job in production to a desk job because of ailments deriving from his physical labor. Despite his transition, however, he did not experience relief but instead started feeling dizzy, his vision became blurred, and he could not concentrate. Through the use of exercise as a form of break for the body, Zhu managed to control and, in the end, improve his condition.[13]

Similar observations held true for physical workers who made more overt use of their energy during their workday and therefore needed (a) to replenish it (through food and rest) and (b) do alternative movements akin to today's physical therapy to avoid stress injuries and an unbalancing of the body. A 1959 article in the *Xintiyu* illustrates the latter by reporting on the exercises physical workers should do in their free time. The author Lin Zhongying 林仲英,[44] himself an avid weightlifter prior to working in the countryside as a physical education instructor, explains how his background in weightlifting helped him in participating in the daily tasks. He emphasizes in his anecdote that "labor cannot replace exercise" (*laodong buneng daiti tiyu* 劳动不能代替体育).[45] Exercise thus served as active rest for both groups of workers, but for different reasons. For one of them it was to undo the sedentary labor-derived aches and pains, the other it was to ease sore muscles and to balance the physically stressed body.

Not only workers but also students were often reprimanded for unhealthy sleeping patterns that would show in their academic performance.[46] Getting up and taking a break from studying was an often-heard recommendation. In the spirit of "Have a healthy body, study well, work well" (*Shenti hao*, *xuexi hao*, *gongzuo hao* 身体好，学习好，工作好), in 1954 Zhou Zuxi 周祖羲 discusses how students improved their health and how important it was for their study success. Apart from gaining physical and mental strength, Zhou identifies rest as a major contributor to success at school. He thus emphasizes the eight-hour period of rest and sleep for students.[47]

Another *Xintiyu* article on the health of students written by Wang Yingjie 王英杰[48] stresses the need for at least eight hours of sleep. The author is convinced that rest is necessary for students' brain health, especially with the increased stress of hard mental and physical work.[49] By making the readership aware of the body's sleep and resting needs during university—a very controlled environment—a base of health awareness concerning sleep was created and certain habits ingrained.[50]

Communicating Exhaustion

The feeling of exhaustion, *pilao*, was explained in popular media as a chemical condition in the body. The authors Jin Jingren 金静仁, Wang Zhanchun王占春, and Du Zhonglin 杜忠林 describe this condition of exhaustion as a threat to the central nervous system.[51] In articles spanning a period from 1962 to 1986, they detail the biochemical reactions within the body (too little oxygen, changes in the muscles, etc.) and the external factors (stress on the muscles, heavy workload, etc.) playing into an assessment of *pilao*. This biochemical explanation was, for example, introduced in 1952 in the small booklet *Suitable Rest* (*Heli de xiuxi* 合理的休息) by Rapoport (translated by Miao Lanqing 苗兰卿).[52] According to him, the need to take a break stems from the need of the cerebral cortex to relax.[53] A similar observation is made in Lukyanov's *Protecting Health and the Ability to Work* (*Jiankang yu laodong nengli de baohu* 健康与劳动能力的保护) translated from Russian in 1955 by Li Guangcheng 李广成. Lukyanov stresses that the physiological need to sleep derives from the impact of sleep on the brain chemistry, on the metabolism, the heart, the respiratory system, and the muscles.[54] Qu Mianyu et al., meanwhile, define sleep as a physiological need (*shengli yaoqiu* 生理要求), making it a top priority for those concerned with the population's health.[55] In this discussion, therefore, sleep is seen as the mechanism to reverse *pilao*. The state of *pilao*—when physical and/or mental capacities were exhausted—resulted in feelings of tiredness, weakness, and listlessness. Combined with too little rest, it was unavoidable, as Qu Mianyu et al. argue.[56] Stress and the wrong exercise routines would aggravate this unhealthy condition, as would environmental factors such as heat, noise, or dirt, further consuming the body's energy resources.[57] Evaluating *pilao* in a biochemical way helped rationalize it in line with the materialist narrative of Mao-era China, and to identify its cause prior to resolving it—for example, if the feeling of fatigue derived from exhaustion of the brain, giving the brain time to rest would solve the issue. This use of rationalized scientific knowledge clarified the condition to the readers and at the same time made use of newly propagated ideas and concepts.

LABOR EXHAUSTION

Since the primary origin of the body's exhaustion in the Mao-era discussion is labor, this topic warrants greater examination, as it is also the driving force of the PRC and of socialism. A world without labor is not feasible, as was postulated by Engels in his aphorism "Labour creates humanity."[58] This puts labor at the very center of what it means to be human, and thus at the center of society. Labor and, by extension, production become the main part of daily life, and though labor creates exhaustion it was welcomed as part of the communist New China. In the PRC constitution the right to work has been present since the first version of 1954, and this also includes the right to rest. Rest, indeed, was seen as part of the improvements brought about by the communist takeover, putting an end to the ruthless exploitation under capitalism.[59] The constitution is thus a place where labor and rest are intertwined: the right to rest follows upon the right to work, as a reminder that humanity does indeed need to refuel and cannot work itself to absolute exhaustion. The first constitution of 1954 stipulates:

> 第九十二条　中华人民共和国劳动者有休息的权利。国家规定工人和职员的工作时间和休假制度，逐步扩充劳动者休息和休养的物质条件，以保证劳动者享受这种权利。
>
> Article 92: The workers of the People's Republic of China have the right to rest. The State stipulates the work time and vacation day system for industrial and office workers, progressively expanding the material prerequisites of breaks and recuperance for workers. [This is to] guarantee that the workers enjoy this kind of right.[60]

Previously, the Soviet Union had adopted a similar passage in its 1936 constitution (Art. 119),[61] regulating the population's free time (if that indeed existed) as well as any other aspects of daily private life. The second version of the PRC constitution from 1975 again defines the right to rest as a basic right of the Chinese population.[62] It is grouped together with the right to work, to education, and the right to get material aid in sickness and old age, giving the concept of rest a wider dimension in connection to labor.

Rest was understood not only in terms of daily rest such as breaks during the workday, but also as resting days, that is, national holidays, that were defined in directives such as the 1949 directive on the "Measure on Taking Off National Holidays and Memorial Days" (Quanguo nianjie ji jinianri fangjia banfa 全国年节及纪念日放假办法). This measure defines all the national holidays and their beneficiaries. During those days work was supposed to be suspended.[63]

Work hours, though not mentioned in the PRC constitution, were defined in various directives to the public and tailored for different places and work environments.[64] In the "Provisional Regulations on the Principles of Production, Work Hours, Wages, Labor Benefits etc. of Privately Run Factories and Shops of the City of Tianjin's People's Government" (Tianjin shi minzhengfu guanyu siguan chang dian shengchan, gongshi, gongzi, ji laodong bao fuli dengxiang yuance zanxing guiding 天津市民政府关于私管

厂店生产，工时，工资，及劳动报福利等项原则暂行规定) of 1952, the working hours are defined according to factory size. Small factories with 50 or fewer workers are subjected to less work pressure and have to work up to ten hours, while larger facilities employing 50 or more workers can limit the daily work time to eight hours. The regulation for days off follows a similar logic, where workers in big factories would get one day a week off, while workers in smaller factories would be off for one day every other week. It is stressed, nevertheless, that labor which harmed the body warranted an even lower number of working hours.[65]

The caution for people working in harmful or dangerous environments that might impact their health is confirmed in a 1965 suggestion by the Ministry of Health concerning workers working with radioactive materials. This suggestion emphasizes that they should be working less than eight hours a day and receive two to four weeks off a year. Given that this line of work needs a high level of alertness, one can understand how longer resting periods and a stricter handling of the number of working hours each day is necessary to ensure safety by upholding the workers' resilience.[66]

Labor Organization, Labor Safety, and Its Meaning for Rest

The labor and production processes were structured so as to make sure that everything went smoothly, avoiding periods of idleness yet with enough time for the workers to rest. Due to bad planning on the factory's side, workers might have found themselves with nothing to do when the workflow was interrupted. The resulting idling cycles, that is, workers sitting around doing nothing, wasted valuable working time that otherwise would have been filled productively, as a 1954 *Laodong* article titled "Improve Labor Organization, Increase Labor Productivity Rates" (Gaishan laodongzuzhi tigao laodong shengchanlü 改善劳动组织提高劳动生产率) pointed out. Another article published in the *Laodong* one year later by Zheng Xingzhi 郑行志 titled "To Improve Labor Organization Attention Needs to be Paid to These Aspects" (Gaishan laodongzuzhi yaozhuyi naxie fangmian 改善劳动组织要注意那些方面) concurs with this argument.[67] The factory head and the state thus implemented various management mechanisms to avoid idling and to improve the continuity of the flow of work, as already discussed by Deborah Kaple and Michael Korzec.[68] Idleness due to a lack of tasks was different to the required idleness during recreational time and rest: it hindered production and output, whereas recreational idleness and rest were supposed to increase the capacity for production. After taking control of the organization of work, authorities thus also had to make room for resting time in the daily and yearly schedule.

The management of the workplace also included labor safety (*laodong baohu* 劳动保护), which is concerned with the safety of the labor environment as well as with the workers' health. A 1951 article in the *Dazhong Yixue* by Yu Wei 郁维 summed up the ways to create a healthy worker and a safe environment: medical supervision was encouraged so as to keep track of overall physical health; the safety and engineering requirements of the work space had to be up to date to avoid accidents and injuries; and the well-being of the workers had to be taken care of so as to ensure a peaceful and happy life. By assessing safety issues in this way, Yu's article recognizes three different spaces the working body acted in: work, life, and personal space. In these spaces the individual ability to work and individual health had to be upheld (*geren jiankang he gongzuo nengli* 个人健康和工作能力). Yu promised that upholding the quality of life would result in higher quality of work.[69] In 1955 Lai Ruoyu 赖若愚 reiterated this,[70] writing that in order for the worker to function at his or her best, physical conditions had to be optimized. By controlling work time and thus limiting overwork, and reminding the workers and leading cadres to take breaks, the optimal state could be pursued.[71] Labor safety tips often remind the workers to take breaks and sufficient rest, which were both deemed important for mental and physical fitness. The workers' concentration was especially affected if they were tired and or lacking in rest. In the newspaper *Laodong* the frequent discussion on the topic of labor safety shows its importance, reminding the readers of the popular media of their responsibility and of the dangers at work.

In this spirit, a 1954 *Laodong* article reports that rehabilitation facilities (*xiuyangsuo* 休养所) had been opened. According to the author Cai Shubin 蔡书彬, the first of these institutions had been established in 1952, and its services had to be paid for. There, workers were not only supposed to sleep, relax, and return to a state of physical balance, but also to take part in recreational activities and receive adequate nutrition. The *xiuyangsuo* were supposed to offer space and assistance for rest and recreation.[72]

PROPER SLEEP HYGIENE

Regularity and a proper sleeping environment were two tiers of the sleep regimen advocated by popular media. In order to induce a healthy state of relaxation, a quiet and non-stimulating atmosphere was suggested to calm down the nerves and guarantee a sound night's sleep. This also included avoiding exercising shortly before going to bed, and no heavy meals just before bedtime (last meal up to two to three hours before). All this was supposed to create a calm and cozy environment that made it possible for the tired worker to relax and find peace at the end of a busy workday. In 1952, Rapoport defined sleep as a personal habit, a phrasing that puts all the control over sleep in the hands of the individual person. He recommended sleeping in a place that was well-aired and not hotter than 16°C to 18°C, and to take a 1.5-hour break after dinner before going to bed. Lukyanov (1955) confirmed these suggestions, stressing that a regular sleeping routine would result in good sleeping habits, which would then help build a strong and healthy individual. Ideally, people would get up at a set time and go to sleep at about the same time every day, thus building a regular pattern the body could get used to. Lukyanov describes the ideal environment for good rest: it should be quiet and calm, dark and warm, and contain a bed to sleep on. In order to calm down the mind and the body enough to achieve a good night's sleep, Lukyanov suggests taking a half-hour walk before going to bed, or a warm bath (*wenshui liaofa* 温水疗法). Sleeping quarters should be well-aired. He reminds the readers that eating too much or eating too close to bedtime will influence sleep negatively, and thus people should not eat for at least two hours before going to sleep. Any stimulating and exciting activities were also dismissed, which includes reading as it might foster vivid dreams and impact sleep quality. Sleeping on the right side of the body, under covers, with the head on a pillow in a darkened and quiet room, and abstaining from caffeine, chocolate, nicotine, alcohol, and other stimulants or oily foods, are advised in Lukyanov's handbook.[73]

Shu Xincheng (1956) concurs by emphasizing—again—the need for regularity in simple daily habits. His recommendations thus are a fixed sleeping routine, a well-aired room with an open window while sleeping, a spacious bed that is padded and supplied with adequately clean and appropriate bedding, as well as wearing pajamas. Shu also advised having a light, early dinner two to three hours before bedtime, and to avoid stimulating drinks, smoking, or reading before going to sleep.[74] In a 1957 *Dazhong Yixue* article on hygiene for mental workers, Song Peihui advises taking time to wind down even before going to bed, so that the mind has time to calm down and one would not be kept awake by thoughts and emotions. This, too, excluded reading in bed and late dinners.[75] Very similar advice can be found in Lan Ding's 蓝宁 1964 publication on improving one's body.[76] He recommends leaving the window open as a way to rid oneself of fatigue, since a closed window or a blanket covering the face may prevent the sleeping person from getting fresh air.[77]

To generate regular and good-quality sleep, Qu Mianyu et al. (1965) suggest quiet surroundings and the avoidance of excitement and stress on the body around bedtime, so as to circumvent the excitement of the nervous system, which would interfere with a good night's sleep. For maximum sleep quality they recommend a period of relaxation for at least 1 to 1.5 hours before sleep, which could be filled with walking as a form of mild exercise.[78] By adhering to these rules about the sleeping environment and hygiene, external parameters were set to an optimal state for resting, as well as inculcating the right internal mindset through the calm down periods. The benefits of these habits and routines for good sleep quality were central to the governance of sleep.

Breaks during Labor

Sleep at night replenishes energy that has been used during daytime, but to enhance individual well-being throughout the workday, as well as to avoid mistakes and injuries in the work process, short breaks were institutionalized. These breaks were evaluated rather positively by Rapoport (1952) and were not treated as a sign of weakness or laziness.[79] Taking frequent small breaks during the day was a way to sustain not only the mental and physical abilities of the workers, but also their mood and morale. Rest (*xiuxi*) and alternative (recreational) activities are at the same time prevention (*fangzhi* 防治) and treatment (*zhiliao* 治疗) of fatigue, taking the individual person out of their work environment and engaging different muscles, which alleviated the stress on overused body parts. Taking a walk and participating in exercises became important resting strategies. According to Lukyanov (1955), rest during the work day had to be organized and structured systematically to benefit the workers and production. These work breaks could either be rest in the form of a nap, some light exercises, or just a walk.[80]

In 1956, Shu Xincheng advocated taking intermittent breaks from work. In his mind, going to a window and taking a deep breath, light stretching, and then returning to one's desk or work place were already sufficient to uphold the workflow.[81] For him, breaks for the mind are as important as breaks for the body as a way to reload the body's energy. Exhaustion for Shu is not a purely internal struggle; on the contrary, external influences such as environmental factors could also influence a worker's need for rest.[82] Thus a change of environment during rest is important, for example, by going outside to exercise. This is a way to rest tense muscles, and the movement would interrupt the work of the mind. An ideal lunch break requires taking a 3 to 5 minute walk after lunch and then a 15 to 30 minute nap.[83]

In a short recollection of Cheng Mingsheng, published in the *Xintiyu* by Xie Bin 谢彬 in 1957, exercise and calisthenics in particular are put in the context of rest. In Cheng's short statement, he emphasizes the positive effect movement has on a worker as a means to extinguish fatigue and alleviate labor strain on the body. Cheng goes into detail specifically about short gymnastic sequences during the workday and their benefits.[84]

An environmental factor that influenced the ability to continue work throughout the day were seasonal changes. Summer heat and winter cold could have direct effects on workers' energy levels. This is the reason for advising for lunchtime naps during the heat of summer, as proposed by Jin Jingren in 1962.[85]

Habitual Rest

As we have seen, the routines pertaining to a healthy body were supposed to develop over time into personal habits which would regulate the work-free parts of the day,[86] and this was also true for sleep and activities during the hours off work. Physical activities deemed good for relaxation included taking a walk, calisthenics, ball games (basketball), or taking up a sensible form of exercise to counteract labor stress and at the same time to strengthen the body.[87]

The expected result of the introduction and implementation of knowledge on sleep was the inculcation of a healthy sleeping pattern in everybody. In this way, sleep knowledge was intended to become a natural and inherent part of the population's thought processes about sleep and rest, as expressed by Sun Yiqing 孙轶青 in his 1953 *Xintiyu* article "From Weakness to Health" (You shuairuo dao jiankang 由衰弱到健康), wherein he tells the story of his own health journey. Sun participated in physical training and adopted healthy habits, including better sleeping routines. He broke his old sleeping patterns of going to bed too late by rigorously pursuing early nights in, and reports feeling much better and healthier.[88]

By establishing good habits, the replenishing of energies was made feasible. In this context, good habits were habits that were deemed healthy and sensible in a labor environment. In order for them to work and take full effect, they needed to become part of the daily practice. In this daily rhythm, time to rest was set aside. The overall consensus on time to rest in the materials examined is that eight hours (at least seven) of sleep a night for adults were sufficient, as Zhou Zuxi affirmed in 1954.[89] One of the habits to achieve enough rest was going to bed early and getting up early (*zaoshui zaoqi* 早睡早起), ideally resulting in eight hours of sleep between 10 p.m. and 6 a.m., as Ke Fan 柯繁 defined in a *Dazhong Yixue* article in 1957.[90] In 1965, Qu Mianyu et al. concurred with the idea of seven to eight hours of nightly sleep.[91] The days were thus divided into one-third of sleep and two-thirds of waking. Only one-third of the day was supposedly used for work, the remaining third being reserved for other daily activities (movement, eating, socializing, and education).[92]

A Matter of Quality

The frequent reference to the scheduling and planning of sleeping hours and resting time might be thought to give insufficient credit to the fact that the quality of sleep is also an important factor in the discussion, but in fact the quality of sleep (depth) is not ignored, and is sometimes even thought to be more important than a set number of hours.[93] Of course, the number of hours available for sleeping guaranteed that people could rest and replenish their energies during that time, but sleep had to be of a certain quality. Several of the previously mentioned guidelines were meant to ensure this deep and relaxing state of sleep.

Not everyone was able to follow these guidelines, and some of the more prominent socialist model workers and heroes did not bow to these rules. Counterexamples to this need of rest and sleep (and self-care) are those who became famous due to their lack of attention to their own well-being for the sake of socialism; for example, Lei Feng, who in his quest to serve the state broke almost all of the health rules that were supposedly necessary to build a strong body to cope with the harsh reality of labor. He saw himself as a small cog in the big system of socialism, and his role as being to keep everything going, but in the narrative of the Lei Feng story, this does not seem to warrant careful handling of one's body. He went to work when he was sick, and gave away his food and even his clothes.[94] Such heroism is not consistent with the paradigm of health and self-care. After all, if the whole of the Chinese population decided to overexhaust themselves in their labor, to freeze and not eat, the whole system would collapse, since their bodies would crumble. In the context of health, Lei Feng can be identified only as a moral example, a vehicle for propaganda, but not as a person to emulate for their medically healthy conduct. The same holds true for the extreme efforts exerted in the model unit of Dazhai and Cheng Yonggui's production successes.[95]

Sleeping in the 1980s

With the opening up of the PRC and the market reforms of the 1980s, the need for sleep is not laid to rest. Instead, a return to old essentially "Chinese" ideas is evident, which shows itself in the sleep discourse, where traditional ideas of sleep hygiene come to the forefront. Furthermore, a broader approach is taken to source materials, and we now find more translations into Chinese from West German, American, and Japanese originals. In the 1980s, all this new input—traditional and transnational—joins the earlier propagated knowledge, and augments the previous framework with additional information on sleep and resting habits.[96] The discussion of health had hitherto always been seen in connection to labor; but now a notion of balance between time spent working and time spent resting becomes more prominent. A well-balanced way of life was advocated in the *Renmin Ribao*, for example, in 1981, to avoid the tragic end of overwork and sickness, by taking up the phrase *laoyi jiehe* 劳逸结合 (combine rest and work).[97]

Earlier, in 1979, Xiao Haoyong 肖浩永 argued for a specific sleeping posture for optimal sleep quality that can prevent snoring. Snoring occurs because air is not drawn into the lungs properly. It often happens when people lie on their backs while sleeping. Xiao advocates sleeping on one's side to avoid snoring.[98] The same year, Peng Shuwu 彭述武 published on the topic of napping during the hot months of the year and puts the focus not only on nighttime sleep, but also on sleep that occurs in the middle of the day. He suggests that during the hot summer months, rest should be scheduled for the hottest time of day to avoid fatigue from summer heat. Workers supposedly work more productively that way.[99]

These different additions to the discourse of sleep are all geared toward balance in daily life, in which a physical space was still reserved for sleep and rest. For the worker to find ideal resting conditions it was not enough to just lie down and sleep. Certain preparations in the sleeping space needed to be undertaken to ensure proper sleep, as I have already shown for the preceding decades. The state was responsible for the framework of sleep (providing time, building houses, organizing labor), but after obtaining knowledge on sleeping conditions from the state it was the responsibility of the individual to execute this knowledge. The authorities could only give space and time to the population by defining a set sleeping time (for shift workers) or by implementing the eight-hour day in factories. They did not enforce this sleep hygiene, but they created a supposedly ideal environment for sleep. The space given for rest includes the living quarters for workers and their families built by factories or the state.[100]

Despite the apparent universal regulation of sleep, proper sleeping habits were still understood to depend on individual moods and feelings. They thus differed between individuals. Whether one is an early bird or a night owl was not influenced by an exact schedule, as Xing Ma 幸马 argued in a 1980 *Jiankang* article.[101] Still, planning ahead was supposed to facilitate a proper universal sleeping routine, which bowed to the dictatorship of production and was adjusted to the rhythm of labor.

Sleep was seen as a way to health and greater vigor for workers, but it was ascribed other feats as well, for example making a human body grow better and bigger. In 1980, Zhang Jiaqing 张家庆[102] claimed that sleep had this additional function: according to his article, children would actually grow into taller adults if they slept well. Notably, through this association Zhang reproduces the Sick Man of East Asia metaphor: a taller population, especially in the younger generation, would come into being supposedly due to an increased level of human growth hormones resulting from proper sleep behavior.[103]

In Wang Deshen's 1982 translation of a Japanese school book by Imamura Yoshio, Kinbara Isamu, Ishiko Toshihiro, and Kuroda Yoshio, exhaustion and fatigue are said to be best resolved through breaks. This observation is in line with its predecessors and links the 1950s and 1960s discussion to reform-era China. The textbook accepts that there are many reasons for fatigue, but it also concurs with previous observations that studying and labor are the main culprits that exhaust a person. If ever a person happens to suffer from fatigue and exhaustion, rest is needed. The book suggests taking ten minutes' rest in each hour. After lunch a longer break of about one hour is suggested, and one day off should be included each week. The suggestion of taking a shower for a break is a new resting activity, which supposedly relaxes the body, while sleep is described as the ultimate way to recuperate from daily life including work and studying.[104] Imamura et al. also recommend exercise to improve on one's exhausted condition, as long as exhaustion due to exercising is avoided. This meant the individual had to be aware of how much exercise was just about enough for their constitution in order to avoid physical injury and *pilao* by default.[105] So, while physical activity was heralded as something rather positive and worth pursuing, exercise as a form of rest could prove a double-edged knife as too much of it may harm the body.

Another incentive for improved sleep hygiene was the introduction of mental exercises. Apart from the routines and habits, which were covered in the earlier discussion of rest, new mental exercises and small rituals were now proposed in the 1980s publications as an aid in falling asleep. Affirmations, self-hypnosis, and purposefully directing the mind toward sleeping are part of these rituals, but are only found in materials from the 1980s onward, as for example in a 1982 article by Xiao Zhenxiang 肖镇祥 in *Changshou* 长寿 entitled "Sleep, Insomnia and Dreams" (Shuijiao, shiyan ji meng 睡觉，失眠及梦).[106]

A return to much older sleeping rituals and knowledge, and thus reminiscences of an ancient tradition, can be witnessed in "Ten Things the Old Chinese Avoided When Sleeping" (Guren shuiyan shiji 古人睡眠十忌), published in 1982 in the magazine *Changshou* 长寿 and then in 1985 in the *Jiankang* 健康. This piece lists ten things the ancient Chinese avoided in order to get a good night's sleep:

1. No facing up when sleeping.
2. No thinking and worrying before going to bed.
3. No intense emotions such as anger before going to bed.
4. No food directly before bedtime.
5. No snoring.

6. No light, instead the surroundings should be dark.
7. No sleeping with an open mouth.
8. No covering of the face.
9. No open windows and wind in sleeping quarters.
10. No facing the stove while sleeping.[107]

The article legitimates the suggested habits by generally referencing traditional medical texts and authorities, such as the medical classics *Huangdi Neijing* 黄帝内经 (the *Yellow Emperor's Classic of Internal Medicine*) or Sun Simiao 孙思邈.[108] This is, for one thing, a return to the roots of Chinese knowledge that may feel more relatable to the readership, while also establishing a longer sleep-practice tradition that is not based merely on a labor discourse but anchored in native tradition as opposed to the previously prevailing biomedical discussion.

Dreaming of a Standard of Sleep

A 1983 article in *Medicine and Philosophy* (*Yixue yu zhexue* 医学与哲学)[109] by Wang Jisheng 王极盛[110] connects sleep, health, and psychology, a new field in the discussion of sleep. Wang focuses especially on the quality of sleep, and dissects how social relations and differences between people influence sleep quality. Apart from connecting sleep with the central nervous system, Wang also elaborates on the length of sleep. He stresses that the ideal length depends on the individual person, and notes that there are people who thrive with only two to three hours or who can function on four to five hours. He observes that a person might even sleep too long. According to Wang, eleven hours of sleep are worse than eight, as in an experiment where the attention span half an hour after waking up of the person who slept for eight hours was better than that of the later risers. Wang furthermore defines insomnia as one factor influencing sleep. Dreams, Wang claims, heavily influence a person's health. They are a depiction of the psychological state and are a part of sleeping and the human experience. Since dreams can interrupt deep sleep heavily, they are not to be dismissed in this discussion.[111] This article shows how psychological thinking and concepts were incorporated into the discourse. It also shows how the perception of dreams evolved over time into something that was necessary for well-being. The fact that the notion of individual problems and needs is taken up and explained in this context shows how it became more prominent, and how the realization that not everybody could be molded into the same shape was expressed.

An article by Zhu Xiao'an 朱小安 in the *Wenhua Yicong* 文化译丛[112] from 1985 describes the difficulty of the previous decades' attempt to define a sleeping standard, and circles back to the question of how many hours of sleep are required. Zhu also reengages with the issue of the depth of sleep, his article being a translation of a West German journal article "Is There a Sleeping Standard?" (You shuijiao de biaozhun ma 有睡觉的标准吗?). It introduces the two categories of quantity and quality, and posits that a good night's sleep does not only depend on the length of sleep, but also on its depth. Depth is reached if a person enters certain sleep phases. Zhu admits that there are different needs at different ages, explaining that after the age of 50 a person supposedly needs less sleep. It ends with the cautious words that sleep can be considered more important to the human being than food, as an American study had shown; according to this study, a person can go 2.5 months without food, but only 121 hours without sleep.[113] This shows how no sleep leads not merely discomfort and a loss of productivity, but in the end to death.

To avoid this end, advice on a good sleep routine and sleep hygiene was disseminated, for example in the 1986 three-piece series by Ruan Fangfu 阮芳赋[114] published in the journal *Jiankang*, which summed up all the sleeping tips that had circulated before:

1. In order to sleep well the environment has to be optimized and a regular schedule needs to be set up.[115]
2. The quality of sleep is as or even more important than the quantity, that is, sleeping a few hours deeply and feeling refreshed is better than tossing and turning and feeling tired in the morning.[116]
3. Loss of sleep can be resolved by different methods, for example, listening to music, drinking a glass of milk,[117] or even taking sleeping pills.[118]

The discourse on sleep in the 1980s was thus blossoming, boosted by the inclusion of psychological aspects, the extension into dreaming, and the realization that sleep was and would always be a part of human life.[119] The reference back to "traditional" practices surrounding sleep is not surprising, but brings another layer into this discourse. While in the 1950s and 1960s the discussion had centered on the biochemical and labor-related aspects of sleep, the mention of essentially Chinese methods and the inclusion of psychological theory now widened the scope of this topic.

In the discussion of sleep in the Mao and post-Mao era, all aspects had revolved around the issue of productivity and the authority of the state; only in the 1980s do we see that psychological categories emerge. The need to uphold the labor force and the national strength required that the individual person fall in line with certain rules that regulated the body, so that it could perform at its peak and ensure production goals were met. Rest and leisure became an integral part of daily life and created a dichotomy between work and leisure activities, space, and time. The state built a knowledge base on the topic of rest and sleep, and designated the needed physical space for these resting practices. Generally, early nights, regular sleeping patterns, a clean environment and clean clothes to sleep in, regular breaks during the workday, and the avoidance of exhaustion were advocated. These observations are part of the third pillar in the grand discourse on individual health. Alongside adequate nutrition and a healthy dose of exercise, enough rest and sleep were seen as nonnegotiable.

This made room for new possibilities for the individual to expand into, which in the end could not be completely controlled by the state, since forcing someone to sleep was not feasible. Sleep as an intrinsically non-violent activity could perhaps only be enforced with sleeping pills and even then with little gain. The necessity for sleep was so important that it had to be ingrained in the individual person in the form of self-care—via an internal authority and an inner voice of reason—to reach where the state could not penetrate, so that the body as the central machine of socialist production was not damaged. With this realization we might want to ask: Why do these points even have to be discussed and explained? Is this not common knowledge? And what were the forces that prevented the population from following a healthy lifestyle, that is, from getting enough rest?

A healthy lifestyle and, in this particular case, good sleeping habits were propagated as part of the scientific assessment and improvement of life. Workers, cadres, and factory owners were reminded of the limited energy resources of the human body. There are reports on workers and cadres overworking themselves because they wanted to do a particularly good job. The promise of more capital and possibly higher social status led individuals to believe that they should outdo themselves in the struggle for socialist revolution and larger production output. Seen from the perspective of the Chinese health discourse, this was not considered sensible. In fact, although the intention behind it was good and well-meaning, the ignoring of human beings' limits might have posed a bigger threat to the production goals than giving the workers adequate time to rest, as Kuang Xiansen 邝贤森 already reported in the *Laodong* in 1959.[120] Ignorance, ambition, and a blind focus on production by the workers and cadres would harm the workers themselves more than was necessary. The factory managers were in need of education to prevent these slipups and stop the development of bad habits. By introducing knowledge about the body's limits, the state intervened in a path that could possibly have been very destructive for the workers. Not only did the state educate, but it also implemented time slots in the workday that were reserved for resting and built housing to supply resting space. By doing so, it intruded on a part of daily life that had not been governed before.

The introduction in the health literature of a perfect resting routine thus shows that the party-state was conscious that continuous war and class struggle were not the path to a socialist future, and that both production and revolutionary zeal had their limits. The stress of both revolution and production itself could not be averted, but it could be accounted for, and by allowing resting time and communicating the need for it, exhaustion could be mitigated. By attaching a health value to sleep and rest, the time set aside for these activities could thus be justified.

NOTES

1. Eluned Summers-Bremner, *Insomnia—A Cultural History* (London: Reaktion Books, 2008).

2. Deborah A. Kaple, *Dream of a Red Factory* (New York: Oxford University Press, 1994), 21–38, 93–100.

3. Frederick W. Taylor, *The Principles of Scientific Management* (New York: Harper & Brother Publishing, 1911).

4. Summers-Bremner, *Insomnia*, 99–100.

5. Although there seems to have been a constant focus on the quantity of workers available, in this context the well-being of the individual is put into focus. Overall health was necessary to pursue the state's needs, but only by helping the individual person to thrive and improve their living quality was a rising health standard possible, as the state cannot permeate all levels of personal life. The quality of the workers' state becomes a new important factor.

6. Sleeplessness was an issue that could have different origins. When eliminating foreign-induced sleeplessness—missing time to sleep due to work and other tasks—which is easily remedied, we are left with the problem of sleeplessness because of the inability to fall or stay asleep. This is a problem if it influences the individual's ability to function in daily life, and thus becomes an abnormal state. In extreme cases the loss of sleep would lead to death, as Song Peihui 宋佩辉 emphasized in 1957 ("Naoli laodong zhe de shenghuo weisheng 脑力劳动者的生活卫生," *Dazhong Yixue* 4 (1957): 137). Reasons for insomnia were overwork, pressure, and the resulting exhaustion, as Xiao Zhenxiang 肖镇祥 reports in the 1982 *Changshou* article titled "Sleep, insomnia and dreams" (shuijiao, shiyan ji meng 睡觉，失眠及梦) (Xiao Zhenxiang, "Shuijiao, shiyan ji meng 睡觉，失眠及梦," *Changshou* 6 (1982): 14–15).

7. See Summers-Bremner, *Insomnia*.

8. Herbert Plügge and Rolf Kohn, "Wohlbefinden und Missbefinden," *Psyche* 12, no. 1 (1959): 38–39. See also "Die objektivierende Hinwendung auf den eigenen Körper und auf das subjektivierende Befinden aber ist der Patientin fremd und unergiebig" (Plügge and Kohn, "Wohlbefinden und Missbefinden," 46)

9. Shock work would influence the energy balance negatively and exploit the body up to the point of utter exhaustion.

10. Rabinbach, *The Human Motor*, 39.

11. Rabinbach, 146.

12. Rabinbach, 152–53.

13. Rabinbach quotes M. Potel and his entry "Neurasthénie" in *La Grande Encyclopédie* (1886, p. 986), see Rabinbach, 154.

14. Rabinbach, 168.

15. Rabinbach quotes Albert Deschamps, *Les Maladies de l'énergie, thérapeutique générale* (Paris, 1908, p. 70), see Rabinbach, 163.

16. Rabinbach, 168.

17. Karl Bücher, *Arbeit und Rhythmus* (Leipzig: Teubner Verlag, 1902), 358; quoted by Rabinbach, *The Human Motor*, 175.

18. Rabinbach, 25–26.

19. Weber, "Die protestantische Ethik."

20. Rabinbach, *The Human Motor*, 31–32.

21. Rabinbach, 20, 21, 46: "[L]abor power became after the discovery of energy conservation the basis of all matter and motion in the physical world. Both a magnitude and a measure, labor was the universal fact of nature assimilated to, and exemplified by, the laboring body in the social world."

22. Rabinbach, 31–32.

23. Kenton Kroker, *The Sleep of Others and the Transformations of Sleep Research* (Toronto: University of Toronto Press, 2007), 4.

24. Kroker, 29.

25. Kroker, 54.

26. Summers-Bremner uses the example of King Wu and his discussion with the Duke of Zhou to illustrate sleep-avoidance: the King is deprived of sleep by his continuous efforts to secure "heaven's support" (Summers-Bremner, *Insomnia*, 32). See also Antje Richter, "Sleeping Time in Early Chinese Literature," in *Night-Time and Sleep in Asia and the West: Exploring the Dark Side of Life*, ed. Brigitte Steger and Lodewijk Brunt (New York: Routledge Curzon, 2003), 33.

A factor influencing rest during sleep was dreaming, especially vivid dreams as those would interfere with sleep quality. Though dreams were not thought unhealthy as such, their ability to infringe a person's resting time was cautioned against by Jin Jingren 金静仁 in 1962 ("Zuomeng yu jiankang 做梦与健康," *Xintiyu* 4 (1962): 15–17.)

27. Antje Richter, *Das Bild des Schlafes in der altchinesischen Literatur* (Hamburg: Hamburger Sinologische Gesellschaft, 2001), 2.

28. Richter, 138.

29. For those persons in classical China who did have to sleep, the classic texts have specific directions for the best sleeping posture, as can also be found in twentieth-century literature: it was best to sleep on the side, not on the back or the belly. As far as the sleeping time was concerned, there seems to have been a consensus on nighttime as the time for sleep, if one really had to do it. Richter, *Das Bild des Schlafes*, 43–44, 94–138.

30. Kroker, *The Sleep of Others*, 70.

31. These observations are remarkable since the Chinese state has on more than one occasion been depicted as ruthless and brutal, as shown on varying topics by authors such as Michael Dutton, *Policing Chinese Politics: A History* (Durham, NC: Duke

University Press, 2005); Edward Friedman, Paul G. Pickowicz, and Mark Selden, *Revolution, Resistance, and Reform in Village China* (New Haven, CT: Yale University Press, 2005); and Susan Greenhalgh and Edwin A. Winckler, *Governing China's Population: From Leninist to Neoliberal Biopolitics* (Stanford: Stanford University Press, 2005).

32. One propaganda example of ruthless exploitation by landlords is that of Liu Wencai, an allegedly ruthless landowner who was made into a symbol of the exploiting class in Maoist lore. Liu embodied all the negative and brutal images of the class of landowners and so illustrated the message of liberation by the CCP. See Wu Guo, "The Social Construction and Deconstruction of Evil Landlords in Contemporary Chinese Fiction, Art, and Collective Memory," *Modern Chinese Literature and Culture* 25, no. 1 (2013): 140–57.

33. Aleksei Stakhanov (1906–77) procured 102 tons of coal within six hours and was made a national hero in the USSR. See Miin-ling Yu, "'Labour is glorious': Model Labourers in the PRC," in *China Learns from the Soviet Union, 1949–Present*, ed. Thomas P. Bernstein (Lanham, MD: Lexington Books, 2010), 232.

34. Miin-ling Yu, "'Labour is glorious,'" 233.

35. This not only meant extremely high output within the normal working time, but workers and factories in the PRC were also encouraged to enter production competitions to push output rates up and reach the fulfilment of five-year-plan goals earlier (Rui Kunze and Marc A. Matten, *Knowledge Production in Mao-Era China: Learning Science from the Masses* (Lanham, MD: Lexington Books, 2021), 167–68.

36. A. Rapoport (Lapopo'ertuo 拉波波尔脱, A.), *Heli de xiuxi* 合理的休息, trans. Miao Lanqing 苗兰卿 (Shanghai: Shanghai weisheng chubanshe, 1952), 12–14. Actual sleeping hours might not have even come close to the suggested eight hours, as Jacob Eyferth reports in his research on home spinning: "For many women, the only way to square the circle was to work ever longer hours, up to the limit of physical endurance. Most women's working days started before sunrise, preparing breakfast while men and children were still asleep. Fieldwork shifts lasted from 6.30 to 8.30 a.m., 10.00 to noon, and 2.30 to 6.30 p.m., or, in busy periods, until sunset—a total of eight to eleven hours. Meals were short and hasty affairs, followed by a nap or a card game for men and household chores for women. After the end of the third shift, women cooked dinner and prepared food for the next day, washed dishes, and put the children to bed; by the time they were done with these tasks, it was close to midnight. It was then, when men and children were asleep, that most textile work was done" (Jacob Eyferth, "Women's Work and the Politics of Homespun in Socialist China, 1949–1980," *International Review of Social History* 57, no. 3 (December 2012): 389).

37. Andreas, *Rise of the Red Engineers*, 162.

38. Andreas, 167.

39. See Mao Zedong, "Shijianlun 实践论 [On Practice]," in *Mao Zedong xuanji* 毛泽东选集 (Beijing: Renmin chubanshe, 1968).

40. Andreas, *Rise of the Red Engineers*, 168ff.

41. Walter Hebeisen and Frederick W. Taylor, *F. W. Taylor und der Taylorismus: über das Wirken und die Lehre Taylors und die Kritik am Taylorismus* (Zürich: Vdf, Hochschulverlag an der ETH, 1999), 119–22. The criticism of Taylor's theory was

directed at the depersonalization of the workers, who were now seen only as laboring hands doing small fragmented work steps in the whole process.

42. Zhang Ruohuang, "Guangbo ticao gei zhuchenglinle jiankang 广播体操给朱成林了健康," *Xintiyu* 8 (1954): 37; "Naoli laodong zhe de xiuxi 脑力劳动者的休息," *Zhi he Zaozhi* 2 (1986): 58.

43. Zhang Ruohuang, "Guangbo ticao gei zhuchenglinle jiankang 广播体操给朱成林了健康," *Xintiyu* 8 (1954): 37.

44. Lin Zhongying edited a book on weightlifting in 1954: Lin Zhongying, ed., *Juzhong lianxi fa* 举重练习法 (Beijing: Renmin tiyuchubanshe, 1954).

45. Lin Zhongying, "Shen qiangli zhuang hao laodeng 身强力壮好劳动," *Xintiyu* 2 (1959): 22. Injuries occurred, for example, in the back and rump (Liu Shisen 刘世森 and Zheng Baoan 郑保安, "He nongcun qingnian tan 'lianyao' 和农村青年谈'练腰,'" *Xintiyu* 6 (1977): 29–30), as already mentioned in the chapter on physical education: rest and exercise as rest was supposed to replenish the workers' bodies (Wang Xuliang, "Zai nongcun zenyang duanlian shenti - jiqiao 在农村怎样锻炼身体–技巧," *Xintiyu* 1 (1977): 55–56).

46. Wang Yingjie 王英杰, "Daxuesheng zenyang guo jiankang shenghuo 大学生怎样过健康生活," *Xintiyu* 23 (1956): 9–10.

47. Zhou Zuxi周祖羲, "Qingnian xuesheng zanyang zuodao shenti hao 青年学生怎样做到身体好," *Xintiyu* 1 (1954): 16.

48. Wang Yingjie (1913–) was a sports pedagogy expert and professor at Qinghua University in Beijing as well as part of many national research committees and institutes on sports pedagogy. (See *Zhongguo dangdai wenhua mingren xiaozhuan* 中国当代文化名人小传 [Shenyang: Liaoning renmin chubanshe, 1993], 34.)

49. Wang Yingjie 王英杰, "Daxuesheng zenyangguo jiankang shenghuo 大学生怎样过健康生活," *Xintiyu* 23 (1956): 9–10.

50. Switching the light off at a sanctioned hour, doing exercises with classmates, having a set lunch break in the middle of the day.

51. Jin Jingren, "Xiatian tan wushui 夏天谈午睡," *Xintiyu* 7 (1962): 26; Wang Zhanchun 王占春, "Zao duanlian yu shuide wan you xunxu zenmeban? 早锻炼与睡得晚有循序怎么办?," *Xintiyu* 5 (1979): 45; Du Zhonglin 杜忠林, "Pilao yu jijixing xiuxi 疲劳与积极性休息," *Hubei tiyu keji*, no. 1 (1986): 45.

52. Rapoport, *Heli de xiuxi*, 7–9.

53. Rapoport, 8; Lukyanov, *Jiankang yu laodong nengli de baohu* 健康与劳动能力的保护, trans. Li Guangcheng 李广成 (Beijing: Renmin weisheng chubanshe, 1955), 68; Shu Xincheng, *Wo zenyang huifu jiankangde* 我怎样恢复健康的 (Beijing: Zhonghua shuju chubanshe, 1956), 121.

54. Lukyanov, *Jiankang yu laodong nengli de baohu*, 66–68.

55. Qu Mianyu 曲绵域, Gao Yunqiu 高云秋, Pu Junzong 浦钧宗, and Chen Jidi 陈吉棣, *Shiyong yundong yixue* 实用运动医学 (Beijing: Beijing daxue yixue chubanshe, 1965), 193.

56. Qu Mianyu et al., 194.

57. Additional to its positive effects on brain chemistry, rest gives the body's muscles a break in order to relax, especially small muscles that are easily affected by

high workloads (jaw muscles, eye muscles), as Shu Xincheng stressed in 1956. See Shu Xincheng, *Wo zenyang huifu jiankangde*, 121.

58. Friedrich Engels, "The Part Played by Labour in the Transition from Ape to Man," in *Beyond the Body Proper*, ed. Margaret Lock and Judith Farquhar (Durham: Duke University Press, 2007 [1876]), 25–29. Sigrid Schmalzer discusses how the phrase "labour created humanity" was utilized in the PRC to paint a picture of human society (Sigrid Schmalzer, "Labor Created Humanity: Cultural Revolution Science on Its Own Terms," in *The Chinese Cultural Revolution as History*, ed. Joseph W. Esherick, Paul G. Pickowicz, and Andrew G. Walder (Stanford: Stanford University Press, 2006).

59. For discussion of the change of system from "feudalism" to socialism and its reception, see Shi Huaibi 史怀璧, "Woguo gongmin huodele laodong de quanli 我国公民获得了劳动的权利," *Laodong* 8 (1954): 5–6; Song Peihui 宋佩辉, "Naoli laodong zhe de shenghuo weisheng 脑力劳动者的生活卫生," *Dazhong Yixue* 4 (1957): 137.

60. "Zhonghua renmin gongheguo xianfa 中华人民共和国宪法," *Renmin Ribao* (21 September 1954).

61. Robert Beard, *1936 Constitution of the USSR, Chapter X* (Lewisburg, PA: Bucknell University, 1996) (https://www.departments.bucknell.edu/russian/const/36cons04.html [accessed July 2, 2018]), chap. X, art. 119: "Citizens of the U.S.S.R. have the right to rest and leisure."

The media commentary on the Soviet "right to rest" in the 1930s underlined the governmental and public awareness of the importance of non-labor time, as argued by Rapoport in 1952 or in Jablovski's 1954 *Xintiyu* article. See Rapoport, *Heli de xiuxi*, 1–3: *xiuxi quan* 休息权. See also I. M. Jablovski 依. 莫. 雅波罗夫斯基, "Tiyu yu changshou de wenti 体育与长寿的问题," *Xintiyu* 10 (1954): 26.

62. "公民有劳动的权利，有受教育的权利。劳动者有休息的权利，在年老、疾病或者丧失劳动能力的时候，有获得物质帮助的权利。" (The citizens have the right to work, [and] the right to education. The workers have the right to rest, in old age, when sick or if they lose the ability to work, they have the right to receive material aid.) Now article 27. See "中华人民共和国宪法（一九七五年一月十七日中华人民共和国第四届全国人民代表大会第一次会议通过）," *Renmin Ribao* (20 January 1975).

63. March 8, Women's Day, was to be one day off just for women, while Qingnianjie was supposed to be a holiday just for middle and high school students. Zhongguo renmin daxue fajiao yanshi bian, *Zhonghua renmin gongheguo laodong fa ziliao huibian* 中华人民共和国劳动法资料汇编 (Beijing: Zhongguo renmin daxue chubanshe, 1954), 50.

64. The eight-hour and thus regulated workday is mentioned by Bucharin in *Das ABC des Kommunismus* (Bucharin, *Das ABC des Kommunismus* (Wien: Kommunist. Partei Deutschoesterreichs, 1920), 605). According to Rabinbach it is a tried-and-tested concept in Europe and the United States, but it was also communicated by the Soviet big brother, which suggested an even shorter workday of seven hours in the constitution of 1936.

65. Zhongguo renmin daxue fajiao yanshi bian, *Zhonghua renmin gongheguo laodong fa ziliao huibian*, 54–55.

66. See this suggestion of the Ministry of Health on the vacation days of workers handling radiation: "Weishengbu guanyu congshi fangshexian gongzuo ren de gongshi he xiujia de yijian 卫生部关于从事放射线工作人的共识和休假的意见," *weiganzi* 卫干字 [1965] *di 106 hao* (April 2, 1965).

67. Zhonghua quanguo zonggonghui gongzibu, "Gaishan laodong zuzhi tigao laodong shengchanlü 改善劳动组织提高劳动生产率," *Laodong* 8 (1954): 10–11; Zheng Xingzhi 郑行志, "Gaishan laodong zuzhi yao zhuyi naxie fangmian 改善劳动组织要注意那些方面," *Laodong* 2 (1955): 21.

68. See for example Kaple, *Dream of a Red Factory*; and Michael Korzec, *Labour and the Failure of Reform in China* (New York: Macmillan Press, 1992).

69. Yu Wei 郁维, "Laogong baohu yao zenme ban? 劳工保护要怎么办?," *Dazhong Yixue* 2 (1951): 143–44.

70. Lai Ruoyu (1910–58) was a CCP politician and engineer. (See *Zhongguo gongchangdan lishi dacidian zonglun. renwu*, 中国共产党历史大辞典 总论·人物 (Zhonggong zhongyang dangxiao chubanshe, 2001), 496.)

71. Lai Ruoyu 赖若愚, "Zhengque guanche dang de laodong baohu zhengce 正确贯彻党的劳动保护政策," *Laodong*, 2 (1955): 1–2.

72. Cai Shubin 蔡书彬, "Zhongguo dian ye gonghui haibin qu laomo xiuyang suo 中国电也工会海滨区劳模休养所," *Laodong* 1 (1954): 22–24. See also Hang Peilan 杭佩兰, "Laodong mofan Hang Peilan laixin tan xihu gongren xiuyang suo 劳动模范杭佩兰来信谈西湖工人休养所," *Renmin Ribao* (December 6, 1951). Treatment in these facilities often led to weight gain, which here is connoted very positively as something the exhausted body can finally achieve thanks to the relaxed and quiet environment.

A lot more research on these facilities is necessary; for the purposes of the present volume, the extent and the availability of materials require that I limit myself only to mentioning them as part of the PRC labor system and its health and prevention methods. In this connection, though, I should mention publications such as a 1950 book titled *Workers' Rehabilitation Facilities* (*Laodong renmin xiuyang suo* 劳动人民休养所) by the Chenguang publishing and editing office (Chenguang chuban gongsi bianji 晨光出版公司编辑) or the 1953 *New China's Workers' Facilitation Facilities* (Xinzhongguo laodong renmin xiuyang suo 新中国劳动人民休养所) of the same publishing house.

73. Lukyanov, *Jiankang yu laodong nengli de baohu*, 70–71.

74. See Shu Xincheng, *Wo zenyang huifu jiankangde*, 130.

75. Song Peihui 宋佩辉, "Naoli laodong zhe de shenghuo weisheng 脑力劳动者的生活卫生," *Dazhong Yixue* 4 (1957): 137.

76. Lan concurs with the call for a well-aired, clean bedroom. He furthermore is in favor of getting up early and going to bed at a reasonable time. Before going to sleep Lan also advises refraining from stimulating activities such as reading in bed, or having tea, or any other activities that excite the nervous system. One should not eat shortly before sleeping either, as this might lead to nightmares. Instead, a light meal

before bedtime was in order (Lan Ding 蓝宁, *Zenyang zaineng shenti hao* 怎样才能身体好 [Beijing: Zhongguo qingnian chubanshe, 1964], 25–29).

77. Lan Ding, 25–29.

78. Qu Mianyu et al., *Shiyong yundong yixue*, 193–94.

79. Rapoport, *Heli de xiuxi*, 29.

80. Lukyanov, *Jiankang yu laodong nengli de baohu*, 92–97.

81. Shu Xincheng, *Wo zenyang huifu jiankangde*, 117.

82. Shu Xincheng sums this up as environmental hygiene, which can include matters of cleanliness (dust, fumes etc.) but also noise and crowded situations. See Shu Xincheng, *Wo zenyang huifu jiankangde*, 125.

83. Shu Xincheng, 121–22.

84. Xie Bin, "Zuocao neng xiaochu pilao 做操能消除疲劳," *Xintiyu* 6 (1957): 20.

85. Jin Jingren, "Xiatian tan wushui 夏天谈午睡," *Xintiyu* 7 (1962): 26. See also Peng Shuwu 彭述武, "Xiatian weishenme yao wushui? 夏天为什么要午睡?," *Xintiyu* 6 (1979): 43.

For a more thorough discussion of midday napping, see Li Yi's 2003 piece in which the labor-related issues and cultural meaning of midday napping are explored. Yi Li, "Discourse of Mid-day Napping—A Political Windsock in Contemporary China," in *Night-time and Sleep in Asia and the West: Exploring the Dark Side of Life*, ed. Brigitte Steger and Lodewijk Brunt (New York: Routledge Curzon, 2003), 45–64.

86. Rapoport, *Heli de xiuxi*, 33.

87. These examples are also made for personal training schedules to improve the body and fitness. For a more detailed discussion see chapter 3.

88. Sun Yiqing 孙轶青, "You shuairuo dao jiankang 由衰弱到健康," *Xintiyu* 31 (1953): 25. For another similar anecdote in favor of exercise for mental workers, see Huang Gang 黄冈, "Zhou Peiyuan jiaoshou tan tiyu duanlian 周培源教授谈体育锻炼," *Xintiyu*, 2 (1957): 6–7.

89. Zhou Zuxi, "Qingnian xuesheng zenyang zuo dao shenti hao 青年学生怎样做到身体好," *Xintiyu* 1 (1954): 16.

90. Ke Fan 柯繁, "Youyi yu jiankang de hao xiguan有益于健康的好习惯," *Dazhong Yixue* 4 (1957): 135–37.

91. Qu Mianyu et al., *Shiyong yundong yixue*, 194.

92. Mao himself advocated a balance between work (*gongzuo* 工作) and everyday life (*shenghuo* 生活) in a 1958 directive (Mao Zedong, "Guanyu gongzuo, shenghuo tongshi bingzhong fangzhen de piyu 关于工作，生活同时并重方针的批语," in *Jianguo yilai Mao Zedong wengao. Diqice, yi jiu wu ba nian yi yue—yi jiu wu ba nian shi'er yue* 建国以来毛泽东文稿. 第七册, 一九五八年一月—一九五八年十二月, ed. Zhongyang wenxian yanjiushi (Beijing: Zhongyang wenxian chubanshe, 1992), 530). A similar view can be deduced from sources calculating kilocalorie needs for everyday tasks, where the activities would be split in a similar 8–8–8 hour pattern, as has already been discussed in the paragraph on labor time and workdays. Rabinbach concurs that historically in the West 8(–10) hours of work have in fact been considered the number of hours feasible and adequate for productive work since the nineteenth century. According to French socialist Edouard Vaillant, eight hours were the "physiological limit" (Rabinbach, *The Human Motor*, 218, 221).

93. Shu Xincheng, *Wo zenyang huifu jiankangde*, 128.

94. Julia Sterzel, *Vom Genossen Lei Feng lernen?: eine Analyse von 50 Jahren Kampagnengeschichte in der VR China* (Bochum: Projektverlag, 2015), 55; Wendy Larson, *From Ah Q to Lei Feng* (Stanford: Stanford University Press, 2009).

95. See Joshua Eisenman, *Red China's Green Revolution: Technological Innovation, Institutional Change, and Economic Development under the Commune* (New York: Columbia University Press, 2018), 8.

96. Due to a lack of materials from the period of the Cultural Revolution, it is hard to fill in the blanks. Nevertheless, the baseline knowledge in other areas was not disputed over this period of time, and it seems likely that knowledge on sleep would not make a 180 degree turn during that time either. We need to keep in mind that experts were publishing and researching before and after the Cultural Revolution. A continuity of ideas is likely given this background.

97. "Jiji tuixing di liu tao guangbo ticao 积极推行第六套广播体操," *Renmin Ribao* (September 1, 1981). Today this is called work–life balance, but this term was not new to the Chinese discourse on labor of the 1980s. The term *laoyi jiehe* has been in use for rather longer: the database *Quanguo baokan suoyin* 全国报刊索引 shows about 150 articles between 1958 and 1986 with the phrase in their titles. There is a peak in the 1960s, when apparently 132 articles on the topic were published in the newspapers catalogued, while according to the *Renmin ribao* online archive the term appeared 22 times in its articles published between 1958 and 1980.

98. Xiao Haoyong 肖浩永, "Jiti sushe li de hulu sheng 集体宿舍里的呼噜声," *Dazhong Yixue* 3 (1979): 24.

99. Peng Shuwu, "Xiatian weisheme yao wushui? 夏天为什么要午睡?" *Xintiyu*, 6 (1979): 43.

100. Yu, "'Labour is glorious': Model Labourers in the PRC," 242.

101. Xing Ma 幸马, "'Bailing niao' yu 'maotouying' yi shuayan zatan '百灵鸟'与'猫头鹰'一睡眠杂谈," *Jiankang* 12 (December 5, 1980): 31–32.

102. Zhang Jiaqing 张家庆, born in 1928, was a doctor of Chinese Medicine native to Shanghai. He was involved with the merging of Western and Chinese Medicine, and was part of the National Chinese Medical Association. (See *Zhongguo Zhongyi renming cidian* 中国中医人名辞典 [Zhongyi guji chubanshe, 1991], 128.)

103. Zhang Jiaqing 张家庆, "Cong 'shui de hao ke cushi ertong shengzhang' tan qi 从'睡得好可促使儿童生长'谈起," *Dazhong Yixue* 4 (1980): 40–41.

104. Imamura et al., *Riben zhongxue baojian tiyu* 日本中学保健体育, 152–56.

105. Imamura et al., 24.

106. Xiao Zhenxiang 肖镇祥, "Shuijiao, shiyan ji meng 睡觉，失眠及梦," *Changshou* 6 (1982): 14–15.

107. Si Hong 思宏, "Guren shuiyan shi ji 古人睡眠十忌," *Changshou* 5 (October 15, 1982): 34.

108. Sun Simiao (581–682) is a central figure in the history of Chinese Medicine. He lived in the seventh century and is considered essential to the formation of Chinese medical thought. See Qiu Keping邱科平, *Shijie dabaike quanshu disanjuan keji tianwen shengwu renti yixue* 世界大百科全书 第三卷 科技 天文 生物 人体 医学. (Beijing: Guangming ribao chubanshe, 2003), 181.

109. *Medicine and Philosophy* (*Yixue yu zhexue* 医学与哲学) has been published bimonthly since 1980 by the Chinese Society for Dialectics of Nature (*Zhongguo ziran bianzhengfa yanjiuhui* 中国自然辩证法研究会). This journal covers ethical topics and psychological issues and lends a new dimension to the previously purely scientific discussion of medicine.

110. Wang Jisheng 王极盛, born in 1937, graduated from the Beijing Daxue philosophy department in 1962 in psychology. He has been publishing extensively on the topic of psychology since the 1980s. (See *Dangdai Zhongguo shehui kexue xuezhe dacidian* 当代中国社会科学学者大辞典 [Hangzhou: Zhejiang Daxue chubanshe, 1990], 13.)

111. Wang Jisheng, "Dibajiang: Shuimeng xinli yu jiankang 第八讲: 睡梦心里与健康," *Yixue yu Zhexue* 4 (1983): 52–54: *ren de geti chayi yeshi henda de* 人的个体差异也是很大的.

112. *Wenhua Yicong* 文化译丛 is a monthly journal published since 1980 by the Tianjin Foreign Language Institute (*Tianjin waiguoyu xueyuan* 天津外国语学院). It is now titled *World Culture* (*Shijie Wenhua* 世界文化).

113. Zhu Xiao'an 朱小安, "You shuijiao de biaozhun ma 有睡觉的标准吗," *Wenhua Yicong* 2 (1985): 57.

114. Ruan Fangfu 阮芳赋, born in 1937, graduated in 1959 from Beijing Health Science University. He was a professor at the history of medicine department there and a permanent member of the China behavioral science association. (See *Dangdai Zhongguo shehui kexue xuezhe dacidian*, 59.)

115. Ruan Fangfu, "Zenyang shuiyan de hao (yi) 怎样睡眠得好(一)," *Jiankang* 1 (January 18, 1986): 16–18.

116. Ruan Fangfu, "Zenyang shuiyan de hao (er) 怎样睡眠得好(二)," *Jiankang* 2 (February 18, 1986): 20–22.

117. Drinking milk to calm down is a Western notion. As with anything dairy-related, this becomes a topic only in the later health suggestions.

118. Ruan Fangfu, "Zenyang shuiyan de hao (san) 怎样睡眠得好(三)," *Jiankang* 3 (March 18, 1986): 16–17.

119. For more articles see: Zhang Kuiyi 张揆一, "Xiuxi de dong he jing 休息的动和静," *Dazhong Yixue* 1 (1986): 32; Yang Youdao 杨友道, "'Ta jing ruci' haoshui '她竟如此'好睡," *Dazhong Yixue* 10 (1986): 18; Sun Jizhi 孙济治, "Jingti hansheng li de xiuzhi yin——shuiyan qi bieqi 警惕鼾声里的休止音——睡眠期憋气," *Dazhong Yixue* 10 (1986): 35; Feng Zhimin 冯致民, "Sanzhong yichang shuiyan 三种异常睡眠," *Dazhong yixue* 10 (1986): 40; Du Zhonglin 杜忠林, "Pilao yu jijixing xiuxi 疲劳与积极性休息," *Hubei tiyu keji* 1 (1986): 45.

120. Kuang Xiansen 邝贤森, "Shuihao xiehao gongxiao gao 睡好歇好工效高," *Laodong* 3 (1959): 22. Zhonggong Shanghai qiche yunshu er chang weiyuanhui, "'Er gong yixiu,' lao yi jiehe '二工一休,' 劳逸结合," *Laodong* 7 (1959): 24–26.

PART III

Disease Government

Part III introduces the discourse of "civilization diseases" (*wenmingbing* 文明病) in socialist China. By the study of two distinct pathologies, obesity and hypertension, the Western impact on the Chinese health discourse in the middle of the twentieth century becomes apparent. These two case studies unveil the measures taken against both conditions, as well as illuminating the continuity of the concern with civilization diseases in China. The research on civilization disease done so far by Sander L. Gilman, Nicolas Postel-Vinay, Paul French and Matthew Crabbe, and Christopher Forth and others has been mostly undertaken from a Euro- and Western-centric point of view, often marked by the remnants of attitudes from colonial times, discussing exoticized colonial bodies, or concentrating merely on nations in the Western hemisphere and the developed world. The focus in these studies on Western nations or countries with former ties to Europe or the Americas is unfortunate, and discussions of other places in the world are often dismissed. Yet the non-Western (European or American) discussions of civilization diseases, specifically obesity or hypertension, are highly significant, since they may offer additional insights into the processes of negotiation between diseases, and into knowledge about and reactions to them.[1] As a non-Western region of the world, the PRC has also been neglected in the studies of civilization diseases by scholars of Chinese studies and of other humanities. There is a widespread conviction that the discourse around the problems of *wenmingbing* only began in the 1980s, after the reform era had established that certain diseases were connected to economic growth and increased consumption.[2] However, a look at the health literature, self-help books, and newspapers and journals dedicated to health shows a different picture.

According to this conviction, furthermore, the emergence and increased perception of civilization diseases was a consequence of the shift of focus from infection-based or communicable diseases, which had previously been the prevalent medical issue of the day, toward degenerative or non-communicable diseases, which now became seen as the main threat to the population. This was coined the "epidemiological transition,"[3] which in China took place in the twentieth century.[4] In fact, however, both issues were discussed in parallel on both sides of the supposed transition. To understand the institutional epistemological perspective that is relevant here, it is important to note that the measures taken to counter non-communicable diseases are very different from programs of vaccination or instilling hygiene habits in the population, since non-communicable diseases do not originate in viruses or bacteria. Instead, medical staff had to determine where these non-communicable diseases originated in the individual patient and devise an action plan that would right the wrong, that is, improve their living situation or take away the negative influences.

WENMINGBING 文明病

The term *wenmingbing* corresponds to the English phrases *lifestyle disease*, *diseases of affluence*, or *civilization diseases*. While the latter may seem to contain connotations of the opposition *civilized versus uncivilized*, which has resonances with colonial history as well as with China's own imperial past, the Chinese *wenmingbing* nonetheless is best translated that way if we conceive of civilization as the mere state of being in a cultivated environment governed by a society and its rules.[5] While *disease of affluence* can be translated as the Chinese *fuguibing* 富贵病, lifestyle disease (*shenghuo fangshi jibing* 生活方式疾病) as a description of the diseases in question is never used in the source material.[6] The decision to use *civilization diseases* was also influenced by the German term for the diseases described, *Zivilisationskrankheiten*, which would be an even more perfect fit for a translation of *wenmingbing* as it is less politically charged.

The research for this book has highlighted the link between health tips for upholding a physical ideal, the meaning ascribed to this information, and the significance of deviations from this ideal. The frequent return to the original admonitions to retain a healthy body has made it clear throughout that physical well-being was of the utmost importance. This happens especially in connection with diseases that were not caused by external threats (bacteria or viruses), but supposedly were caused by not adhering to certain rules. Accounts of diseases of affluence are already present in the contemporary health care magazines, self-help books, and pamphlets, and this presence shows the awareness of professionals and authorities of these problems, as well as their desire to use education as a way to help the population avoid falling into, for example, the obesity trap. It also shows how previously published health knowledge, training, education, and cautioning words had not been effective in preventing a health crisis from happening. Civilization diseases were already present in the public mind in the 1950s, despite the continuing efforts of the government to perfect the population's living standard and physique.

Here I focus on obesity and hypertension, these being two civilization diseases that concerned experts and the population alike, according to reports and medical publications in the PRC. These documents demonstrate the persistence of the pathological discourse from the middle of the twentieth century until China opened up to the world.

I propose to take an epidemiological approach, investigating the descriptions of the diseases and the ways they were diagnosed and treated, thus adopting the standpoint Adrian Wilson refers to as historicalist-conceptualist, as part of a retrospective epidemiology. At the same time, I do not dismiss the realist view on the subject matter, in so far as there is a biological condition as the basis for the epidemiology in the case of both diseases. Due to the lack of patient information and the incomplete statistics of the time, the study focuses on the concepts rather than the real numbers of patients.

NOTES

1. For an account on obesity culture, and a discussion of obesity in non-Western countries, see, for example, Mohamed Rguibi and Rekia Belahsen, "Fattening Practices among Moroccan Saharawi Women," *Eastern Mediterranean Health Journal* 12, no. 5 (2006): 619–24; WHO, *Obesity in the Pacific: Too Big to Ignore* (Noumea, New Caledonia: Graphoprint, 2002); WHO and IASO, *The Asia Perspective: Redefining Obesity and its Treatment* (Australia: Health Communications Australia, 2000).

Postcolonial, sociological, and medical studies of Pacific and African ethnicities and their reaction to a Westernized diet discuss their descent into obesity and other kinds of civilization diseases brought about by "the contact with the West." This can also be confirmed by reference to the *Encyclopedia of Obesity* by Kathleen Keller (Los Angeles: Sage, 2008). For a historical discussion of fat in colonial times, see Christopher Forth, *Fat—A Cultural History of the Stuff of Life* (London: Reaktion Books, 2019), 207–35, on the topic of "savage desires."

2. See Sander L. Gilman, *Obesity: The Biography* (Oxford: Oxford University Press, 2010); Paul French and Matthew Crabbe, *Fat China: How Expanding Waistlines are Changing a Nation* (London: Anthem Press, 2010); Libin Zhang, "A Multilevel Study of Effects of Socioeconomic Status, Income Equality, and the Built Environment on Adult Obesity in China" (PhD diss., University of Illinois, 2012).

3. Nicolas Postel-Vinay, *A Century of Arterial Hypertension 1896–1996* (Chichester: John Wiley & Sons, 1996).

4. See Bridie Andrews and Mary Brown Bullock, eds., *Medical Transitions in Twentieth-Century China* (Indiana: Indiana University Press, 2014).

5. A big thank you goes out at this point to Marta Hanson who advised me to stay as true as possible to the original wording of the Chinese authors and authorities.

6. This is not because the term *lifestyle* is absent. "Lifestyle" appears frequently in the advice and admonitions of professionals to care for one's body.

Chapter 5

Overweight and Obesity

A study of the pathology of obesity (*feipangbing* 肥胖病) and how it was approached in China not only offers insights into the workings of contemporary medical research, but also into the way the Chinese state responded to the changing environment after rising living standards began to result in a decline in individual health.

The academic discussion of obesity as a body form and health problem accepts that obesity has not always been such a serious issue as it is today.[1] Paul French and Matthew Crabbe reviewed the issue of weight gain in China from the 1980s until the 2010s and summarized the issues the state has thus been facing:

> 1982—Three years after its initiation, a partial survey on diet and nutrition finds 7 percent of China is overweight.
>
> 1992—A national nutrition survey clocks 15 percent of the country as overweight—double the figure of a decade ago. Some 30 million Chinese are now clinically obese.
>
> 2002—The China Academy of Medical Science conducts the most comprehensive national diet study to date, surveying 270,000 people countrywide. Some 22.8 percent of Chinese adults are found to be overweight (200 million people) while 7.1 percent are clinically obese (60 million). Within a decade, the prevalence of the overweight has increased by 39 percent and the obese by 97 percent.
>
> 2005—Xinhua reports that 70 to 90 million Chinese are now clinically obese—one-third of the total number of obese people worldwide. Between 6 and 10 million adult Chinese become obese each year.
>
> 2008—China's largest and most shocking survey of obesity and diabetes to date finds that the prevalence of diabetes and pre-diabetes to be nearly 10 percent and 16 percent, respectively, across China, accounting for 92.4 million adults with diabetes and 148.2 million adults with pre-diabetes.

> 2015—Predictions indicate that as many as 200 million Chinese will be morbidly obese within five years. China's heavyweights still lag behind the US, where two out of three people are overweight or obese, but China is on course to be exactly like the US in approximately 10 to 20 years.[2]

This summary shows two things: first, we see that there is a rapid increase in weight over the forty years since the PRC recovered from famine and political upheaval; second, and less directly, we also see that the socialist era is not included in this survey. In past research, Socialism was mostly equated with poverty and a lack of resources, which manifested at the time in a slim population; thus the socialist state is never included in historical obesity discussions. Yet despite its perceived slow economic growth and lack of wealth, obesity did have a place in the socialist health discourse. Indeed, the literature contains warnings and teachings on obesity's dangers to the national body.

On a global scale, being fat, or "well-nourished," used to be a sign of affluence, financial means, and health. A change in this perception took place when fatness became related to laziness, being criticized from the perspective of the Protestant work ethic and seen as evidencing the inability to perform daily tasks in a context of production.[3] Suddenly, what once was an outward reflection of a person's standing, and their ability to amass enough calories to be healthy, now acquired a moral framing as a sin and a medical framing as a physical deviation in a labor-centered world where a body's function and power were its greatest assets. Fatness and obesity are intriguing subjects from a social perspective, since the biochemical process of gaining weight is a natural process of the body that used to help early humans and any other mammals to store energy for times when food was scarce. This mechanism is necessary to ensure survival, but in a world where food and shelter are plenty it is no longer essential. Nowadays—especially in developed countries—there is generally no scarcity of food or warm housing and clothing,[4] and the Chinese state shares this narrative in which a modern and advanced nation no longer has to worry about possible famine. However, making the population fat leads to earlier death—just as starvation does. In the resulting medical as well as sociopolitical discourse, obesity is framed as a disease, as opposed to a visual clue of prosperity, when it is recognized how harmful and debilitating a fat body can be to the individual and to society. Obesity, thus, is categorized as a non-communicable civilization disease that occurs in specific social and cultural environments.[5]

Understanding and acknowledging the process by which diseases are defined is central to this chapter's observations. Diseases, like any other social and cultural element of our lives, are time- and place-sensitive. The act of defining or identifying a set of symptoms as belonging to a disease can be termed "framing a disease," in reference to Charles Rosenberg's approach, and is culturally specific. This means that diseases need to be named in order to be identified as such, and that they exist in a social context. Rosenberg uses the term "framing" for this process and not "(social) construction," as the latter "invokes [. . .] a particular style of cultural criticism and particular moment in time—the late 1960s through the mid 1980s—and a vision of knowledge and its purveyors as rationalizers and legitimators, ordinarily unwitting, of an oppressive social order." "Framing of disease" simply includes the "fashioning of explanatory and classificatory schemes of particular diseases."[6] Adrian Wilson disagrees, however, noting that this simple switch from the concept of construction to that of framing does not elicit the "programmatically charged" air such diseases carried with them. He emphasizes that diseases are not identical with their names, and that in fact a construction of the named entity of disease does take place.[7] For Rosenberg, diseases remain social phenomena and are social actors and mediators at the same time.[8] A disease is always structured and framed by its social environment, but at the same time it also has structuring attributes and impacts its surroundings. In the case of obesity, basic daily activities such as eating and working are witness to this impact; it also influences routines at the doctors' office, such as the introduction of weigh-ins, nutrition information, physical training, and so on. I maintain the term "framing" as a way to describe what a specific disease term encapsulates (such as symptoms, testing, diagnosis, etc.) and also to underline the framework that is built up around the pathology. For the present case study, it is first and foremost the medical link between health, obesity, and productivity that is important.

There is evidence of fat bodies as far back as in ancient Greece. Medieval physicians were also aware that an overly voluminous body entailed a number of issues and sicknesses.[9] For the closer examination of this issue, Sander Gilman revisits the *History of Sexuality*, where Foucault comments on the Greeks' awareness of the physical repercussions of an unhealthy lifestyle.[10] By the age of industrialization, the body had been rationalized in such a way that being fat was no longer a moral sin but a scientific category. This leads to the question of how a specific body shape can be defined as "normal" or "healthy."

Paul French and Matthew Crabbe's *Fat China* and Zhang Libin's doctoral dissertation on adult obesity in China[11] are helpful in informing us about how obesity has fared in Chinese history. The Republican era represents a time when the issue of obesity made an entrance into popular media such as the *Shenbao* 申报 (*Shanghai News*), the *Funü Shibao* 妇女时报 (*Women's News*), or the *Xin Nüxing* 新女性 (*New Women*);[12] the Mao period, on the other hand, is dismissed by most researchers on the grounds that it does not have much to offer to the discussion of obesity, implying a lack of affluence.

While in the Chinese empire there was a clear trend toward more voluptuous figures, the start of a discourse on obesity, that is, an awareness that overly heavy bodies suffered certain repercussions, can only be found in postimperial China. This is particularly interesting since, at the time, the Republic of China was fighting against the stigma of the Sick Man of East Asia.[13] The media at the time discussed the thin and weakened Chinese body, yet in parallel warned against overweight, since a state of sickness could befall those who were not careful in this regard.[14] The Sick Man of East Asia was thus seen as weak and defenseless not only in his skinny state, but also in his overweight body, lacking muscle definition and strength. According to Gilman, the issue of obesity was discussed during the republican era, but was then vanquished by the coming of famine in Communist China. As the Great Leap famine impacted upon the Chinese, the fear of malnutrition became widespread. It remains to be explored whether Mao's Great Famine was the only famine that traumatized the Chinese population, or whether past experiences of severe hunger in the imperial and republican periods also contributed to this trauma.[15] Gilman does not inquire deeply enough into the physical state of bodies in the Mao era: he claims outright that there were no cases of obesity at this time.[16]

French and Crabbe have also studied the development of this issue in the twentieth century, and address the environmental, logistical, social, and political changes related to the changing bodies of the Chinese population during the Republican era and post 1980.[17] The time period between 1949 and 1980 is missing from their considerations, however, for they consider that the famine in the Mao era made it impossible for people to be fat.[18]

While this choice of focus is valuable in indicating the major issues of the period, in particular the nutritional transition to post-Mao times, it nevertheless overlooks the fact that the previous discussion of obesity did not simply fade away and was not recovered only when economic growth and rising consumption resurfaced. During the Mao era the expert discussion of obesity did in fact continue, contrary to the widely accepted supposition in the scholarship on that era that it vanished. The discourse was indeed kept alive, and there are reports of patients suffering from overweight and accompanying symptoms. Nevertheless, the conviction that obesity as an epidemic is a rather new phenomenon in China cannot be refuted. It is verified by reports on the different increases in weight, bringing with it the introduction of the BMI (Body Mass Index) (weight in kg/(height in m)2) as a standardization tool, and the introduction of its Asia-specific interpretations, as well as its meaning for the overweight threshold of China at the end of the twentieth century.[19]

Zhang Libin introduces the social and cultural view of the body in twentieth-century China and remarks on how these aspects impacted the physical weight of the Chinese, suggesting that the plump figures in Chinese history attribute a positive connotation to overweight due to their link to prosperity.[20] However, this is a generalized assumption, since not all dynastic periods favored overweight women, as Cho Kyo and Kyoko Selden have shown in their *The Search for the Beautiful Woman* (2012): they even go as far as claiming that "[in] China, slim women were considered beautiful from ancient times."[21]

When touching upon the Mao era, Zhang is convinced that "obesity or overweight was a foreign concept in China in the days when the masses were still threatened by hunger and malnutrition."[22] Zhang repeats the famine argument as a reason for there having been no awareness of obesity in mid-twentieth-century China. The lack of coordination and mindful economic planning during the Great Leap Forward led to severe health problems and malnutrition.[23] The situation today is very different, however, since the PRC has come to shoulder "the double burden of malnutrition,"[24] that is, the case where there is at the same time an issue with over- and underweight due to unequal demographic development. The cultural and environmental contexts of obesity not only influence its spread but also its definition, expanding it from a merely biomedical issue to a cultural and economic one. Indeed, the perception of what is obese and what is normal is influenced by both culture and environment.[25] The Western standard is one way to form such a definition, but it is not the only one and can be perceived in some sense as relative to different cultural environments.[26] According to Zhang, this cultural relativity of obesity extends to studies that examine differences in ethnic physical reactions to obesity risk factors such as the susceptibility of Asians to cardiovascular disease and type 2 diabetes, suggesting an inherent difference between the Chinese and Western bodies.[27]

The factor that is most often blamed for China's obesity problems today is the nutrition transition; this transition has been experienced in many developing countries, and it is the most important factor for this book's considerations. By shifting activity and eating patterns, a change in body form can be observed.[28] In a sense, this is exactly what the twentieth-century Chinese experts and interpreters of foreign knowledge wanted to achieve: a change from traditional to modern, scientific nutrition, so as to foster strong and well-nourished bodies, although they were nevertheless aware of the problems of inactivity and overfeeding. It may be considered ironic that, by adopting a more Western diet rich in wheat, animal proteins, and fats, the Chinese authorities hoped to strengthen their nation, but by adopting that foreign diet, production methods, and food culture, the same health issues as plagued the West now reached the People's Republic.[29] Instead of strong bodies, the nutrition transition led to chubby bodies, contrary to the ideal—the image of the muscular and slender European body.[30]

THE CALCULATED BODY

Scientific knowledge concerning the precise needs for food was established during the Republican and Mao eras, leading to a rationalization of body and food.[31] The required physical education and standardized tests pointed out the bodies that lay in the "healthy" range, while they marked those that fell outside this range as "not-healthy." The issue with civilization diseases falls into the category of a body lacking certain abilities, meaning that there is a need for improvement, but unlike in the case of viral or bacterial infections the bodies suffering from civilization diseases have to invest individual efforts to improve their situation.

Why is excessive weight gain even deemed a problem? In the early years of the PRC the paradigm of "labor creating humanity" was stipulated throughout the country to foster development and emancipate China from the past.[32] As excessive weight gain impacts a person's ability to partake in labor, causing a loss of vigor and restriction of movement, its prevention was just as important to the process of labor as was the strengthening of the working bodies. Since obesity obstructed production and labor, it, too, impacted the socialist revolution and the process of national rejuvenation. By communicating the need for a rigorous diet structure, for the good of the individual and the nation, a major incentive is given to gaining plentiful nutrition so that the body is perfectly able to withstand the daily pressures and stresses. The "plenty" in this equation becomes an issue in an environment that makes overconsumption possible. Here the mere control of diet seems not to have worked to keep the population healthy.

In the 1950s we already find short articles and anecdotes on the issue of "fatties" (*pangzi* 胖子), obesity (*feipangzheng* 肥胖症, or *feipangbing* 肥胖病), "puffiness" (*xupang* 虚胖), and so forth.[33] Quite a few of the articles examined from the 1950s through to the 1980s categorize bodies into four different weight stages: underweight, normal, overweight, and obese, which are further subcategorized. A person's ideal bodyweight is measured through different calculations that include a ratio of height and weight. There are calculations that are adjusted to sex and age, acknowledging differences between bodies. Oftentimes the BMI is used as a means to establish whether a person is in the ideal weight range, but the most widely advocated and easiest way to figure out one's ideal weight is the simple calculation of subtracting 100 centimeters from one's height (in cm), to come up with an "ideal" (in kg). In a 1954 article on a structured life for patients with high blood pressure, translated by Wu Zhongbi, the Russian author Kondratiev suggests the same equation to arrive at an ideal weight. On top of this Kondratiev introduces a tolerance margin of +/– 6–7 kilograms.[34] This may encompass fluctuations due to the muscle-fat ratio, fitness levels, sex, or age. The simple calculation of an ideal weight (in kg) by subtracting 100–105 centimeters from one's height is still used in the 1980s. The excess was often equated with excess body fat, as Li Bingcheng 李秉诚 demonstrates.[35]

A *Renmin Ribao* article from November 1957 titled "Can You Have Fatties Slim Down?" (Nengrang pangzi xiaoshou ma 能让胖子消瘦吗?) by Mu Feng 木风 even suggests that there are different requirements between the Chinese and foreigners. The formula to calculate an ideal weight of the Chinese is altered slightly from the above-mentioned basic calculation to only 90 percent, which was claimed to be the Chinese ideal weight.[36] Nevertheless, this article concedes that there needs to be a tolerance margin of +/– 5 percent for weight fluctuation.[37] These considerations hint at a basic anatomical difference between Chinese and non-Chinese people that can nowhere be confirmed, but which probably emerged from the Republican discussion of military nutrition, as Michael Shiyung Liu has shown in his article "Diet for War." The lower ideal weight for Chinese people can be interpreted as the conviction that there was a unique feature about them, or that they could do with less. In no place is this backed up with studies and empirical data by Mu Feng or any other contemporary author,[38] yet similar calculations are found in a *Dazhong Yixue* article from 1979.[39]

Instead of letting the readership figure their ideal weight out for themselves, a short article in the *Xintiyu* from 1979 offers a table of the correct height-weight ratio.[40] It shows both extremes of the accepted weight range: the lowest and the highest acceptable weight correlated to a certain height.[41] Heights range between 141 centimeters and 190 centimeters and the acceptable weight ranges per height are a spectrum of 15 kilograms to 20 kilograms. The table is another tool that standardizes and normalizes human bodies, or, in case of deviation from this standard, marks them as not normal.

This simplistic view of the weight-height correlation does not take into account muscle mass—which is heavier than fat tissue—or bone density, or other factors, similar to the BMI calculation. It would render most athletes and overly fit and muscular people obese. This was also acknowledged in Yi Jian's 伊坚 1977 piece on height and weight,[42] as well as by Li Yulin 李玉琳, who in 1985 also notes that water retention, muscle gain, or even tumor growth might influence a person's weight.[43] One way of countering this misunderstanding is the introduction of an ideal weight range instead of a fixed weight per height.

The +/– 10 percent margin used in some of these articles gives an appropriate range within which to situate people found in different living conditions (physical or mental labor, age, fitness level, etc.), and shows how relative this calculation can be: the ideal, therefore, is a spectrum. This can be attributed to muscle mass, age, sex, bone structure, and so on. What this highlights is that not every body can be expected to be identical, and so it gives each body wiggle room for its own unique moment in time and space.[44]

These calculations are also directed by sex, as different discussions of female weight emphasize.[45] A *Dazhong Yixue* article from 1982 offers two different calculation modes for women and men:[46]

For men:

$$height\ in\ cm - 100 - \frac{(height - 150)}{4}$$

For women:

$$height\ in\ cm - 100 - \frac{(height - 150)}{2}$$

From this weight baseline, ideal and not-ideal bodies can be defined. Additionally, the differentiation between the two sexes again emphasizes a perceived physiological difference between male and female bodies.

Another correlation chart showing weight expectations in relation to age and height was published in Xu Pingji's 徐平吉 and Lu Dingxi's 陆定熙 1986 article on how weight increases (a) with height and (b) with age. They offer overlapping margins, which constitutes a fuzzy continuum of age-related weight gain. A 29-year-old at 147 centimeters can be at the margin of overweight at 50 kilograms, but be underweight with the same weight at age 60.[47]

The categories of age and sex show how bodies are treated differently depending on a person's life situation. A different set weight for different age groups was implemented, since younger people tend to weigh less due to their earlier development (height and muscle mass) and the metabolism of middle-aged to elderly people slows down, which often results in higher body weight.[48] Babies, on the other hand, are the only group of the population that are supposed to be "fat." This may derive from the fact that babies (1) do not have to be productive except for growing into healthy adults, and that (2) a plump baby was considered well-fed and healthy.[49]

Discovering Deviations: Fat Bodies

Now that thanks to these measurements and calculations bodies could be categorized as "ideal weight" and "nonideal weight," the nonideal category was split into "over- (the ideal) weight" and "under- (the ideal) weight." Anything not conforming to the aforementioned weight margin fell into either one of these categories.

In the 1950s' health discourse, being fat or "puffy" is no longer seen as healthy, but rather as a sign of weakness and a pathological state. A healthy appearance, on the other hand, often is equated with a strong appearance (*zhuang* 状/*qiang* 强), this—nevertheless—should not be equated with a big body mainly made up of fat, that is, weight gain due to over-intake of energy. Being "strong" (or sturdy) describes the muscle and fitness of a person, not sheer bodily girth. In order to achieve the desired physique, people would sometimes supplement their diet to gain weight and breadth. This approach would result in weight gain, but not necessarily in gain of muscle. Supplements (*bupin* 补品) (also labeled medical foods) included fish oils or eggs: they were often thought to be a cure-all, so that no additional treatment or training to gain healthy weight was implemented, even though it was only the latter that was sanctioned by experts to improve the body's quality, as Mao Zhongyao 毛中耀 emphasizes in 1954.[50]

Overweight (*feipang* 肥胖) bodies were identified as up to 20 percent heavier than the "ideal weight." If the excess was 20 percent or more of the ideal bodyweight, this was considered to be obese (*chao feipang* 超肥胖), as put forward by Mu Feng in 1957.[51] Later, in 1985, it is suggested by Li Yulin that "obesity points towards the excess of body fat that results in excess body weight."[52] Li includes a tolerance of up to 20 percent of weight on top of the ideal weight as still acceptable, but anything more than that is considered obese and dangerous to the body. Here a gender-specific distinction is presented once more, where males are considered obese (*feipangzheng*) if they are 20–25 percent over their suggested ideal weight whereas females are considered obese starting at 30 percent of additional weight.[53] In all these calculations there is never a reference to the reason why these percentages are used, and the authors do not quote studies or sources.

The other extreme was being underweight, also a nonideal state, that is, unhealthy. Being underweight—especially in the 1950s till the 1970s—was declared malnutrition and not considered a disease in its own right. Later, in the 1980s when anorexia nervosa and similar eating disorders made an appearance in popular media, being too skinny was treated as a sign of the specific pathology of underweight as opposed to being a comorbidity of an underlying disease or bad nutritional condition.[54]

The diagnosis of over- or underweight impacted daily life at different levels, since any deviation from the ideal was considered a deviation from ideal function and thus an obstacle for daily life, production, and revolution. In the medical discussion of obesity, it is not the workload (energy needs) that defined the treatment of the overweight body. In production and labor, a body has to be supplied with adequate amounts of various nutrients to function, since when the nourishment breaks down, function breaks down—not only if there is a lack, but also if there is too much. In the discussion of civilization diseases and obesity, height is the decisive quality that governs weight and in turn energy intake. If a body is judged too heavy for its height (and age and sex) it has to be adjusted and returned to a weight within the acceptable margins. This differs from the considerations in nutrition sciences where daily workload energy expenditure is given more emphasis. Here the focus is clearly placed on the height-weight relation, sometimes coupled with what is considered age-related weight gain and an excess of consumed calories or a lack of activity.

THE VARIETIES OF OBESITY

Different kinds of obesity with different causes are acknowledged in the discussion of healthy weight. All these varieties present outwardly merely as overweight bodies and do not visually indicate their cause. The interpretation of their pathologies mostly follows the Western discourse of the biomedical, biochemical, and external causes of obesity. Three different kinds of overweight anomalies are defined:

1. Simple obesity (*danchunxing feipang* 单纯性肥胖): Due to a higher energy intake than output, weight gain is unavoidable.[55] It is also called "external obesity," as its causes are purely external (food, beverages, lack of activity).[56]
2. Obesity as a medical condition: Due to medical factors there can be hormonal reasons for weight gain, while medicines or the presence of other diseases can also cause weight increase. This kind of obesity is also called "internal obesity," as it occurs due to internal causes.[57]
3. Inherited obesity: This will make it difficult for the individuals to lose weight.[58] One possible solution for those suffering from "bad genes" is continuous exercise and a regulated lifestyle.

Neither Xu Shengwen 许胜文[59] (writing in 1959), Wei Xiesen 魏协森 (writing in 1960), nor Wei Kaiyuan 魏开元 (in 1986) concludes that the Chinese population is especially prone to gaining weight or that there is any essential risk that the Chinese as a nation might fall victim to this condition more easily than the rest of the world. In their eyes, obesity is a deviation from the norm, that could (a) be prevented, and, in case it was not, could (b) be reversed by practicing a healthy lifestyle.

Simple obesity is the most common form of obesity: here, the patient takes in more energy, that is, food, than his or her body actually needs, which results in accumulated fat storage. The excess intake may be due to different factors, either a change in activity levels—the person spends less energy daily, but eats just as much as before—or the person eating more than necessary and so not using up all this energy. The excess is stored as fat in the body's fat cells. This kind of obesity happens especially when living circumstances change, for example, in relocating from the countryside to the city, as in the story of Sun Ke 孙克 reported in the *Xintiyu* in 1954. Before 1949, Sun was living in the countryside and felt healthy while doing a lot of manual work outside. This changed when moving to Beijing after 1949 and starting work at a local administration office. His new living and working environment included mental work and a rather sedentary lifestyle, with the result that he found himself gaining weight. In the beginning he still thought this to be a good thing, as his formerly lean body gained mass, but the additional health problems that often accompany weight gain soon made him aware of the problems attached. Suffering from high blood pressure, he finally consulted a doctor who then explained that the lack of physical activity resulted in weight gain and this in turn produced cardiovascular problems. Sun then decided to take his recovery in his own hands in order to avoid further health issues and started a workout regimen to successfully lower his body weight.[60]

While Sun's weight gain was due to a changed living situation, medical conditions were also a reason for added weight, where the resulting obesity is thus often a symptom of another pathology. In 1959, Xu Shengwen lists encephalitis as one such illness that may result in weight gain. As this disease influences part of the brain, it leads to changes in brain chemistry and causes the body to fatten. A body can store excess fat or water due to a number of different diseases or internal problems. Bodily functions may be impaired due to metabolic, endocrinological, or nervous problems. Externally caused injuries like a concussion or brain damage due to a fall can also cause changes in brain chemistry and influence a person's appetite, taste, and so on, as was suggested in Xu's pamphlet on exercise treatment for overweight patients.[61] In 1980, Wei Mingyan notes two reasons for being overweight, which were discovered in experiments with rats: (1) the part in the brain that controls the absorption of food is not working properly; and (2) due to metabolic issues, the amount of fat cells increases, leading to what Wei calls metabolic fat, which is hard to get rid of.[62] In 1984, Li Bingcheng emphasizes that endocrinological problems can cause weight gain, pointing specifically toward the pituitary gland and low thyroid function.[63] In the same year, Cui Bozhong 崔伯重 refers to metabolic reasons for weight gain in the *Journal of Postgraduates of Medicine* (*Yishi jinxiu zazhi* 医师进修杂志).[64]

On top of excessive weight, other comorbidities have an effect on overweight patients and their ability to function. Comorbidities that are connected to obesity include heart diseases, diabetes (type 2), arteriosclerosis, kidney stones, fatty liver, high blood pressure, high blood fats, and high blood sugars, among others.[65] Some of the sufferers also admit experiencing low energy and difficulty in finishing work tasks. This influences the worker drastically and thus reduces labor power and production rate, and in the most extreme cases will lead to death. These are health issues that need to be addressed and avoided so as to keep up labor and not put any extra strain on the nation. With these consequences in mind, it seems arguably rather simplistic to declare that all the information on how to build a healthy body was already available, and hence that the application of said health knowledge should have been possible. Obviously, this was not what in fact happened, or else the continuing admonitions to train the body and avoid a fattening lifestyle would have disappeared. As it is, the PRC discourse on obesity and its prevention has continued until the present day, even in the face of rising patient numbers.

Over time, additional reasons to avoid obesity were brought forth. Apart from the physiological problems that overweight poses, in the 1980s the question of aesthetics arose. Especially in post–Cultural Revolution texts, the argument for a slim and trained body turns from being a purely functional ideal to one being connected to looks.

The ideal look is connected to the question of obesity by the discourse of health, but also by the propagated beauty standards. In the context of the Mao-era and post–Cultural Revolution health discourse, being obese does not conform to the desired physique. In both time periods, for women this meant a slim body, and for men a strong, muscular body. But in the post-Mao period there is a turn away from the androgynous looks of the Mao era, when women started to work in the same domains as men, marking their bodies as like men's.[66] In the post-Mao era, femininity was rediscovered. Yet in both cases looking attractive could be achieved and interpreted in two ways: (1) by being healthy, which leads to being slim due to adequate exercise and nutrition, where the result is considered attractive, that is, health is attractive;[67] or (2) by being slim, a form which is considered attractive regardless of the method by which this state of the body is reached. For the purposes of my research, I adopt the first consideration as being the more reasonable way to understand attractiveness as linked to health.

The fact that prior to the 1980s, strength and functionality were ascribed to the healthy body can already be seen in a 1956 discussion by Wu Zhuzhong 吴柱中 of fat and skinny people's problems. He notes that in neither case does a person look particularly good. Instead, he defines an aesthetic body as being muscled and vigorous (*jirou jieshi, jingshen baoman* 肌肉结实，精神饱满).[68] This gives a very specific idea of what is considered not ugly (*bu nankan* 不难看) but acceptable and visually pleasing and at the same time functional. The idea of *jianmei* 健美, meaning strong and handsome, as a way to reach good health but also a good exterior, was used in the description of the process of building a strong and beautiful body only later, in the 1980s.[69]

A 1987 article in the *Jiankang*, part of a five-part series, connects the wish to be trim and healthy with the idea of building an aesthetic physique: "If one is determined to make oneself into a strong and beautiful person, then one has to deal with both of them [diet and exercise], only then will one be successful."[70] Fitness is turned into a hobby,[71] which opens the new possibility of talking about it not as an obligation to the state, but as an activity one personally enjoys. Prior to this, physical exercise was described as a means to a very specific end: vigor and endurance for the goal of production. Now, it turns into a concept similar to the idea of *l'art pour l'art*: doing exercise because of the fun of exercising, breaking with the purely spartan idea of steeling the body for a higher purpose. Instead, physical fitness becomes part of an individual's expression, while also playing into the hands of the national strengthening plans.

TREATING OBESITY

To ensure continued economic and national growth, obesity had to be defeated—if it was not avoided in the first place—in order to maintain a productive national body. The paradigm of prevention and the vision of health propagated by the PRC authorities should, in theory, have prevented the decline of bodies, but since this was not achieved, different ways to negotiate the new situation were implemented. Measures depended on the kind of obesity in question, and included dieting, exercising, or even Chinese Medicine.

Exercising the Weight Away

In 1957, the First Shanghai Hospital (*Shanghai diyi yiyuan* 上海第一医院) introduced new training methods for people who had to lose weight in order to regain their health. This hospital published its new methods for curing their patients of ill health and included an exemplary case study in the *Xintiyu*. The patient in this study was a woman who at 80 kilograms and a circumference of 113 centimeters was unable to get out of bed. She was diagnosed with simple obesity by the hospital's doctors and put on a calisthenics routine twice daily. Additionally, it was suggested to her to practice sit-ups.[72] The article lists her weight as 76 kilograms and circumference as 112 centimeters after two months on this program, as 74.5 kilograms and 100 centimeters after four months, and 63 kilograms and 90 centimeters after six months. Reportedly, the lady was not recognizable by her acquaintances after finishing treatment, but was fully able to go about her daily life again. The article's author, Xu

Shengwen, emphasized the role of medical staff in the weight loss process and their authority over the new life structures.[73]

In the same year, Wu Rongfen 邬荣芬 reports that she herself had suffered from being overweight her whole life. According to her own assessment, she had been eating too much since she was a child. She had thought of herself as too fat, but over the years had always had different excuses as to why she could not change her habits. She finally changed her ways and started incorporating more exercise into her daily routine, with the end result of slow but steady weight loss. Wu chose to follow Soviet female gymnastics as a daily activity to burn more calories and improve her physique.[74] Most of the lifestyle-change case studies and personal anecdotes include the notion that a change in diet and exercise improved the suffering person's quality of life, as does Wei Xiesen's short 1960 article "Do You Want to Lose Weight?" (Ni xiang xiaochu feipang ma 你想消除肥胖吗).[75]

To make the prescribed exercise routines accessible to the readers and patients, very specific training methods are at times introduced, for example in the *Xintiyu* in 1979 when a reportedly successful training method from Japan is introduced by Lin Xiaofeng 林笑蜂. This method used predefined sets of exercises that burn 300–500 kilocalories at a time. By monitoring the pulse during these exercises, the sets were adjusted to the individual participant and were meant to aid in losing weight and lowering blood pressure. According to the article, this training was quite successful for those who took part in it, even over a relatively short time.[76]

In 1980, Huang Meiguang 黄美光[77] agrees that exercise is the treatment of choice for overweight patients, combined with adjusted nutrition. It is not only the way to prevent obesity and related diseases, but is also the solution to these issues. As exercise builds up muscles, it strengthens the formerly weak body, improves metabolism, and finally results in more vigor and power. By doing easy exercises to start with, the body is slowly built up and can endure more and more pressure. Walking, slow jogging, or ball sports are all valid ways to exercise, but daily chores or field work also already function as a way to control weight, as they burn off energy.[78] Another 1980 *Dazhong Yixue* article by Peng Shuwu puts physical education directly in the context of civilization diseases: "Physical Education and Civilization Diseases" (Tiyu yundong yu "wenmingbing" 体育运动与'文明病'). Peng reassures his readership that physical education is an easy treatment for the central health problems of the time.[79]

In the series "Fat People Have to Read This" (Pangren bidu 胖人必读), published in the journal *Jiankang* in 1987, several different aspects of weight gain and weight loss are discussed. The fourth part of this series includes suggestions on how to lose weight not unlike the previous publications in the series. It also repeats the admonition that just because one increases one's activity level, energy intake should indeed stay balanced and not be increased. Exercises to lose weight suggested in this piece include walking for an hour each day, cycling for 45 minutes, or swimming for 15 minutes. These exercises would burn 350 kilocalories, and in order to burn half a kilogram of fat, 3,500 kilocalories would have to be burned. The article urges that by doing these exercises 1 kilogram could be lost in a month.[80] This way of exercising depicts the importance of predictability for this process. It gives a time frame and becomes a plannable activity. This particular series on desired behavior in obese patients demonstrates that the authorities' nudging of the population in the right direction was occurring both pre- and post-reform.

While all these authors stress how important it is to exercise for fitness and well-being, there are also cautious voices on the topic of physical activity. Gao Qiang 高强, for example, cautions the readers of the *Xintiyu* in 1977 that when exercising to lose weight comes to a halt, so does the weight loss and burning of energy. The end of exercise is a critical point in the process, as it can lead to new weight gain. If a person stops their fitness training, there is the real risk of "piling on the pounds" again, especially when they continue to eat as if they were still active. Gao Qiang emphasizes that in this case the body will store the excess energy in its fat storage. This has to be kept in mind if one stops participating in physical activity.[81]

Eating Yourself Slim: A Return to the Nutritionist Paradigm

Apart from adequate activity levels for shedding the kilos, a dietary plan is incorporated into weight loss plans and obesity prevention tips, for example in Sun Zhiming's 孙知明 1958 article "Discussing the Origin of Overweight and its Treatment Problems" (Tantan feipang de yuanyin yu zhiliao wenti 谈谈肥胖的原因与治疗问题). Sun advises the adoption of a diet low in carbohydrates and fats, and even suggests hunger treatment.[82] During this procedure only 1,000–1,400 kilocalories per day were to be consumed. He agrees that this is hard for many patients, especially at the beginning, so he refers to Soviet sources which suggest a three-phase approach: First, the patients should take some days to prepare themselves by consuming protein-rich food (meat) and should eat less carbohydrates (rice) and fats and compensate with an array of vegetables and fruit. Then, food intake had to be controlled strictly so that the patients get used to the treatment. This could take ten to fifteen days. In the third phase, patients were only supposed to have a little tea and fast for three to five days depending on their physical condition. Sun notes that young patients tended to have problems with this.[83]

The idea that an appropriate diet aids in keeping the body healthy is reiterated in 1985 when Li Yulin gives a brief rundown of how obesity has developed over time. He recounts the story of obesity: before the Second World War obesity was considered a "rich men's disease" (*fugui bing* 富贵病) as it was identified as a disease of advanced economies and societies. Li explains that weight control is managed by combining exercise with a suitable diet, such as a high-carbohydrate, low-fat diet, or the high-fat, high-protein, low-carbohydrate diet.[84]

Culprits that countered the healthy intent were the new and increasingly available sweets and snacks which entered China especially after the Cultural Revolution. Gao Qiang[85] and Zhou Wenquan 周文泉 et al.,[86] for example, advise strongly against them, as well as against oily and greasy foods, too much starch (carbohydrates), and big portions. It seems that after an era of shortage the era of plenty overwhelmed the population so that advice on these new kinds of snack foods, that had not been available before, finds its way into the discourse of health.[87]

All of these solutions are described in simple terms and, apart from a visit to the doctor, are low-cost approaches. There are no references to expensive supplements in this process, or to expensive treatment recommendations.[88] The only access needed was to hospitals and information to implement preventive measures. One should also not dismiss the propaganda impact when reading the anecdotes or testimonies, since most of them glorify a basic farmer's life which included plenty of daily activity and the most basic (pure) food, that is, an ideal way to structure life in a healthy manner.[89]

Treating the New with the Old

During and after the Mao era, Chinese Medicine experienced a renaissance and transformation, not least thanks to Mao Zedong's description in 1958 of Chinese Medicine as a treasure trove.[90] Traditional medicine was applied cheaply and practically, especially by "barefoot doctors" and farmers who were also trained as medical staff. The financial aspect of training a part of the population in traditional medical practices was a big driving force of the Chinese Medicine revival, since at the time it was much cheaper to deliver this training than to engage a large number of people in the study of biomedicine.[91] Accordingly, for the treatment of obesity there were not only Western treatments in the medical press: Chinese Medicine also offered alternative treatments of obesity as a specific health problem.[92]

While Chinese Medicine and other Chinese traditions only played a very marginal role in nutrition sciences and physical education—for example, the incorporation of Chinese martial arts elements in the *Guangbo ticao* sequences—in the realm of actual disease treatment they played a bigger role. In the second half of the twentieth century, Chinese Medicine returned as a standardized system that incorporated rationalized views of the body: a patient was first thoroughly measured and weighed in order to assess the sick body,[93] then basic medical diagnosis techniques (measuring, weighing, taking temperature, etc.) were integrated and directly linked to the creation of *zhongxi jiehe* 中西结合, which describes the combination and incorporation of Chinese and Western medical practices to form a new medicine.

To aid an overweight patient with Chinese Medicine, they were examined using the traditional diagnosis techniques (observing visually, smelling, listening, and pulse taking [*sizhen* 四诊]) as well via as a biomedical assessment, and then given a prescription for herbal concoctions that had to be ingested over a period of several weeks, sometimes months.[94] Most of the time these techniques were supported by adding other metric data, such as height, weight, blood pressure, and so on, and by relating the biomedical data to the Chinese medical observations.

To illustrate these treatments, I want to introduce Mrs. Zhao and her recovery story printed in a 1965 *Zhonghua Yixue Zazhi* issue. Mrs. Zhao was examined for the first time in September of 1963. She was 27 years old at the time and had rapidly gained weight, especially around the belly. Originally, she had weighed 80 pounds (40 kg) at 133 centimeters, but then her weight shot up to 117 pounds (58.5 kg). Other symptoms she observed with the weight gain included dizziness, bad memory, an inflamed larynx, lack of strength, and difficulty in movement. She was diagnosed with simple obesity and latent diabetes. The suggested treatment involved an herbal concoction made from ten different Chinese medical herbs of which she took 23 doses in the following weeks. The patient lost 17 pounds (8.5 kg) and felt more vigorous and stronger. Additionally, the patient was directed to practice Qigong to accompany the treatment. In January of 1964 the patient had managed to get down to 99 pounds (49.5 kg) and two months later she weighed 95 pounds. By July 1964 she was able to return to do her normal work.[95]

Another example, published in 1979, shows the continuity of these kinds of case studies and their treatments. After giving birth in 1976, Mrs. Lü kept gaining weight. She was a primary school teacher and was examined for the first time in May 1977. After giving birth she had weighed 120 pounds (60 kg) and would continue gaining weight until the first visit to the Chinese doctors, when she was 172 pounds (86 kg). Before consulting with the article's author, Liang Guoqin 梁国卿,[96] she had already been to different other hospitals but treatments never worked. When she started to use Chinese Medicine, her body evened out: she ate normally and her bowels also moved regularly. Her diagnosis was a depletion of Yuanqi (*yuanqixu* 元气虚), which led to insufficient digestive activity, resulting in insufficient nourishment of the body and manifesting in fat and phlegm stored in the skin and muscles. In order to cure this condition, an elimination of dampness and heat was attempted as this would help to digest foods and stimulate energy flow. Liang suggests here a decoction of ten different Chinese medical herbs, called *Pingchentang* 平陈汤.[97] The treatment seems to have been successful, as at the following meeting the patient weighed 160 pounds (80 kg), at the next visit she only weighed 150 pounds (75 kg), and then in the end slimmed down to 142 pounds (71 kg).[98] All this was attributed to the doses of the herbal concoction she was taking regularly during this period.[99]

These articles show how measurements are incorporated into Chinese medical treatment and how a treatment for a biomedical pathology was generated. The regular measuring of the patients as well as the continuous considerations of their pulse, facial color, and so forth, show how a connection was established between all those symptoms.

The ultimate goal of these treatments is the return to work and productivity, which is why relatively quick and sustainable cures are highlighted by these case studies. The sick body needed to be restored to a state of equilibrium and comfort, so it could return to productive labor. This is the mark against which the body's health is measured. Chinese Medicine in this context is a means to an end: it helps in long-term weight loss as it eliminates blockages and stimulates the flow of energy so that the body can find its balance and return to a state of health.[100]

Apart from the medicinal herbs which were administered during a Chinese medical treatment, not many other drugs seem to have been used at the time. Unlike the drugs involved in hypertension treatment, obesity treatment did not rely on chemical stimulants for its success.[101]

To recap the argument and observations in the present chapter, we have seen how an examination of the discussion of obesity in mid-twentieth-century China yields interesting results, especially regarding the conviction, common in the scholarship, that there is nothing to be found on this topic for this period of time. It shows how a medical discourse on overweight bodies did in fact prevail during a period which is mostly known for its scarcity, famine, and lack of material goods. This chapter has traced the discussion in the popular media from the Republican period until the 1980s, and has tried to correct the false assumption that obesity was not a topic in the Mao- and reform-era health discourse.

Obesity, we have seen, was categorized into three different types: simple obesity (external obesity), internal obesity (medical causes), and hereditary obesity. As they all are the result of different causes, treatments vary as well. Simple obesity was cured by a change in lifestyle, increased exercise regimen, a structured diet, and medical supervision if necessary. External obesity was cured by tackling the underlying issue or sickness. Hereditary obesity could only be influenced by adhering to a strict and healthy lifestyle. In the treatment of obesity, the combination of Chinese Medicine and biomedicine comes into play, and its successful application is demonstrated by case studies which show the merging of the different ways to diagnose and treat. By involving Chinese Medicine in the treatment of biomedical diseases, a medical development is effected which opens the way to the emergence of the Chinese New Medicine.

The discourse of obesity in the PRC also shows how the paradigm of prevention is widened to encompass an understanding of a sickness which was the opposite of the contemporary burning issues of malnutrition and famine. It engaged the idea of self-treatment, involvement of experts, and opened a new arena for integrated Chinese-biomedical treatment.

The increasing relevance of this topic for the PRC today might indeed be read into the increasing number of articles that we find written on the subject, but that would be a false assumption, based on an epistemological fallacy. Due to the logistics of publishing in the timeframe examined and the contemporary political events, there is no certainty as to how many articles, handbooks, or papers were written on the subject of obesity, and no conclusions about the increase in significance can be drawn from the change in the numbers of sources found. The continuous importance of the topic, nevertheless, can be assumed because of the continuous appearance of works in different media on the width, weight, and size of the body.

The evolution of the discourse in the periods under discussion can again be seen to lead to a change in the way the body was perceived. The body as a machine was nothing other than a power plant and the muscles were the little engines that made it run. Thus, the idea of muscularity emerged more strongly. Muscularity in a Chinese socialist context fed the revolutionary rhetoric and displayed the population's and the party's ability to bring about change. The machine metaphor specifically points to its production value and the function the human body had to fulfil in a labor environment. This is where obesity, as a new and drastic change in the body, comes into play. A body too frail and weak to work was no option for the Chinese workers, and a body that was too fat was not able to function either. And we have seen that the idea of function in production was later supplemented by ideas about aesthetics.

Obesity was not the only deviation from the idealized body form that emerged with the increase in general affluence. The pathology of a sickly thin body deriving from eating disorders such as anorexia nervosa made an entrance in the 1980s. Here psychological issues are introduced as a cause for the disease: whereas before being skinny indicated a lack of food, now the unwillingness to ingest food marked this skinny condition as a sickness. The malnourished state arose from a pathological state of the mind, not from a circumstance of food shortage.[102] The discussion of obesity, health, and skinniness swings between the two extremes and the experts and authorities had to establish an equilibrium to ensure that the nation's body was in the middle range.

Different layers of authority can be identified in this discussion. On top is the state that is building the basic infrastructure and supervising knowledge production. Through the established medical institutions, personnel and experts are trained who then in turn publish their knowledge and by doing so make it available to the population. Doctors publish their own findings and are talked about in anecdotes by former patients. In this dynamic the doctors often are the ones who make the diagnosis and then offer treatments, supervising the road to recovery. The patient has the power to choose whether to consult a physician, and if so which doctor to see. They can also choose to read the published information and decide whether to follow the advice or not. If they choose to follow the advice, they can then implement some lifestyle changes and follow the doctors' advice and treatment plans as well. This falls in line with the Maoist aspiration of making everybody an expert; the expectation that people would read what experts and the party published can be traced back to Liu Shaoqi and his description of the way to be a good communist.[103]

All of the collected materials were meant to prevent bodies from deteriorating into the state of obesity. Although they brought together health tips and prevention ideas from the Soviet Union, the United States, Europe, and even Japan, they did not change the course of history or avert the obesity epidemic that is continuing to grow today.

NOTES

1. See French and Crabbe, *Fat China*; "Obesity: The Big, Fat Problem with Chinese cities," https://www.theguardian.com/sustainable-business/2017/jan/09/obesity-fat-problem-chinese-cities (accessed February 25, 2019); UNICEF Obesity Report on China, http://www.unicef.cn/en/uploadfile/2018/0423/20180423114400165.pdf (accessed February 25, 2019); Benjamin Shobert, "China's Growing Obesity Problem," *Forbes*, 11 January 2017, https://www.forbes.com/sites/benjaminshobert/2017/01/22/chinas-growing-obesity-problem/#7f8b3ca86ecf (February 25, 2019).

2. French and Crabbe, *Fat China*, 37.

3. See Gilman, *Obesity*; Weber, "Die protestantische Ethik"; and Forth, *Fat*.

4. Anne Scott Beller, *Fat and Thin—A Natural History of Obesity* (New York: McGraw-Hill, 1977), 4–5.

5. For a more in-depth discussion of fat and its historical relevance, development, and meaning to life, see Forth, *Fat*.

6. Charles Rosenberg, "Introduction," in *Framing Disease*, ed. Charles Rosenberg and Janet Golden (New Brunswick: Rutgers University Press, 1997), xv.

7. Adrian Wilson, "On the History of Disease-Concepts: The Case of Pleurisy," *History of Science* 38, no. 3 (2000): 281f.

8. Rosenberg, "Introduction: Framing Disease," xvii.

9. Gilman, *Obesity*, 21ff.

10. Michel Foucault, *Die Sorge um sich (Sexualität und Wahrheit 3)* [*History of Sexuality*] (Frankfurt: Suhrkamp Verlag, 2012), 55–93.

11. Zhang Libin's dissertation has to be approached carefully. It sports a few generalized expressions that need to be reviewed and researched in more detail, and not taken as given, since the unreflective manner of presentation is quite problematic. The basic observations in this work were, nevertheless, helpful to complete a view of overweight issues in the PRC.

12. Gilman, *Obesity*, 135–36.

13. The Sick Man of Asia was mostly depicted as weak and skinny, unfit for the accelerated modern life and without any resistance to external influences.

14. Gilman, *Obesity*, 136ff.

15. See Walter H. Mallory, *China—Land of Famine* (New York: American Geographical Society, 1926).

16. Gilman, *Obesity*, 142.

17. French and Crabbe, *Fat China*, 135.

18. French and Crabbe, 135–36. See also Zhang, "A Multilevel Study of Effects."

19. French and Crabbe, *Fat China*, 30, 37. For this see also Zhang, "A Multilevel Study of Effects."

20. Zhang gives no text reference here. She refers to the Tang dynasty's beauty ideal without quoting any source. Zhang, "A Multilevel Study of Effects," 33.

21. Ko Cho and Kyoko Iriye Selden, *The Search for the Beautiful Woman: A Cultural History of Japanese and Chinese Beauty* (Lanham: Rowman & Littlefield, 2012), 29.

22. Zhang, "A Multilevel Study of Effects," 34. In this case, the expression "the masses" is complicated. Here the author does not distinguish between her own phrasing in describing the situation and the ideological subtext of expressions like this. A lack of distinction between political rhetoric and academic language is thus displayed by this choice of words.

23. Frank Dikötter, *Mao's Great Famine: The History of China's Most Devastating Catastrophe, 1958–1962* (New York: Walker & Co., 2010); Kimberly E. Mannings and Felix Wemheuer, eds., *Eating Bitterness: New Perspectives on China's Great Leap Forward and Famine* (Vancouver: UBC Press, 2011).

24. Zhang, "A Multilevel Study of Effects," 30. See also Ana Carden-Coyne, *Reconstructing the Body—Classicism, Modernism, and the First World War* (Oxford: Oxford University Press, 2009).

25. Zhang, "A Multilevel Study of Effects," 11.

26. Zhang, 12.

27. P. Deurenberg, M. Deurenberg-Yap, and S. Guricci, "Asians are Different from Caucasians and From Each Other in Their Body Mass Index/Body Fat Per Cent Relationship," *Obesity Reviews*, no. 3 (2002): 141–46.

28. Zhang, "A Multilevel Study of Effects," 40. These shifts are also observed and described in James Watson, "China's Big Mac Attack," in *The Cultural Politics of Food and Eating*, ed. James L. Watson and Melissa Caldwell, 70–79 (Oxford: Blackwell Publishing, 2005); and Jing Jun, ed., *Feeding China's Little Emperors: Food, Children, and Social Change* (Stanford: Stanford University Press, 2000).

29. Zhang not only takes this transition as a deciding factor for obesity, but considers income inequality and socioeconomic factors, which will not be considered here as they cannot be measured by the materials I am examining. I am, after all, focusing on the fact that despite the introduction of healthier ways of eating and a modern job structure, the body is, nevertheless, overwhelmed and oftentimes treated unhealthily, which then results in obesity. For a discussion of the issue of introducing Western cuisine to China, see also Gilman, *Obesity*, 131f.

30. Post–World War I, there was an effort to ingrain habits by showing hygienic, clean, healthy, and strong bodies which were able to shoulder responsibility and military tasks. See, for example, Forth, *Fat*, 236–73.

31. See chapters 1 and 2; see also Seung-Joon Lee, "The Patriot's Scientific Diet: Nutrition Science and Dietary Reform Campaigns in China, 1910s–1950s," *Modern Asian Studies* 6, no. 49 (February 2015): 1–32; and Michael Shiyung Liu, "Diet for War: Military Nutrition in Republican China," *Journal of Modern Chinese History* 14, no. 2 (2020): 240–54.

32. See Sigrid Schmalzer, *The People's Peking Man: Popular Science and Human Identity in Twentieth-Century China* (Chicago: University of Chicago Press, 2008).

33. *Feipangzheng* / *Feipangbing* are descriptions of a pathological condition, whilst *feipang* / *pang* just hint at the fact that a body weighs more than it should, no pathological symptoms being involved other than the visible weight gain and encasing of fat. Still, this is considered unhealthy and a marker for ensuing symptoms (high blood pressure, diabetes, difficulty moving etc.).

34. Kondratiev, B. A. (B.A. 康德拉季也夫), "Gaoxueya bing huanzhe de shenghuo zhidu (xuwan) 高血压病患者的生活制度 (续完)," trans. Wu Zhongbi 武忠弼, *Dazhong Yixue* 2 (1954): 103–6.

35. Li Bingcheng 李秉诚, "Kepa de wenmingbing 可怕的文明病," *Shandong tiyu keji* 1 (1984): 25–27.

36. This can be co-referenced with the overall lower BMI of the Chinese at the time and also the fact that diabetes occurs much earlier in the Chinese population as opposed to Western populations. See Deurenberg, Deurenberg-Yap, and Guricci, "Asians are Different from Caucasians," 141–46.

37. Mu Feng 木风, "Nengrang pangzi xiaoshou ma? 能让胖子消瘦吗?" *Renmin Ribao* (November 3, 1957).

38. Michael Shiyung Liu noted in his article on the Republican war diet that a decreased energy need in the Chinese soldiers was discussed at length by Li Tingan in the 1940s, who "explained that the physique and digestion of the Chinese soldier was weaker than that of Westerners, and that the smaller Chinese body could be an evolutionary consequence due to the long history of food scarcity in China" (Liu, "Diet for War," 247). This different experience resulted in a lowered calorie need on the side of the Chinese. Liu supposes that the young Chinese Republic could simply

not supply the Western standard of calories and nutrients, and that the assumption that Chinese could do with less helped in keeping up morale (pp. 247–48).

39. The author Shen Qianglin calculated: body height in cm—105 cm = ideal weight. He includes a 10 percent tolerance margin. Anything more than 10 percent above this ideal weight he considered overweight. See Shen Qianglin 沈强霖, "Feipang yu yinshi 肥胖与饮食," *Dazhong Yixue* 7 (1979): 29–32.

See also Zhu Zhiming 朱志明, "Tixing jiankang shouming 体型 健康 寿命," *Dazhong Yixue* 5 (1983): 4–5.

40. "Zhengque dui de feipang 正确对得肥胖," *Xintiyu* 8 (1979): 30.

41. Similar tables can be found in Wei Kaiyuan 魏开元, "Feipang ji qi fangzhi 肥胖及其防治," *Shengwuxue tongbao* 2 (1986): 21.

42. Yi Jian 伊坚, "Zhangde tinggao, tingpang jiu jiankang ma 长得挺高□挺胖就健康吗?" *Xintiyu* 4 (1977): 47: Yi Jian notes that it is difficult to measure how much the ideal weight of a person is, as height and muscles also play an important role. As muscles are much heavier than fat, athletes would often be considered too fat by just looking at the scales, whereas they are heavier than average people due to more developed muscle groups.

43. Li Yulin 李玉琳, "Feipang zheng ji tizhong kongzhi 肥胖症及体重控制," *Tiyu jiaoxue yu keyan* 4 (1985): 33–37.

44. Li Yulin, 33–37.

45. In the case of young women in a 1980 *Xintiyu* article "Talking about young women getting overweight" (He nüqingninan tan fapang 和女青年谈发胖), the author Xu Xuzhi徐勖志 also employs a margin and defines it as +/– 10 percent of the ideal body weight (in kg), which he calculates as height minus 100 centimeters as well.

46. Yan Ke 严克, "Feipang he xiaoshou 肥胖和消瘦," *Dazhong Yixue* 3 (1982): 35–36. The same equation is also published in Du Xixian 杜希贤, "Naxie ren rongyi fapang 哪些人容易发胖," *Dazhong Yixue* 3 (1986): 48. This article also shows a way to calculate the amount of fat in a body: (body weight in kg / (height in cm)2) x 100.

47. Xu Pingji 徐平吉and Lu Dingxi 陆定熙, "Jianfei yao——fenfulaming pian 减肥药——芬氟拉明片," *Dazhong Yixue* 8 (1986): 40.

48. Xu Shengwen 许胜文, "Cong zhongnian fapang tanqi 从中年发胖谈起," *Xintiyu* 5 (1979): 26–27.

49. Xu Xuzhi 徐勖志, "He nüqingnian tan fapang 和女青年谈发胖," *Xintiyu* 3 (1980): 36.

50. Mao Zhongyao 毛中耀, "Xupang bushi zhuang 虚胖不是壮," *Xintiyu* 4 (1954): 28.

See also Beijing yiyuan, *Laoren baojian bidu* 老人保健必读 (Beijing: Renmin weisheng chubanshe, 1982), 24; and Gao Qiang 高强, "Shouren lian changpao hui yuepao yueshou ma? 瘦人练长跑会越跑越瘦吗?" *Xintiyu* 1 (1980): 44.

51. For the different considerations on how to term different stages of overweight, see:

Mu Feng, "Nengrang pangzi xiaoshou ma? 能让胖子消瘦吗?," *Renmin Ribao* (November 3, 1957). There is also the notion of +20 percent being 轻度肥胖症 and +40 percent being 中度肥胖症.

Xu Shengwen, *Feipangbing de yiliao ticao* 肥胖病的医疗体操 (Shanghai: Shanghai kexue jishu chubanshe, 1959), 2–3. Xu even distinguishes between 25–35 percent of additional body weight as slightly overweight, 35–50 percent as moderately overweight, and anything of more than 50 percent on top of ideal weight as heavily overweight.

Xu Xuzhi 徐勖志, "He nüqingninan tan fapang 和女青年谈发胖," *Xintiyu* 3 (1980): 36. Anything up to +20 percent of weight is considered overweight (*chaozhong* 超重) and anything more than 20 percent of weight is considered obese (*feipang* 肥胖).

Zhou Xiaohan 周小寒, "Gao, duan, pang, shou—jizhong changjian de yichang tixing 高，短，胖，瘦—几种常见的异常体型," *Dazhong Yixue* 4 (1982): 15–16. Obesity as a disease manifests when the weight of the body exceeds 20 percent of the normal body weight.

Zhu Zhiming 朱志明, "Tixing jiankang shouming 体型 健康 寿命," *Dazhong Yixue* 5 (1983): 4–5. Normal weight: anything in the +/– 10 percent range of the ideal weight. Anything more than 10 percent is seen as relatively fat (*jiaopang tixing* 较胖体型), but anything that exceeds an additional 20 percent of body weight is considered obese (*feipang tixing* 肥胖体型). On the other end of the scale, less than 10 percent is seen as relatively skinny (*jiaoshou* 较瘦) and less than 20 percent as emaciated (*xiaoshou* 消瘦).

See also Ke Fu 柯夫, "Pang ren bi du (yi) 胖人必读（一）," *Jiankang* 11 (1986): 58–59.

52. Li Yulin 李玉琳, "Feipangzheng ji tizhong kongzhi 肥胖症及体重控制," *Tiyu jiaoxue yu keyan* 4 (1985): 33–37: 肥胖症是指由于体脂过多而引起的体重过重.

53. Li Yulin does not explain where he gets these numbers from, but he adds that being overweight may also be caused by other factors apart from body fat, for example water retention, tumors, or well-developed muscle mass.

54. Wang Ruilin 王瑞麟 and Liu Qipei 柳启沛, "Xiaoshouzhe de yinshi 消瘦者的饮食," *Dazhong Yixue* 7 (1983): 43.

Liu Shaojing 刘韶景, "Cong jianfei dao shenjing xing yanshi 从减肥到神经性厌食," *Dazhong Yixue* 4 (1985): 14.

55. Wei Xiesen, "Ni xiang xiaochu feipang ma 你想消除肥胖吗," *Dazhong Yixue* 2 (1960): 77. See also Wei Kaiyuan, "Feipang ji qi fangzhi 肥胖及其防治," *Shengwuxue tongbao* 2 (1986): 20–23.

56. Xu Shengwen, *Feipangbing de yiliao ticao*, 3.

57. Xu Shengwen, 3.

58. Wei Mingyan 魏铭炎, *Jiankang. Yukuai. Changshou* 健康。愉快。长寿 (Guangzhou: Kexuepuji chubanshe guangzhou fenshe, 1980), 16. See also Cui Bozhong 崔伯重, "Feipang zheng 肥胖症," *Yishi jinxiu zazhi* 1 (1984): 20–21; Wei Kaiyuan, "Feipang ji qi fangzhi 肥胖及其防治," *Shengwuxue tongbao* 2 (1986): 21, who includes family background and behavior into the examination of the patient. Oftentimes unhealthy habits are learned from the parents and influence the younger generation's weight.

59. Xu Shengwen, born in 1933, was a professor of sports medicine at the Shanghai Medicine and Science University. He graduated from the Medical Institute of the

Shanghai First Medical School in 1956. He is on the editorial board of the *Zhongguo yundong yixue zazhi* 中国运动医学杂志. (See *Yundong jiepouxue, yundingyixue dacidian*, 运动解剖学、运动医学大辞典 [Beijing: Renmin tiyu chubanshe, 2000], 490.)

60. Sun Ke 孙克, "Wo you xupang biande jiankangle 我由虚胖变得健康了," *Xintiyu* 4 (1954): 34.

61. Xu Shengwen, *Feipangbing de yiliao ticao*, 4. See also Cao Wujun 曹武君, ed., *Yinshi yu jiankang* 饮食与健康 (Guangzhou: Guangdong keji chubanshe, 1981), 63.

62. Wei Mingyan, *Jiankang. Yukuai. Changshou*, 16–17.

63. Li Bingcheng, "Kepa de wenmingbing 可怕的文明病," *Shandong tiyu keji* 1 (1984): 25.

64. Cui Bozhong, "Feipang zheng 肥胖症," *Yishi jinxiu zazhi* 1 (1984): 20–21.

65. Yi Jian 伊坚, "Zhangde tinggao, tingpang jiu jiankang ma 长得挺高□挺胖就健康吗?" *Xintiyu* 4 (1977): 47. See also Liu Rong 刘嵘 and Liu Weimin 刘为民, "Feipang you naxie haichu 肥胖有哪些害处," *Dazhong Yixue* 10 (1984): 5; Xu Aihua 徐爱华, "Feipang yu changshou 肥胖与长寿," *Dazhong Yixue* 10 (1984): 43.

66. Bret Hinsch, *Masculinities in Chinese History* (Plymouth, UK: Rowman & Littlefield, 2013), 154.

67. Wu Zhuzhong, "Pangren yu shouren de wenti 胖人与瘦人的问题," *Xintiyu* 22 (1956): 21.

68. Wu Zhuzhong, 21.

69. See Ke Fu 柯夫, "Pangren bidu (yi) 胖人必读（一）," *Jiankang* 11 (1986): 58. See also Ke Fu 柯夫, "Pangren bidu (si) 胖人必读（四）," *Jiankang* 2 (1987): 36.

70. Ke Fu, "Pangren bidu (si) 胖人必读（四）," *Jiankang* 2 (1987): 36: 有决心要使自己健美的人，必须二者兼顾，才能奏效.

71. Wang Peiqin 汪佩琴, "Yu guniang tan pangshou 与姑娘谈胖瘦," *Dazhong Yixue* 7 (1980): 23.

72. This would have helped with core strength and built up the stamina for moving and getting up from the bed.

73. Xu Shengwen, "Xin de yiliao jigou 新的医疗机构," *Xintiyu* 7 (1957): 16–17.

74. Wu Rongfen 邬荣芬, "He feipang zuo douzheng 和肥胖作斗争," *Xintiyu* 3 (1957): 23.

75. Wei Xiesen 魏协森, "Ni xiang xiaochu feipang ma 你想消除肥胖吗," *Dazhong yixue* 2 (1960): 77.

76. Lin Xiaofeng 林笑蜂, "Weile zhiliao fapang he gaoxueya 为了治疗发胖和高血压," *Xintiyu* 7 (1979): 37.

77. Huang Meiguang, born in 1929, was a doctor and professor of sports medicine. He graduated from Kirov Military Medical College in the Soviet Union in 1959 and has since published on sports medicine and Qigong. (See *Yundong jiepouxue, yundingyixue dacidian*, 485.)

78. Huang Meiguang 黄美光, "Tong feipang zhe tan yundong liaofa 同肥胖者谈运动疗法," *Dazhong Yixue* 1 (1980): 34.

79. Peng Shuwu, "Tiyu yundong yu'wenmingbing' 体育运动与'文明病,'" *Dazhong Yixue* 8 (1980): 30.

80. Ke Fu, "Pangren bidu (si) 胖人必读（四）," *Jiankang* 2 (1987): 36.

81. Gao Qiang, "Duanlian tingxialai ren jiuhui fapang ma 锻炼停下来人就会发胖吗," *Xintiyu* 7 (1977): 45–47.

82. Sun calls this treatment *ji'e liaofa* 饥饿疗法: starvation treatment.

83. Sun Zhiming 孙知明, "Tantan feipang de yuanyin yu zhiliao wenti 谈谈肥胖的原因与治疗问题," *Dazhong Yixue* 6 (1958): 228–29.

84. Li Yulin 李玉琳, "Feipangzheng ji tizhong kongzhi 肥胖症及体重控制," *Tiyu jiaoxue yu keyan* 4 (1985): 33–37.

85. Gao Qiang, "Duanlian tingxialai ren jiuhui fapang ma 锻炼停下来人就会发胖吗," *Xintiyu* 7 (1977): 45–47.

86. Zhou Wenquan 周文泉 et al., "Feipang zheng de zhongyi zhiliao 肥胖症的中医治疗," *Yunnan Zhongyi Zazhi* 1 (1984): 56–60.

87. For the evolution of Chinese snack foods, see James L. Watson, "Food as a Lens: The Past, Present, and Future of Family Life in China," in *Feeding China's Little Emperors: Food, Children, and Social Change*, ed. Jun Jing, 199–212 (Stanford: Stanford Universtiy Press, 2000), and Watson, "China's Big Mac Attack."

See also Ke Fu, "Pangren bidu (san) 胖人必读（三）," *Jiankang* 1 (1987): 53. This article targets luxury items such as coffee, alcohol, and chocolate and their negative influence on the body, advising that they be consumed with utter care.

88. One article by Mao Zhongyao in 1954 even stresses that students who tried to improve their physique by taking supplements (*bupin* 补品) without proper exercise routines would only gain weight and worsen their physical state. See Mao Zhongyao, "Xupang bushi zhuang 虚胖不是壮," *Xintiyu* 4 (1954): 28.

89. This becomes obvious when the narrative of most anecdotes confirms that the protagonists' health was normal while living in the countryside and everything turned bad after moving to urban areas, as Sun Ke describes.

90. See "Zhonggong zhongyang ba weishengbu dangzu baogao pishi gesheng shi qu dangwei zuzhi xiyi xuexi zhongyi shi jian dashi fanshi you tiaojian de, dou yinggai ban xiyi li zhixuexi zhongyi de xuexiban 中共中央把卫生部党组报告批示各省市区党委 组织西医学习中医是件大事 凡是有条件的，都应该办西医离职学习中医的学习班," *Renmin Ribao* (20 November 1958): "*ta* [*Zhongguo yiyaoxue*] *shiyige weida de baoku* 它 [中国医药学] 是一个伟大的宝库."

For a deeper discussion of Chinese Medicine in Maoist China and its establishment as a national medical system, see Kim Taylor, *Chinese Medicine in Early Communist China, 1945–63: A Medicine of Revolution* (London: Routledge, 2011).

91. On the topic of barefoot doctors, see Xiaoping Fang, *Barefoot Doctors and Western Medicine in China* (Rochester: University of Rochester Press, 2012).

92. Guo Jinyuan 过晋源, "Duzhong gao xueya bing de chubu baogao 杜仲高血压病的初步报告," *Zhonghua Yixue Zazhi* 9 (1954): 704–7.

93. Measured parts include height, weight, age, and assessment of the face, skin, and pulse.

94. This points to a slow and long treatment which would ensure a steady and sustainable weight loss.

95. Yang Shuqian 杨树千 and Leng Fangnan 冷方南, "Danchun xing feipang bing yili zhi yan 单纯性肥胖病一例治验," *Zhongyi Zazhi* 965, no. 1 (1965): 25.

96. Liang Guoqing 梁国卿, born in 1902, was a doctor at Liaoning Chinese Medical School. (See *Zhongguo Zhongyi renming dacidian*, 252.)

97. This decoction contains betel palm, bark of magnolia officinalis, cooked rhubarb, orange peel, rhizome of Chinese atractylodes, tuber of Pinellia ternata, Wolfiporia extensa, dried fruit of citron, white mustard seeds, and dried hawthorn fruit.

98. Liang Guoqing 梁国卿, "Feipangbing zhiyan 肥胖病治验," *Liaoning Zhongyi* 6 (1979): 5.

99. This article mentions slight discomfort during the process of weight loss, but it was connected to another birth. The patient felt rather tired and sluggish after the second birth. Apparently, these symptoms disappeared after some time and she could even go back to work.

100. The basic idea of using a long-term solution is in contradiction to today's numerous quick-fix diets, but actually follows medical advice: slow and long-term weight loss is more sustainable as it is connected to a change in lifestyle and habits that will support the individual in keeping the weight down.

101. The 1984 article "Chinese Medical Treatment of Obesity" [*feipangzheng de zhongyi zhiliao* 肥胖症的中医治疗] by Zhou Wenquan et al. supposes that medical treatment of obesity with drugs or even surgery were methods that were used abroad: see Zhou Wenquan 周文泉 et al., "Feipang zheng de zhongyi zhiliao 肥胖症的中医治疗," *Yunnan Zhongyi Zazhi* 1 (1984): 56–60.

In 1987, Ke Fu mentions appetite suppressants as pills that can control energy intake and by doing so influence a person's weight: see Ke Fu, "Pang ren bi du (wu) 胖人必读（五）," *Jiankang* 3 (1987): 54–55.

102. Liu Shaojing 刘韶景, "Cong jianfei dao shenjing xing yanshi 从减肥到神经性厌食," *Dazhong Yixue* 4 (1985): 14.

103. Shaoqi Liu, "How to be a Good Communist," in *Sources of Chinese Tradition, vol. 2*, ed. William Theodore de Bary et al. (New York: Columbia University Press, 1960).

Chapter 6

Hypertension

Civilization diseases come in many shapes and degrees of severity. While obesity is a fairly obvious pathology, others are less visible. One of the non-communicable and for the most part invisible pathologies is hypertension, that is, abnormally high blood pressure. It derives from environmental, lifestyle, and hereditary pressures. Pinpointing the state of hypertension was for a long time—in China as elsewhere—rather difficult. Its specifics were hard to define despite the fact that it was a growing problem in populations. Nevertheless, experts attempted to explain and treat it. The Chinese discourse of hypertension plays out in medical and popular medical media, and finds its way into the actions of the PRC government and health experts who sought to combat a disease that was invisible and hard to detect.

Cardiovascular diseases, of which hypertension is a part, are one of the main killers in today's developed society, yet despite their recent rise they are not new diseases if viewed through retrospective diagnosis, and in fact have a long history in human civilization. So, contrary to appearances, the nineteenth and twentieth centuries do not represent the beginnings of hypertension and a look into the past can unveil its historical impact and convey a deeper understanding. So far, this historical impact has not been widely researched. To circumscribe the "age" of hypertension, or rather to find the point in time when it was first framed as a pathology, Jeremy Greene refers to a publication from 1956 that contains a collection of a few primary sources on hypertension: *Classics in Arterial Hypertension* by Arthur Ruskin. In it, Ruskin refers back to the *Huangdi Neijing* as one of the first written sources discussing hypertension, before he takes a look at Caelius Aurelianus (ca. 400 CE), who theorized about the condition of *apoplexia*, the fall that can often follow upon a stroke. Retrospectively, Ruskin pulls together a list of Western authors to demonstrate that hypertension, or post hoc identified equivalents thereof, is an old illness and has been discussed since antiquity.[1]

Is hypertension a normal disease that occurs due to certain circumstances? Or is it triggered more by modern civilization, which would imply a responsibility within society for the outbreaks, just as hinted at by the designation "civilization disease"? Hypertension can have different origins and appear in different contexts. It is either a comorbidity of another disease (even of other civilization diseases such as obesity,[2] heart diseases, diabetes, etc.),[3] or a disease in itself.[4] Its origins influence the way it is treated and framed. Whichever the case, hypertension is not a disease that just happens to occur, but can be considered "a disease of cultural adaption," which means that the human genetic makeup cannot keep up with changes of the environment and with cultural practices. This manifests in problems in everyday life.[5] While this is an interesting observation, looking at hypertension through a lens of nostalgia may not be beneficial to its treatment, as surely nobody wants to forsake modern, affluent life and its luxuries.

The Chinese hypertension discourse shows how the supposedly new pathology was examined by the medical and political authorities and how treatments were negotiated at a time when major epidemics such as tuberculosis, the plague, or schistosomiasis had just been defeated. In this sense, hypertension is new to the period as a rising problem for a bigger part of the population, even though the pathology itself is not new. By opening up the discussion of hypertension the discussion on civilization diseases in the PRC is broadened, coming to focus on diseases that are not contagious but are spreading like wildfire in the modern world, not limited to times of hardship or to underdeveloped countries.

HYPERTENSION: A BRIEF HISTORY

Historically, hypertension has always been very hard to diagnose, not because blood pressure is hard to measure, but because of the difficulty of recognizing the issue, since it is invisible in its early stage. Furthermore, the definition of a standardized threshold for when blood pressure can be called high has been engaging experts for a century.[6] To get a closer look at the medical attempts to understand this curious pathology, Nicolas Postel-Vinay in his *A Century of Arterial Hypertension 1896–1996* (1996) traces the development of hypertension as a disease from the late nineteenth until the end of the twentieth century. This covers the present book's era of interest in the Chinese discussion. Postel-Vinay also unveils possible inconsistencies within the discourse, of which the biggest problem is the agreement of when hypertension starts. How does blood pressure, a property that has to exist for an organism to survive, turn pathological? This process shows how health and disease are negotiated by experts in order to frame hypertension as a disease in the context of civilization diseases.[7] The example of hypertension depicts how framing a disease happens not only when a doctor diagnoses a patient, but also via the medical and social context that influences the picture of the sickness to be diagnosed. The patient's experiences and symptoms, the doctor's ability to identify and put them into context, as well as society's ability to perceive the patient's symptoms and the doctor's diagnosis as a disease, all play a role in its identification. In the case of hypertension, one issue in its framing lies with its visual perceptibility. Without methods to measure blood pressure, it is impossible to make it visible to the patient and to society.[8] The scientification of the subject matter becomes apparent when looking at hypertension's history: it is defined, measured, and data is amassed for future use. Throughout the twentieth century it proved difficult to define parameters for hypertension due to its obscurity; after all "the most common forms of heart disease are those of which the patient is unaware."[9] Two important factors in the framing of new pathologies arise here: (1) the importance of awareness in the population and experts and (2) the measurability that ultimately improves the awareness. For the latter, technical requirements had to be met. American physicians started routinely measuring blood pressure in the beginning of the twentieth century.[10] At this time, degenerative and cardiovascular diseases were becoming more common and widespread, resulting in an increasing number of registered deaths due to non-communicable diseases.[11]

Defining what actually ailed patients when they were diagnosed with hypertension was closely linked to the definition of a standard. In the case of hypertension, this problem hailed from the different theories on the origin and the process of hypertension as well as the different perception of this illness.[12] The uncertainty is made all the more obvious in the experts' varying understanding of hypertension as a disease that is treatable in itself or rather as a mere symptom of another condition. This defines how the sickness is diagnosed, treated, and cured.

Historically, not only the diagnosis but also hypertension's variation is remarkably random in different publications and discussions.[13] The unclear line between normal and pathological confirms Canguilhem's discussion of Claude Bernard's continuum of the normal and pathological, namely that there are no specific lines between the two that will separate healthy from unhealthy.[14] In general, the sources reinforce George Pickering's notion that the higher the blood pressure, the more severe a patient's condition and the shorter their remaining lifespan.[15]

The issue with hypertension and its diagnosis is, for one thing, its obscurity and the oftentimes different temporal onset of symptoms in different patients, as well as the doctors' decision over when to locate the pathological onset, even while the individual may not yet perceive it. The imbalance of medical observation and individual experience displays the switch of authority over the physical state. It takes away from the perception of individual suffering and coping with illness and superimposes medically sanctioned concepts.[16]

A body was judged and assessed by routinely conducted biomedical examinations during which medical authorities could determine a body to be ill by measuring it against a standard. All the while, what "Leriche elegantly defined in the past as '*the progression of life in the silence of the organs*' was losing ground. With experimental medicine, a patient with glycosuria or albuminuria, irrespective of his complaint, lost his state of health and became not ill, but 'abnormal.'"[17] The new ways of diagnosing, examining, and putting those results into context marked, for example, asymptomatic patients of hypertension or patients in the earlier stages as sick despite the lack of feelings of unwellness. In this process, the responsibility to identify a sick state is taken out of the hands of the individuals caring for themselves and put onto the shoulders of professionals, who are able to assess and provide explanations for the sick state. A shift in power occurs in this process, where the power of decision is taken from the patient and given to the medical professionals.

CHINESE BLOOD PRESSURE

The definition of hypertension is not simply a matter of medical science, but is shaped by various social, political, and economic actors. Can the same definition and approach be applied to China as well? Can hypertension even be considered an issue for the population of the PRC at the time? It apparently was, since it caused death rates to rise as patients died of hypertensive cerebral hemorrhage[18] or strokes,[19] as shown by late-1970s articles in the *Zhonghua Yixue Zazhi* and the *Dazhong Yixue*. In the middle of the twentieth century, any disease that impacted daily life and the population at large was considered by the Chinese government to be a threat to the national development.[20]

Chinese authors faced the same difficulties as Western authors when describing hypertension to patients and the public. They too encountered the difficulty of setting a standard for pathological hypertension and of understanding the cardiovascular system as the problem's location. The discussion made use of the previously established body discourse and fell back on the body-machine metaphor; in 1953, a *Dazhong Yixue* article equates the cardiovascular system to a system of water pipes, and blood pressure to water pressure in those pipes.[21] This lent the story an air of familiarity.

Finding the Beginning

In 1954, Wu Xingye 吴兴业 tries to answer the difficult question of normal and abnormal blood pressure in primary hypertension in a *Zhonghua Yixue Zazhi* article. The article, titled "Discussion of a Primary Hypertension

Standard" (Yuanfaxing gaoxueya biaozhungzhi shangque 原发性高血压标准之商榷), is an answer to readers' questions on hypertension. It is the printed reaction to the public's need to know more about this health problem. Wu admits to not being able to define the starting point of hypertension, and thus specifically shows that there was no standard at the time. This issue was examined at a 1953 meeting at the Hypertension Conference (*Gaoxueyabing zuotanhui* 高血压病座谈会),[22] where after thorough discussion 150/90–94 millimeters of mercury (mmHg) was defined as the threshold for hypertension. This marker was important for future treatments, as it made the evaluation of a patient's health status possible, that is, it marked one set of blood pressure as normal while the other became abnormal.[23]

At the conference, a possibly racial component in hypertension research and treatment emerged, suggesting that blood pressure values between Europeans and Chinese may not be the same due to external factors (nutrition, height, habits, environment).[24] This takes into account the environment's influence on body and health, and suggests that there is a fundamental difference due to environments and their influence on bodies, as Wu reports. In the conference discussions, the temporal component also played a role in the work on hypertension since it may have been different in former generations. Here Wu especially notes the economic and social development of China, which, according to the conference, may influence bodies negatively. Another problem verbalized in the discussion was the lack of data and research. Age as a factor was seen as influencing the perception of hypertension. At this point of his report, Wu quotes a study in which students in Guangzhou were tested for hypertension, but he criticizes the limitations of the research and the research methods used. This study did not find any hypertension in the students, and thus it was concluded that the Chinese as a whole did not suffer from it. In the end, Wu stresses the bias within the material used for hypertension work, much of which derived from insurance company archives and had an economically driven agenda. All of these considerations shape the perception of blood pressure. To measure hypertension and thus diagnose the disease, Wu advocates the use of objective measuring methods and devices like the sphygmomanometer as well as large-scale trials.[25]

The way blood pressure is measured and categorized includes different parameters to assess different parts of the population. Apart from the measured value, assessment, and treatment of the patients' condition as well as their sensitivity toward heightened blood pressure was impacted by their individual situation. Since natural blood pressure varies in different age groups, the individual effect hypertension has on the bodies made it even harder for doctors to set down hard limits and thresholds. One patient might feel the effects of hypertension much sooner than another: this, coupled with altogether asymptomatic hypertension, blurs the lines not only for the experts but for the patients.

The various publications on hypertension between 1949 and 1986 do not give a simple or clear answer to the question "Where does hypertension start?"[26] Different journal articles give different values over time, that is, the threshold is not assigned the same value (see table 6.1).

The different onset points of hypertension can be identified by a close reading of contemporary journals. Table 6.1 shows the varying starting points sorted chronologically. Note that this does not take into account the three different stages of hypertension with their different thresholds.

The late consultation with a doctor in the case of asymptomatic hypertension makes it possible for the disease to progress quite far without treatment and without clear identification of its onset. Asymptomatic patients prove the point that hypertension is a medical problem that has to be clinically measured in order to be traced and documented. If symptoms show in later stages because of their severity, the damage has often already been done and the condition is harder to reverse. Xu Zhanfei 徐展飞 notes in 1986, as a case in point, that according to a study there existed a 7.8 percent hypertension

Table 6.1. Values of hypertension in Chinese medical publications 1950s–1980s.

Issue Year	*Onset of Hypertension in mmHg*	*Journal*
1954	150/90–94	*Zhonghua Yixue Zazhi*
1954	>160	*Zhonghua Yixue Zazhi*
1955	>200	*Zhonghua Yixue Zazhi*
1955	176/102	*Zhonghua Yixue Zazhi*
1955	198/100	*Zhonghua Yixue Zazhi*
1955	185/80	*Zhonghua Yixue Zazhi*
1957	>135	*Dazhong Yixue*
1974	250/140	*Zhonghua Yixue Zazhi*
1978	150~244/74~105	*Dazhong Yixue*
1978	150–160	*Zhonghua Yixue Zazhi*
1980	>140/90	*Xintiyu*
1980	>160/90	*Xintiyu*
1980	140/90	*Xintiyu*
1980	160/90	*Xintiyu*
1981	160/90	*Zhongyi Zazhi*
1981	210/140	*Zhongyi Zazhi*
1981	160/105	*Zhonghua Yixue Zazhi*
1982	200/110	*Dazhong Yixue*
1983	210/130	*Zhongyi Zazhi*
1983	129/77	*Dazhong Yixue*
1983	170–200/100–130	*Dazhong Yixue*
1983	170–200/70–90	*Dazhong Yixue*
1986	160~190/100–120	*Dazhong Yixue*

disease rate among the Chinese in the 1970s. He compares this number to the US occurrence of hypertension and the fact that 40 percent of US citizens suffering from hypertension did not know about it. With increased age this disease is detected more often and the number of undiagnosed patients may rise even higher.[27]

An issue that makes identifying hypertension even more difficult is the changing pressure throughout the day.[28] Blood pressure is not even and stable throughout the day, but naturally changes due to activities, resting time, and meal times. In the morning blood pressure tends to be low. It rises in the afternoon and after large meals.[29] This is a natural process in the body and makes the definition of "normal" for blood pressure even more difficult.

A late diagnosis leads to more severe impact on the cardiovascular system. Some examples for this observation can be found in a 1956 article in the *Zhonghua Yixue Zazhi*, which covers the renal impact of hypertension, harming the renal glands with increased pressure, or in the article by Jin Beiwen 金蓓文 et al., who in 1980 stress the impact on the blood vessels of the tongue.[30]

Primary and Secondary Hypertension

The two different kinds of hypertension that are predominant in the medical publications are primary and secondary hypertension. These two designations profoundly impact the framing of hypertension. Chinese authors and translators adopted the distinction of primary (*yuanfaxing* 原发性) and secondary hypertension (*jifaxing* 继发性), as Xu Kaisen 余开森 described as early as 1956 and which 22 years later, in 1978, Du Shihua 席时华[31] et al. would reaffirm.[32] The two descriptions hint at the origin of the condition and include all forms of pathologically high blood pressure.[33]

Primary hypertension, which according to Du Shihua et al. is the most frequent kind of hypertension in patients (up to 90 percent of cases),[34] encompasses all conditions of high blood pressure that arise due to a hereditary disposition, diet, climate, environment, or a disposition of the nervous system as discussed by Xu Kaisen, Zhou Guanhong 周冠虹, and Zhang Chongde 张崇德.[35] It is a disease in its own right and not a comorbidity or a mere symptom of other pathological factors. Nevertheless, with primary hypertension the cause is often unclear, as a translated 1984 article from the US magazine *Science Digest* in the *Dazhong Yixue* by Qian Qiyuan 钱启源 emphasizes.[36] The actual origin of primary hypertension is hard to make out. Contemporary materials offer different assumptions as to why and when it manifests, including hereditary factors or environmental influences. There are certain anatomical occurrences that appear in the case of hypertension or which contribute to it: a rise in nervous stimulation was observed by Shen Zhonggui 沈仲圭

(in 1956), Bertschnikov (in 1956), Xu Kaisen (in 1958), Zhou Guanhong (in 1978), and Zhang Chongde (in 1983);[37] the narrowing of the arteries as a cause for hypertension was observed by Bertschnikov (in 1956);[38] Tu Yuanshu 涂沅淑 and Tong Etang 童萼塘[39] (1978) observe atherosclerosis as caused by hypertension, but sometimes a rise in renal, cerebral, or coronary blood pressure is also noted.[40] In any case, whether a patient remains asymptomatic or displays symptoms is not predictable, according to their consensus.

Secondary hypertension, on the other hand, is caused by other diseases. It is the symptom of these diseases and can be cured by treating the underlying illness, but not by treating the raised blood pressure. Diseases that may cause hypertension are kidney diseases, brain diseases, poisoning, endocrinological or metabolic issues, heart disease, and atherosclerosis, among others, as Xu Kaisen (1958) and later Zhou Guanhong (1978) discuss. Secondary hypertension is also called symptomatic hypertension (*zhengzhuangxing gaoxueya* 症状性高血压).

The treatment of primary hypertension is not as straightforward as the treatment of the secondary kind. Primary hypertension and blood pressure–lowering treatments are structured into three stages that describe different progressions of the disease. They all entail different degrees of severity and damage to the organs.

The different stages' onsets are a source of uncertainty for experts. The three stages of hypertension display an arbitrariness in their starting points, which is in line with the general problem of onset definition. Hypertension values from the *Zhonghua Yixue Zazhi* and the *Zhongyi Zazhi* at three different times (1956, 1980, 1981) show great differences in their perspective on the issue. For Stage I, one value from 1980 goes up until 110 mmHg systolic pressure while another only starts at 160 mmHg (1981). This displays a huge discrepancy in the same publication—*Zhongyi Zazhi*—only one year apart, which shows that there was no consensus about the absolute values, thus no authority seems to have existed over it.

Stage I

Stage I is the lightest and mildest stage of hypertension. At this stage there is no need for medical treatment. Liu Minying's 刘民英 1954 translation of a decision by the Soviet Institute for Medicine and Science (*Sulian yixue kexue yuan* 苏联医学科学院) titled "General convention in the treatment of hypertension patients" (Gaoxueya binghuanzhe zhiliaode yiban changgui 高血压病患者治疗的一般常规) even claims that at this stage antihypertensive drugs can prove harmful, and nor do patients need to stay at the hospital or stop working.[41] Instead, they should be examined by a doctor and start with basic changes in their lifestyle. The issue with an assessment at that stage is the already mentioned often-asymptomatic progress of hypertension and the ignorance of the condition on the part of the patients. If, due to the lack of symptoms, no harm or pain can be detected, as Dan Shouzhun 单守谆 describes in his 1981 book *Hypertension* (*Gaoxueya* 高血压), it is difficult to convince a patient of their sick state.[42] In this case the measuring of blood pressure values makes the sick state visible and warrants treatment to avoid further deterioration. Lifestyle adjustments suggested at this point include dietary changes, taking up exercising, and taking care of proper sleep hygiene. The change presumes the cooperation and acceptance of the diagnosis by the patient. If that is not the case, treatment will prove difficult.

Dan further divides Stage I hypertension into two different groups: in the first group, diastolic pressure situated somewhere between 90–100 mmHg may drop down to normal at times. The systolic pressure is higher than normal, but with no harm to the brain, heart, or kidneys. In the second group, diastolic pressure is higher than 100 mmHg, but there is no harm to the brain, heart, or kidneys either.[43]

Stage II

The levels of Stage II are more elevated than Stage I. It is more severe, but can be improved quickly with good treatment and under supervision. Liu's 1954 translation suggests that Stage II patients should sleep at least 12 hours a night to bring down their blood pressure. Apart from sleep therapy, the incorporation of plenty of rest during the day is highly recommended. Additionally, the reduction of salt as well as an increase in vitamin intake was suggested. Different diets were proposed for this effect by Liu Minying (1954), Zhou Guanhong (1978, 1979), and Song Baosen (1982), for example, a rice diet[44] and a diet high in potassium.[45]

In the first two stages, treating hypertension with exercise is still possible, as advocated in 1980 by Zhou Guanhong and Zhao Guangsheng 赵光胜.[46] The treatments prescribed seem to be easily implemented, but their impact was to be big enough to prevent a worsening of the situation. That is especially important as at Stage II, damage to the brain, heart, and kidneys was common. Some symptoms, such as an enlarged left heart chamber, narrowing of the blood vessels, excess proteins in urine (proteinuria), or creatinine in the blood plasma can be observed, as Du Shihua et al. (1978) and Dan Shouzhun (1981) mention.[47] These deviations from a healthy body were recognized as signs of physical problems.

Dan defined Stage II hypertension as a diastolic pressure higher than 90 mmHg and a raised systolic pressure. At this stage, organ damage became visible, which is why Dan suggested that diagnosis be performed via physical examination or X-ray, so that an enlarged left heart chamber could be detected. Other harm that might be uncovered could include organic brain damage that changes the fundus oculi. He also subscribes to testing for too much protein (proteinuria) and red blood cells in urine.[48]

Stage III

The third stage of hypertension is the most severe condition of this disease. Dan Shouzhun talks about the many pitfalls and symptoms that show and manifest at this stage: (a) in the heart (weakening of the left heart chamber), (b) in the brain (hemorrhage and other vascular issues), and (c) a worsened eyesight (retinas bleed, swelling occurs). These often-seen symptoms are not necessarily introduced by hypertension. They may also stem from coronary heart disease, inner cranial arterial thrombosis, kidney failure, and so on.[49] The third stage is characterized by continuously rising blood pressure. This brings about the above-mentioned organ damage. Diastolic pressure rises higher than 130 mmHg and may cause bleeding in the fundus oculi and swelling, as Dan sums up in his book.[50]

At this stage patients' nutrition practices and daily structures had to be monitored closely. Their diet had to be low salt, low fat, and low animal protein to avoid cholesterol. Another way to lower blood pressure in Stage III were breathing exercises. The reference to breathing exercises occurs frequently in treatment suggestions throughout the second half of the twentieth century.[51] The distinction of the treatment approaches in each stage are specified by experts. This forms a basis not only for individual treatments but for broad scale trials.

Risk Groups

Not everyone belongs to the group of potential hypertension patients, but there are some people who are more at risk of developing a hypertensive condition than others. Groups who are very susceptible to hypertension include the elderly, the urban population, obese patients, and high-stress patients. An interesting observation is the increasing divide between the urban and rural population, the former manifesting more cases than its rural counterpart. As there was an increased mobility between rural and urban areas in the second half of the twentieth century, peasants became physical workers and then mental workers, the latter supposedly suffering the highest rates of hypertension. Zhou Guanhong and Li Bingcheng mention this phenomenon in the late 1970s and the early 1980s.[52] This trend shows how social mobility can function as a catalyst to introduce sickness into formerly seemingly untouched parts of the population.

Age contributes to a higher risk factor in this context, since blood pressure rises with age. The age threshold for increased risk of hypertension is 40 years or "middle age," after which people are at higher risk than the younger generations, as Zhou Guanhong, Shi Yongde 施永德 and Tang Zhensheng 唐镇生, and Song Baosen note.[53] A much earlier article in the *Zhonghua Yixue Zazhi* from 1954 by Guo Jinyuan 过晋源[54] claims that the group between 50 and 60 years of age have the highest occurrence of hypertension,[55] followed by the "elderly" (people aged 60 years or older).[56] All of them are supervised more frequently and closely than the younger population. In 1978, Tu Yuanshu and Tong Etang suggest preventive check-ups in those 40 years old and above who have not suffered from hypertension before.[57] Zhou agrees with the evaluation of elderly as the highest risk group. For their treatment, Zhou admonishes doctors to be careful since if blood pressure drops too low during treatment, this would also cause further issues, such as stroke or coronary heart disease. A cautious approach is thus recommended to avoid brain damage or other impairments.[58]

Patients suffering from hereditary hypertension are a distinct risk group. Where a genetic predisposition engenders the development of elevated blood pressure, it is to be soothed by lifestyle adjustments, as Li Guanglian 李广镰 reports in 1986.[59]

The third risk group are sufferers of other diseases that entail hypertension as a symptom (secondary hypertension). Even more at risk are patients who work in high stress environments, eat the wrong diet, lack rest, suffer from nervousness and overstimulation, or are sensitive to climate and other environmental factors that make blood pressure rise. They make up the fourth risk group. Patients in high-stress environments are mostly mental workers, students, and cadres, as in those cases the individuals have no means to alleviate mental stress by physical exercise or movement, as discussed by Kondratiev in 1954.[60] A 1980 article in the *Xintiyu* defines desk work and any mental work as high-stress jobs which can bring about hypertension, confirming earlier observations. A parallel to obesity research exists in this context, where physically taxing labor meant a lower probability of succumbing to it. In the case of hypertension more physical relief of stress, that is, physical labor, was linked to lower occurrence of elevated blood pressure. It is not directly explained why hypertension was more common in mental workers, but from the treatments suggested and the changed load of responsibility in mental labor, it seems that a lifestyle of sitting the whole day, working in a high-pressure environment while carrying heavy responsibility was thought to be causing hypertension. This is an observation already made by Bertschnikov in 1956.[61] The sedentary lifestyle hinders natural processes and leads to changes in the body. The increased work stress may lead to less rest and insufficient sleep, which results in an increase in blood pressure, not to mention an insufficient diet. To top it all off, in 1982 Song Baosen includes social settings and exercise as origins of primary hypertension, as they increase nervous stimulation and can result in stress.[62]

DIAGNOSING HYPERTENSION: CASES TO STUDY AND TREAT

To get a deeper understanding of actual treatments, medical case studies from the realm of Chinese Medicine yield interesting observations,[63] illustrating how patients were examined, diagnosed, and then treated individually. Medical case studies show the standardization of contemporary medical treatments. Additionally, they detail the physicians' diagnosis and give a rundown of the prescribed treatments. Here, I discuss three case studies to show disease assessment and interpretation in three different decades. They are published in the *Zhonghua Yixue Zazhi* and the *Zhongyi Zazhi*, both Chinese medical journals. The nature of the Chinese medical tradition brings with it the frequent use of individual case studies to illustrate pathologies and treatment. They show a comprehensive picture of the case, and in socialist China display the sum of what is called *New Medicine*, that is, they contain references both to the traditional knowledge system of Chinese Medicine as well as to biomedicine, which are thus working in tandem. The case studies display how theoretical knowledge was implemented practically. They were meant as examples to other physicians and for the audience to gain insight into the practice of established experts. Generally, they contain information on the patients' person (age, gender, sometimes occupation), their medical history, the symptoms they suffered from, and observations by the doctors. They also include the treatments prescribed to them, which are revisited at the end of this chapter.

Case 1: Mrs. Jiang (1955)

In 1955, Mao Gongde tells of a Mrs. Jiang, 51 years old, no mentioned occupation, who had at the time of examination been suffering from hypertension and its symptoms for about ten years. In 1953, she was reexamined and put on a different treatment than before. The results of the renewed examination showed that her blood pressure was 176/102 mmHg. This is, according to the previously examined materials, a case of not severe but clear hypertension. Apart from this elevated hypertension, she was in good condition and only suffered from dizziness, back pain, and numbness in the hands at night.[64]

Case 2: Male (1977)

The second examined case study is a blood pressure diagnosis from 1977. In this case a male worker (*gongren* 工人) of 56 years came to the hospital for an eight-hour observation and was found to suffer from aphasia and a coma after having had a headache, followed by vomiting and the worsening of symptoms. He had been suffering from hypertension before but did not have any further history of disease. At the hospital his blood pressure was measured at 220/130 mmHg.[65]

Case 3: Mrs. Huang (1981)

The third case study from the *Zhongyi Zazhi* from 1981 introduces a 62-year-old Mrs. Huang who had been suffering from hypertension for two years and was measured at 180–220/100–110 mmHg. Her symptoms included headaches, dizziness, chest distress, and palpitation as well as numb hands and feet. She was diagnosed with Stage II hypertension.[66]

By examining these cases, it becomes obvious that hypertension symptoms, the part of the disease that patients feel more or less acutely, vary in severity according to the hypertension stages. Early symptoms of hypertension include headaches, dizziness, fatigue, inability to concentrate, getting out of breath easily, and low stress resistance.[67] All of those influence a person's daily performance, especially in later stages when hypertension can result in exhaustion or strokes. This makes it hard to work in physically demanding jobs, and at the same time it changes the physical makeup of the body and influences concentration negatively so that sedentary work also becomes more difficult.

All of these case studies display the characteristics of contemporary medical ideals: standard measurements and observations of the body are noted in a seemingly standardized order. The physical diagnosis as well as the later mentioned treatments constitute a mixture of Chinese and biomedical approaches, which is typical at the time. The treatments that are put forward in these three case studies include a range of cures.

TREATING HYPERTENSION

The contemporary discussion of antihypertensive treatment is extensive and shows the urgency that was attributed to the road to recovery and the cure of hypertension. The different recovery plans were published in detail, but treating hypertension did not obviate the major leaps an individual had to make to stay healthy. Treatment built on the idea of healthy living, reinforcing the importance of an adequately healthy and good life that would reduce the risk of *wenmingbing* and other diseases. Again, exercise and being active, a healthy and sufficient diet, and plenty of rest and relaxation were heralded as the basic solutions to this particular deviation from the ideal state of health. Actual clinical treatments and medication are only used if absolutely necessary, so as to distribute resources in the most beneficial way.

A Change in Lifestyle

Changing one's lifestyle is a common practice today, and it, too, was considered to be one way of improving one's life quality in the Mao era. Choosing a healthy way of living (*jiankang shenghuo fangshi* 健康生活方式) was seen as an option to lower the risk of hypertension and considered a cheap way of self-treatment after diagnosis. This included adjustments in the forms of exercise, nutrition, rest, and labor.

I have already introduced the story of Sun Ke in previous chapters. His autobiographical case from 1954 lends itself to a short discussion of secondary hypertension as well. Sun Ke started to suffer from hypertension in the wake of gaining weight due to city life. By his doctor-approved change of habits, all the symptoms and issues disappeared. This story shows how secondary hypertension can be reversed with a change of specific habits and the addressing of the original cause, in Sun's case weight gain.[68] A lifestyle change encompasses the strict and thorough regulation of daily life and personal habits, as Sun demonstrated. This also included the regulation of active and resting times. Starting with sleep and rest, patients were recommended to go to bed early and get up early. The nudging toward better sleep hygiene is linked to the notion that hypertension is caused by an overstimulation of the central nervous system. Calming the nerves, thus, was the logical conclusion.

In a similar fashion, Kondratiev's 1954 two part report addresses regulations for hypertensive patients and their situation, including their workload and productivity.[69] Starting with the work schedule, Kondratiev emphasizes in the first article from January 1954 that hypertensive patients should avoid night shifts as those interfere with regular sleeping patterns. A regular schedule is important for the central nervous system. Even farther-reaching recommendations include that patients should not choose jobs that are too mentally challenging, as they can overly stimulate the mind. Instead, they should engage in jobs that are interesting to them but do not burn them out. Stress due to labor should be avoided, and job suitability must be assessed beforehand. In daily life, patients had to pay attention to exhaustion and its symptoms: heaviness of the head, dizziness and headaches, and diminishing eyesight while reading. If these occurred, a short break might help them recover, as would physical exercise. [70]

The follow-up article from March 1954 turns toward specific areas of daily life that can be adjusted and improved for the well-being of hypertensive patients, focusing on ideal sleep and sleeping habits. These suggestions repeat what has been published on sleep in a different context: at least eight hours of regular sleep are recommended. Additionally, the article suggests taking one day off a week, during which patients should sleep even more. Patients were to take advantage of regular breaks during the day in order to avoid overwork. To counter exhaustion, Kondratiev advises patients to go outdoors to the park or into the gardens. Regular vacation days were part of this resting routine. These regular rests are essential to calm down in order to regulate blood pressure. Another form of treatment and regulation for daily use is exercise. Either napping after lunch or partaking in light exercise was to help regulate their blood pressure. A little exercise in the morning improves the metabolism, and breathing exercises would aid in lowering their blood pressure. During these exercises the breath should flow freely and the whole body had to be relaxed. A qualitatively and quantitatively good diet supplemented the physical training with adequate nutrition. To extinguish the diseases and the harm they did to the population, harmful habits had to be kicked. For patients of hypertension those included smoking or drinking alcohol, but sexual intercourse was also something to be wary of as it puts a heavy strain on the nervous and cardiovascular systems.[71]

The regulation of daily life is a lingering theme in the literature on hypertension. Creating good and practicable habits would change a person's life for the better and ensure the right conduct, as shown in the 1957 translation of Sberianski's article "Hypertension" by Zheng Yiliu 郑依柳.[72] This idea remained strong during the following three decades.

In 1954, a translation by Liu Minying suggests sleep therapy for patients in Stage II. Patients of this stage should sleep for about 12 hours a night, which exceeds the average 8 hours for the healthy population. During sleep therapy, the first night aims at 14–16 hours. This needs to be repeated for the following 10 to 15 days and should be supplemented by medication, according to Liu. By inducing this amount of sleep, the natural blood pressure–lowering potential of sleep was called upon.[73] During sleep, blood pressure drops naturally, and this can be utilized as a noninvasive, drug-free, antihypertensive blood pressure–lowering treatment.

Regarding Exercise and Hypertension

As Kondratiev had already observed, the incorporation of physical activity and the change toward a healthier lifestyle was part of the hypertension treatment. Adapted exercise plans were created for hypertensive patients to suit their physical needs. This included discussions of what was the most befitting activity for hypertensive patients without aggravating their condition. In some experts' eyes, exercise was one of the ways to improve bodily health in order to prevent or regulate hypertension. Since physical training was acknowledged for its strengthening and health-improving effect, it is no wonder it was also applied to the pathology of hypertension to prevent the onset of disease. Most patients were encouraged to engage in exercise but not to overdo, that is, the patients needed to balance movement and rest according to their condition. For this, they had to know their individual limits, especially when physical culture pushed hard for greater effort.

This growing self-awareness is evident in articles such as the 1956 piece by Bertschnikov "Can People with High Blood Pressure Take Part in Exercise Activities?" (Xueyagao de ren keyi canjia tiyu yundong ma? 血压高的人可以参加体育运动吗?). It categorizes people with elevated blood pressure into four groups and judges their exercise potential. The first group's highest blood pressure is measured at 85–105 mmHg systolic pressure; this is the low blood pressure group. It consists of athletes and people who can work very well. Their blood pressure does not interfere with bodily functions.[74] The second group's highest blood pressure level is measured at 106–25 mmHg systolic pressure. It includes most healthy people and can be described as normal blood pressure group. Everyone in this group could participate in exercise without problems. For the third group—the elevated blood pressure group—the highest blood pressure is measured at 126–45 mmHg systolic pressure, which is a little higher than the norm, but cannot yet be counted as sick. The fourth group displays blood pressures higher than 145 mmHg systolic pressure, which is defined as hypertension. At this point processes in the body take place causing a rise in pressure, especially in situations of excitement and stress, after too much food or too little exercise. This last group's blood pressure is not stable and can randomly spike or drop. This does not mean that a member of the fourth group cannot do their work or partake in physical exercise. According to Bertschnikov, patients are able to do heavy work and exercise, as it positively impacts the central nervous system and the circulatory system and regulates blood pressure. This marks physical exercise and labor as forms of curative and preventive activity. Bertschnikov notes further on, however, that hypertensive patients should adjust their training by cutting down on intensity, speed, and competition.[75] He affirms that such measures can cure hypertension within a timeframe of one to two months, after which workers could return to work.

Another *Xintiyu* article published in 1957, titled "Physical Exercise Therapy of Hypertension Patients" (Gaoxueya bingren de tiyuliaofa 高血压病人的体育疗法) and written by Lea Bernaya, shows how a controlled and unstressful environment, including breathing techniques, could improve the exercise regimen and benefit patients' blood pressure. Avoiding hectic and forceful movements but accompanying each one with one's breath would yield the best results in slowing heart rates and lowering internal pressure. In this respect, radio calisthenics are a less suitable way of exercise for hypertensive patients, as they contain movements that are executed fast and are meant to invigorate the cardiovascular system. Bernaya suggested patients partake in activities that take place outside to benefit from the fresh air. Especially suitable were exercises and activities where the head stayed above the heart, such as ice skating, fishing, boating, and anything that did not put stress on the body. To provide the most beneficial exercise plan, a medical exam had to be completed to assess the patient's condition. Doctors and medical staff then sanctioned the right kind of exercise.[76]

A follow-up article in the same 1957 *Xintiyu* issue even presented specific exercise suggestions. Being a translation from a Soviet source written by Moskov and translated by You Dajun 游达钧 from the Russian journal *Health* from September 1956, it proposes exercises that utilize a chair as prop and avoid overly stimulating the body. Paired with explanations of what movement the body had to execute, advice on the best breathing method is included. Breathing is not identical in each movement but changes according to the exercise performed. There is a prescribed number of breaths one should take in specified positions, but at times natural breathing is enforced.[77]

A few years later, in 1962, Ding Haochuan 丁浩川 published his own personal story of hypertension. His prolonged fight with hypertension resulted in its curing by alternative methods. Ding had been suffering from hypertension for a while and had been treated with traditional methods before (acupuncture, tonics, etc.) to no avail. Since he lacked understanding of the reason for his disease, only after an examination at a hospital did he make the connection between symptoms. Due to a lack of money Ding decided that he had to self-treat his condition to keep it at bay, thus taking responsibility for his condition. He started with easy calisthenics for ten minutes and fifteen minutes of running every day. In 1954, he was finally diagnosed correctly and received treatment in the form of resting treatment (taking a year off from work), a low-sodium diet, acupuncture, and some drugs. When his hypertension flared up again in 1960, he finally entered Beijing Hospital and got in-house treatment that also included *Taiji Quan*. In the end, this practice resolved his condition.[78] Ding's story is one of trust in medical staff and an urge to find prevention measures that would avoid the worsening of the hypertensive condition, and it also displays a trust in traditional methods that are intertwined with scientific medical thinking.

Dietary Treatment

Another non-invasive lifestyle-change method to treat hypertension was a change of diet. Certain factors in nutrient intake were acknowledged to influence patients' blood pressure. The diets proposed to resolve hypertension were often described as bland and ascetic, yet still on a medical level they showed (positive) effects. The idea of blandness does not factor into the suggestions of Chinese experts such as Liu Minying (in 1954), Ding Haochuan (in 1962), Zhou Guanhong (in 1978), Song Baosen (in 1982), or Li Guanglian (in 1986) and their discussion of an appropriate antihypertensive diet. For them the results were more important than the appreciation of taste. Patients were advised to adopt a low-sodium, low-cholesterol, and high-vitamin diet. This was seen as effective in early stages of hypertension but not in Stage III, when more intense measures such as drugs or even surgery often yielded the only results.

Kondratiev argues that four to five meals a day which contain all major nutrients, especially in the form of vegetables, ensures that the body is provided appropriately. Ingesting lean meats, yogurt, cheese, and fish are deemed viable protein sources, while high-fat animal products and eggs should be avoided, as should white breads, which might be replaced by small amounts of dark bread.[79]

In 1978, Zhou Guanhong briefly points out the link between hypertension and dietary sodium, noting that doctors advise their patients to lower their salt intake since salt, due to its chemical properties, is linked to heightened blood pressure.[80] A follow-up article by Zhou gives simple rules for an adequate diet:

1. Individual nutrition requirements have to be met.
2. The patient needs to feel satisfied after each meal so as not to feel hungry.
3. The amount of food needs to be controlled to avoid weight gain.
4. The diet needs to take into account the economic situation of the patient.

These rules repeat the diet tips discussed in the context of nutrition sciences. Zhou becomes rather specific in his further advice: patients should avoid excessive animal fats and high-cholesterol foods (lard, fatty meat, eggs, pig's brain, pig's liver, pig loins, fish roe, etc.). They should eat a lot of fresh vegetables and fruits for their vitamins and minerals and not limit their protein (lean meat, chicken, fish, as well as soy milk, tofu, and other bean products). To control energy intake, eating fewer carbohydrates like rice, noodles, or sugar is promoted. Additionally, patients are discouraged from overeating and encouraged to have lighter and less salty meals.[81]

These suggestions promote a high-vitamin, high-protein, and low-fat diet. There were ongoing discussions in the context of ideal dietary habits concerning health and the correct way of eating, as a 1979 *Renmin Ribao* article by Cong Linzhong 丛林中 shows. Cong gives insight into the wider discourse of hypertension and the awareness of its risks. He relays knowledge from foreign experts who stress how a standard Western diet high in fat and a lot of protein with little carbohydrates leads to a plethora of health problems (heart disease, diabetes, hypertension, obesity, and even some kinds of cancers). The above-described hypertension-approved diet varies greatly from the Western diet. While hypertension did not yet exist in many parts of China, Cong assumes that areas with a high amount of animal husbandry needed to be monitored. Other risk areas were places where plant oils were produced, and thus more frequently consumed. The author warns about the risks of increased consumption, since it might lead to severe health problems in the future.[82]

A rather specific dietary suggestion was the consumption of milk, introduced by a short review from a Japanese journal called *My Health* from 1984. The article is titled "Milk Prevents High Blood Pressure" (Niunai yufang gaoxueya 牛奶预防高血压). In 1985, Gong Xianzhong 龚宪中 discusses the original Japanese text which made the suggestion that milk consumption could help in the prevention of hypertension, due to its calcium and protein content. According to this study, rat experiments had shown that the amino acids in milk control the sympathetic nervous system. It was also found that protein in milk lowered blood sodium levels and prohibited the hardening of the blood vessels, keeping them elastic.[83]

Drug Treatment

When a "simple" lifestyle change was not enough to heal a patient, either due to the stage of the disease or the fact that their condition had worsened quickly, more drastic methods of treatment had to be chosen, such as blood pressure drugs or surgery.

According to Liu Minying, writing in 1954, medical drugs to widen coronary, cerebral, and kidney blood vessels were effective in treating the more progressed stages of hypertension. The use of antihypertensive drugs was dependent on the availability of medical staff, the pharmaceuticals themselves, and financial means. The first drug of choice was magnesium sulphate, suggested by two articles in 1954. It was described as having controlling and anaesthetizing effects on the central nervous system. By injecting magnesium sulphate intramuscularly or intravenously, blood pressure could be lowered. Liu suggests 15–20 injections of varying amounts depending on the target area (muscle or veins).[84] Another article by O. H. Afanaseva translated by Ye

Zhixiu 叶知修 is concerned with a study of 200 patients and their reaction to magnesium sulphate. It thoroughly examines the different stages of hypertension and the different applications of the drug. The subjects were injected with different rounds of magnesium sulphate at different stages of the disease, both intramuscularly and intravenously. The rounds held different amounts of the injectant. Overall, this study was evaluated positively, since a majority of the patients found their blood pressure lowered after treatment.[85]

Another drug used to treat hypertension was Novocaine. It was introduced in the *Zhonghua Yixue Zazhi* via translations from Russian texts in 1956. Originally used as an anesthetic in tooth treatment, it was—by chance—discovered to also resolve headaches caused by hypertension, as Chitarev reported in 1956.[86] In the same year, Mirikumova and Streitova showed that Novocaine regulates the central nervous system. In early stages 3–5 milliliters of a 1 percent solution Novocaine is injected, which will first increase the pulse and then slow it down. This is not advised in severe cases of hypertension, for which smaller dosages should be used (1.4–2 ml).[87]

Surgical Treatment

The most invasive and extreme treatment for very severe cases of hypertension was surgery. In the case of hypertension, which often led to cerebral hemorrhage, this method is even more risky. Surgery suggestions included drilling a small hole in the skull bone to relieve pressure and extract the hematoma or hemorrhage.[88] A 1978 article by Luo Zuyi 罗祖贻 emphasizes that surgical treatment of cerebral hemorrhages in China emerged relatively late (in the wake of the Cultural Revolution).[89] A translation from the American *Science Digest* by Qian Qiyuan, published in the *Dazhong Yixue* in 1984, introduces a similar surgical treatment.[90]

Traditional Treatments

Apart from biomedical drugs and surgical solutions, a turn to physical activity was encompassed by the lifestyle change that supposedly aided in preventing and curing mild cases of hypertension. Not only did the experts suggest exercise in the modern sense of the term, that is, gymnastics, walking, swimming, and so forth, but also activities that nowadays are gathered under the term traditional Chinese exercises: Taiji and Qigong. (These activities will here be referenced to as "traditional," although that term is highly debatable, as David A. Palmer has established.)[91] The "traditional" way of exercising refers to practices that are perceived to be of Chinese origin and are classified as "traditionally Chinese" from the 1980s on.[92] This category is highly problematic as it ascribes a homogeneity to an array of practices that were grouped together retrospectively. For the following section I concentrate on body practices that are claimed to be examples of the *traditional Chinese method*.

As Bernaya has already shown, breathing exercises could benefit hypertensive conditions since they calm down the central nervous system. The mastering of breathing was part of the traditional approach to curing hypertension. By control over the breath, blood pressure was lowered and the body's resilience increased. When harsh exercise could not be done, the lower-impact and more balancing practices of Taiji and Qigong as well as different sets of calisthenics and gymnastics were preferred. Qigong was a rather popular method in therapeutic practice in the 1980s, as Palmer notes, for the treatment of anything from headaches to chronic pain.[93] It was a way of exercising and at the same time influencing the body toward lower blood pressure, seen as a national treatment that controls the breath, the heart, and the body.[94]

An article from 1978 by Zhao Guangsheng introduces Qigong as self-healing practice. The quiet and calm demeanor of Qigong and Taiji practice relaxes the body, resulting in lowered blood pressure levels. By mixing Chinese Medicine and traditional body practices, patients had a set of tools at hand that would help them lower blood pressure without the aid of expensive drugs or medical experts. According to Zhao, it was possible to improve the individual's physical condition under the correct and scientific introduction of these practices and the correctly chosen training form. These improvements are most efficient if one approaches the practice gradually, step by step, and if they are incorporated into daily life, turning into a sustainable habit.[95]

The topic of Qigong and hypertension is discussed in a study by Jiang Minda 蒋敏达 from 1980. Jiang followed groups of test subjects through their first one or two years of Qigong practice and examined them before and after their Qigong sessions. Most of the examined subjects were 40–60 years of age and categorized as Stage II hypertension patients. The results when comparing the values from before Qigong practice and after show that, on average, blood pressure dropped.[96] According to Jiang, these case studies demonstrate the calming and controlling effect that Qigong and its deep breathing techniques have on the central nervous system.[97]

Another way to treat—and diagnose—hypertension was Chinese medicinal methods (*Zhongyao fangfa* 中药方法). Treating hypertension with Chinese herbal concoctions, acumoxa, or massage is suggested in several articles and considered quite useful. They serve as alternative and additional methods of treatment. These treatments for a scientifically assessed disease such as hypertension were not only based on the twentieth-century "New Medicine," the merging of new and traditional medicines, but were often founded in descriptions of traditional medical literature as a way to validate their use. Shen Zhonggui, for example, writing in 1956, refers back to the

Huangdi Neijing Suwen in his quest to explain hypertension.[98] Shen observes that pathologies are named differently in the Chinese medical tradition than they are in biomedicine. Due to the differences between the two medical systems the rationale behind each diagnosis method varies fundamentally. This means that first one must examine which pathology of Chinese Medicine actually corresponds to the disease that in Western terms is called "hypertension." One term that is introduced by Shen Zhonggui is *zhongfeng* 中风, which today is often translated as "stroke." Its preconditions show similarities to the symptoms associated with hypertension, such as dizziness, unclear sight, bad memory, and red cheeks. Shen specifically states that what occurs before *zhongfeng* displays similar symptoms to hypertension, which is why he postulates a correspondence between the two: "That is why I consider the pathologies of *zhongfeng* and hypertension to be the same."[99] The interesting point here is the similarity in symptoms which makes the merging of treatment and diagnosis possible, hence making the pathology of "hypertension" accessible to Chinese medicinal treatments.

This description and use of equivalents in articles on treatment of hypertension by Chinese Medicine is very revealing for contemporary discourse. In the Chinese medical system there are several varying diagnoses which can all describe the biomedical pathology of hypertension.[100] While in biomedical diagnosis the measurable blood pressure in the vessels in certain body parts is crucial for diagnosing the state of tension in the vessels, in Chinese Medicine the balance of Qi within the body takes center stage and depending on its disbalance different ways of treatment are prescribed. The different diagnoses all point to a varying set of disbalances. The resulting different pathologies all need different treatments, as they describe different conditions, although they all describe the same biomedical phenomenon.

In order to reconcile these two ways of diagnosing the (biomedical) pathology of hypertension, especially in the field of the "New Medicine" in China, experts had to negotiate the respective terms of diagnosis, treatment, and recognition.[101] Medical experts in the field of medicine used a very pragmatic approach, namely incorporating scientific measuring and diagnostics into methods of Chinese Medicine, resulting in quantitative, experimental trials such as the one described by Li Zhensheng 李震生in the *Zhongyi Zazhi* from 1980. In his trial, 40 hypertensive patients were monitored and categorized into different groups according to their Chinese Medicine diagnosis.[102] The study was intended to show the mutual influence and relevance of biomedical and Chinese Medicine.[103] The Chinese medical treatments of hypertension refer to hypertension (*gaoxue ya*) and not specifically to the related Chinese diagnosis. This merging of concepts occurs in the spirit of *zhongxi jiehe*, the integration of Chinese and Western medicine.

When a patient came to a practitioner of Chinese Medicine at the time, the practitioner would take a number of vitals to analyze their state of sickness (weight, height, blood pressure, and pulse).[104] From after the middle of the twentieth century the assessment method of patients in Chinese Medicine was changed from the traditional four diagnostic methods (seeing, hearing, feeling, and smelling) (*sizhen* 四诊) to the combined method of "New Medicine" or the combination of Chinese and Western medicine.

To illustrate this combined approach, I now return to two of the three cases discussed earlier and look at the incorporation of the different systems, starting with Mrs. Jiang, 51 years old. Her case was published in 1955 and focused on her hypertensive state and the treatment she received. Gong Maode, the article's author, gives insight into her treatment by first adding up all the symptoms she experienced, such as dizziness, palpitation, pain in the neck and the back, pain in the left hypochondrium, and so on. She had already received Chinese medical and other treatments without any success. Her vitals read: 176/102 mmHg blood pressure, normal lung function, no enlarged heart, heart rate normal, normal cardiac sounds. She was diagnosed with hypertension. Mrs. Jiang's treatment had consisted of daily administered doses of a pharmaceutical treatment, but this treatment was abandoned after yielding no positive results. She then was treated with acupuncture four times using the *fengchi* 风池 point. The latter treatment made her symptoms vanish and dropped her blood pressure down to 130/94 mmHg.[105]

In the case study of 1981, the patient Mrs. Huang was diagnosed on the basis of her blood pressure (180–220/100–110 mmHg) and the assessment of her symptoms: dizziness, palpitation, loss of sleep, numbness of hands and feet. Furthermore, her face color, pulse, and color of the tongue were examined according to Chinese medical principles. Summing up all the findings, the diagnosis reads: "Western medical diagnosis: hypertension (stage II)." Coupled with the assessment of tongue color, pulse, and other factors, the biomedical diagnosis is complemented by the employment of Chinese Medicine. Mrs. Huang was cured by relieving her internal heat using a concoction called *huayu qingsan tang* 化瘀清散汤.[106]

The case studies published in the *Zhongyi Zazhi* and the *Zhonghua Yixue Zazhi* are exemplary of the merging of the two medical systems. Patients are assessed first according to their biomedical vitals and then examined according to the Chinese diagnostics. They are treated with varying approaches, including herbal and acupuncture approaches. "Traditional" herbal treatments propagated in health magazines and newspapers included, for example, the bark of *Duzhong* 杜仲, Eucommia ulmoides. *Duzhong* was described by Guo Jinyuan in 1953 in the *Dazhong Yixue*. He evaluates it as a valid alternative to expensive antihypertensive drugs as it was a national product. And while it grows in the PRC, this treatment also had ties to the Soviet Union: in the

Soviet Union the medical attributes of this tree bark now aiding in the scientification of Chinese Medicine had already been examined and catalogued. By using the scientific method and testing the bark's effect on lab animals its effectiveness was proven. *Duzhong* was easier to procure than biomedical drugs, and also cheaper, so that patients of hypertension could apply it more easily.[107] One year after this short introduction to *Duzhong*, Guo published another article on this treatment, this time in the *Zhonghua Yixue Zazhi*. Due to the more academic nature of this journal, the article is much more detailed in its descriptions of the clinical trials and the treatment with *Duzhong*. Patients receive a solution of 10 grams of *Duzhong* in 100 milliliters of 70 percent alcohol, and were to take 30 drops of this solution three times a day. They were monitored for a period of three to four weeks. This treatment eased or eliminated some of the symptoms of hypertension (dizziness, headaches, numbness, etc.) for more than half the test subjects. It furthermore lowered the patients' blood pressure and, in the end, cured about 42 percent of the patients, which Guo calls a satisfying outcome.[108]

In the following years more herbal treatments were introduced in the popular and medical literature. In 1956, Shen Zhonggui very thoroughly describes four different kinds of herbal concoctions to treat hypertension:

1. *Yangxin anshenji*养心安神剂[109]
2. *Qianyang xifengji* 潜阳熄风剂[110]
3. *Zigan yishenji*滋肝益肾剂[111]
4. *Pinggan jiangyaji* 平肝降压剂[112]

In 1957, there is an article in the *Dazhong Yixue* by Jia Qian 嘉千 who introduces Ophiorrhiza japonica or *shegencao* 蛇根草. This herb stems from India and is said to lower blood pressure.[113] It is discussed again in a 1958 article by Xu Kaisen, where he presents Ophiorrhiza japonica, also called devil pepper or Rauwolfia, as an effective treatment, especially for primary hypertension.[114] For treatment he suggested that devil pepper should be used under the supervision of a doctor. Its effects are slow, with a two- to four-day margin until there is a response to the treatment. It has a calming effect and can be ingested orally or by injection.[115] After the Cultural Revolution other herbal concoctions were advertised that lowered elevated blood pressure levels. For example, radish seed (*laifuzi* 莱菔子) and *ziqianlifufang shengyapian* 滋潜利复方降压片. Both of these herbal medicines were tested in clinical trials and on animals and were considered alternative treatments to conventional drugs.[116]

Herbal treatments were often an integral part of a treatment which also involved acupuncture and moxa, as Gong Maode 公茂德 described. In his study, 38 people with hypertension were subjected to a blood pressure–lowering acupuncture method, with the researchers observing improvements after said treatments. Similar results were found in 1983 in a treatment trial which was published in the *Zhongyi Zazhi*. The trial included 60 test subjects who had acupuncture, which successfully lowered their hypertension.[117]

An easy self-treatment was self-massage (*ziwo tuina* 自我推拿), which Fan Xingfa 范兴发 introduces in 1985 in the *Dazhong Yixue*. By following this sequence, a person's blood pressure could be lowered. It can be seen as a quick-fix, self-help tool that enables the individual person to take charge of their blood pressure at home and at a time when they felt they needed it.[118]

The way hypertension was pathologized, measured, and diagnosed in the PRC over four decades shows a continuing engagement with the problem, and a grappling with issues similar to those found in the Western discourse. The scientific understanding of hypertension also included a standardization of the body. This was important for the contemporary project of biopolitical population management. The discussion of hypertension reveals the relevance of the pathology of hypertension in a production-driven socialist society, and the dangers this poses. It furthermore confirms the observation made in the context of our discussion of other health issues in previous chapters, that authorities sought to make knowledge about hypertension widely accessible to the population, and emphasized the need for prevention.

Hypertension became a scientific category, a pathology that needed to be diagnosed by experts. The engagement of experts is indeed vital for its diagnosis, as hypertension can only be detected by the act of measuring, giving medical personnel a very specific task on the road to recovery. The detection occurs via interpretation of these measurements by the trained physician. Still, its threshold is set differently by different experts and by the institutions which possess the power to identify the otherwise invisible sickness. Discussion about the difficulty of diagnosing the condition appears in many medical publications as well as articles in the popular media, ensuring the involvement of the whole population.

Nowadays hypertension, just like obesity, is widely considered to be a "new disease." This assumption disregards the simple fact that the human organism has historically succumbed to it. It also ignores the fact that as a disease of civilization, hypertension had existed prior to the twentieth century. While hypertension, for the most part, is interpreted as the response of the body to a high-intensity and stressful environment, few contemporary authors acknowledge the long history of hypertensive diseases. In China, hypertension-like cases seem to have long existed in the medical literature. In the Mao era and under the paradigm of the "New Medicine" in New China, the pathology of hypertension was explored and paired with Chinese medical pathologies that were then treated with a mixture of "old" and "new" approaches. These approaches and treatments were also thoroughly entrenched within the discourse of civilization diseases that emerged especially after the epidemiological transition in post-Mao times. To interpret the physical reaction represented by heightened blood pressure as a response to the fast rhythm of economic development might be read as a hidden critique of the times, or indeed as a fair and realistic view of the status quo. This puts civilization diseases, hypertension included, in the role of a rite of passage through which developing countries must pass in order to enter into the ranks of the developed countries.

The historical continuity of the discussion of hypertension and its associated pathologies is worthy of note in this respect. The new "spin" which hypertension gained from the introduction of Chinese Medicine demonstrates the practical application of the New Medicine. However, the questions of why hypertension has not been kept at bay, and why today cardiovascular diseases are still widely suffered from and are nowhere close to being cured, cannot be answered. What this discussion has shown, if anything, is therefore the prevalence of attempts to tackle civilization diseases through the transmission of knowledge from experts to the wider population, and through the translation of medical knowledge—both from other countries, and between the different medical paradigms.

NOTES

1. Jeremy Greene, *Prescribing by Numbers: Drugs and the Definition of Disease* (Baltimore: John Hopkins University Press, 2007), 55; Arthur Ruskin, *Classics in Arterial Hypertension* (Springfield, IL: Charles C. Thomas, 1956).

2. Zhou Guanhong 周冠虹, "Gaoxueyabing fangzhi changshi wenda (3) 高血压病防治常识问答 (3)," *Dazhong Yixue* 1, 1979: 28–29.

3. This link is not unique to the PRC and its health discourse, but is also noted by Postel-Vinay (*A Century of Arterial Hypertension 1896–1996* (Chichester: John Wiley & Sons, 1996), 141, 149–50).

4. For a very clear definition of this, see Pickering's categorization of hypertension: George Pickering, "Hypertension—Definitions, Natural Histories and Consequences," in *Hypertension Manual*, ed. John H. Laragh (New York: Yorke Medical Books, 1974), 21–22.

5. Postel-Vinay, *Century of Arterial Hypertension*, 153; S. B. Eaton, M. Konner, and M. Shostak, "Stone Agers in the Fast Lane: Chronic Degenerative Diseases in Evolutionary Perspective," *American Journal of Medicine* 84, no. 4 (April 1988): 739–49.

6. This has already been discussed at length by the doctors and researchers on hypertension and the cardiovascular system, as shown by Pickering, "Hypertension."

7. Rosenberg, "Introduction."

8. The visible and invisible signs of hypertension can be a cause of tension in this discussion. Arterial and renal sclerosis, for example, have been known since the nineteenth century as causes for hypertension, but the role of arterial pressure as actually measured was not identified until long after. There was no perceived distinction between the symptom, the reaction, and the disease in the understanding of hypertension at the time (Postel-Vinay, *Century of Arterial Hypertension*, 63). Here, seeing is believing, as Miriam Gross and Marc Matten have remarked (Miriam Gross, *Farewell to the God of Plague—Chairman Mao's Campaign to Deworm China* (Oakland: University of California Press, 2016); Marc A. Matten, "Coping with Invisible Threats: Nuclear Radiation and Science Dissemination in Maoist China," *East Asian Science, Technology and Society* 12, no. 3 (2018): 235–56).

9. Postel-Vinay, *Century of Arterial Hypertension*, 40f.

10. Postel-Vinay, 45. In the beginning of the twentieth century Theodore Janeway, a professor at Johns Hopkins, started the habit of measuring blood pressure in his patients and in this way contributed to the development of routinized measuring in insurance applications and health check-ups. These measurements gave the insurance companies a baseline of patient information which they could later draw from for future contracts.

11. Postel-Vinay, 50.

12. Postel-Vinay, 58: "[C]linicians view Conn's syndrome as a disease while epidemiologists define essential hypertension as a risk factor. As for biologists and geneticists, they emphasise the diversity of situations that come under the heading 'arterial hypertension.'"

13. Postel-Vinay, 139: The lowest value of 120/75 mmHg and the highest at 180/110 mmHg are far apart on the chart Postel-Vinay offers to the readers. This shows how unclear the actual value of hypertension was at the time, he even calls it arbitrary. Additionally, he observes changes in several studies (including a National Health Survey from 1966) over time, including differences between genders, and the age-related increase in blood pressure.

14. Georges Canguilhem, *The Normal and the Pathological* (New York: Zone Books, 1989), 72.

15. Pickering, "Hypertension," 19–20: "The higher the arterial pressure when initially measured, the greater the mortality [. . .]. The relationship is quantitative. There is no sudden break." Sir George Pickering's essay "Hypertension. Definitions, Natural Histories and Consequences" is part of the *Hypertension Manual* edited by John H. Laragh in 1974. In it, Pickering introduces the pathology of hypertension, its reception in medical circles, and the research into it. His approach is rather skeptical and he emphasizes the difficulty of pinpointing when a case of hypertension is actually present and when it is not. That being said, Pickering does recognize the increasing fatality rates with increased blood pressure, making hypertension research medically necessary.

16. Postel-Vinay, *Century of Arterial Hypertension*, 141–42. This is also argued by Canguilhem, *The Normal and the Pathological*.

17. Postel-Vinay, *Century of Arterial Hypertension*, 142.

18. Luo Zuyi 罗祖贻, "Gaoxueyaxing naochuxue de zhiliao 高血压性脑出血的治疗," *Zhonghua Yixue Zazhi* 5 (1978): 312–14.

19. Tu Yuanshu 涂沅淑 and Tong Etang 童萼塘, "Gaoxueya yu Zhongfeng 高血压与中风," *Dazhong Yixue* 12 (1978): 5–7; Zhou Guanhong, "Gaoxueya bing fangzhi changshi wenda (4) 高血压病防治常识问答（4）," *Dazhong Yixue* 2 (1979): 18–19.

20. The PRC had already vanquished communicable diseases such as tuberculosis, the plague, leprosis, and so forth. by activating the population in mass movements such as the Patriotic Health campaign. After eliminating these threats, more pervasive ones had to be destroyed, including non-communicable and lifestyle diseases.

21. Zhi Ge 止戈, "Tantan gaoxueya 談談高血压," *Dazhong Yixue* 3 (1953): 104–5.

22. This conference was hosted by the Chinese Medical Association (Zhonghua Yixuehui 中华医学会) on April 6, 1953, in Shanghai.

23. Wu Xingye 吴兴业, "Yuanfaxing gaoxueya biaozhun zhi shangque 原发性高血压标准之商榷," *Zhonghua Yixue Zazhi* 11 (1954): 929–30. Wu summarizes the discussion of a 1953 meeting of the conference on hypertension *gaoxueya bing tanzuohui* 高血压病座谈会.

24. Similar discussions of physical standards were prevalent in the Republican era, as Jia-chen Fu has demonstrated.

25. See Greene, *Prescribing by Numbers*. For a thorough study of the kinds of methods and apparatuses invented, tested, and used over the twentieth century, see Postel-Vinay, *Century of Arterial Hypertension*.

26. The question was also asked by Chen Mingde 沉明德 in his 1960 *Jiankangbao* article: Chen Mingde 沉明德, "Rang gaoxueya ditou 让高血压低头," *Jiankangbao* (June 1, 1960).

27. Xu Zhanfei 徐展飞, "Gaoxueya bing shi yizhong xinshen jibing 高血压病是一种心身疾病," *Dazhong Yixue* 5 (1986): 7–8.

28. Here a short note on the perceived difference between *gaoxueya* 高血压 and *gaoxueyabing* 高血压病 has to be made. Elevated blood pressure levels do not necessarily warrant the diagnosis of hypertension. High blood pressure may occur due to different reasons and for a limited time period; it becomes pathological only if it is constantly elevated and does not show signs of decreasing on its own, in which case it needs to be corrected to avoid health problems.

29. Bertschnikov, "Xueya gao de ren keyi canjia tiyu yundong ma 血压高的人可以参加体育运动吗," trans. Zou Shunhe, *Xintiyu* 11 (1956): 6–7; I. Y. Sberianski (伊·伊· 司别兰斯基), "Gaoxueya bing 高血压病," trans. Zheng Yiliu 郑依柳, *Dazhong Yixue* 12 (1957): 485–86; Zhou Guanhong, "Gaoxueya bing fangzhi changshi wenda (1) 高血压病防治常识问答（1）," *Dazhong Yixue* 11 (1978): 25–27. Also, the pulse and blood pressure will change during sex, and this is not hypertension but a temporal change. See Tie Ying 铁英, "Guanxin bingren kangfu qijian de xingshenghuo 冠心病人康复期间的性生活," *Dazhong Yixue* 11 (1982): 36–37.

30. On the renal impact of hypertension, see M. I. Rutterer (М.Я. 拉特聂尔), "Gaoxueya bing shi de shenzang xunhuan 高血压病时的肾脏循环," trans. Jiang Mingxing 江明性, *Zhonghua Yixue Zazhi* 3 (1956): 281–83 (originally published in the *Zhiliao Xuewenxian* 治疗学文献 in 1953); Jin Beiwen金蓓文, Xu Daosheng 许道声, and Lin Jiesheng 林捷生, "275 lie gaoxueya bing de shece xueguan yu yandi

xueguan bianhua de yanjiu 275 例高血压病的舌侧血管与眼底血管变化的研究," *Zhonghua Yixue Zazhi*, 4 (1980): 242–44 (tongue blood vessels).

For hypertension's impact on the body, see also Luo Wenyi 罗文一, "Gaoxueya bing de yixie qingkuang 高血压病的一些情况," *Zhonghua Yixue Zazhi* 12 (1974): 760; Di Shangda 翟尚达, "Gaoxueya huanzhe pifu xiaodongmaiya de yanjiu 高血压患者皮肤小动脉压的研究," *Zhonghua Yixue Zazhi* 9 (1981): 541; Yuan Zhaokai 袁肇凯, "Gaoxueya bing xueyu bianzheng yu shejian weiguan bianhua de chubu yanjiu 高血压病血瘀辩证与舌尖微观变化的初步研究," *Zhongyi Zazhi* 11 (1982): 65–67.

31. Du Shihua 席时华, born in 1935, was a professor at Henan Chinese Medical School and assistant head doctor. He graduated in 1955 from Nanjing School of Medicine. (See *Zhongguo Zhongyi renming cidian*, 606.)

32. Xu Kaisen 余开森, "Shegencao zhilia gaoxueya bing de zhishi 蛇根草治疗高血压病的知识," *Dazhong Yixue* 2 (1958): 57–59; Du Shihua, Li Zhensheng 李震生, Lü Jingzhong 吕敬中, and Wang Rukun 王汝琨, *Gaoxueya bing* 高血压病 (Henan: Renmin chubanshe, 1978), 21.

33. This excludes the resulting temporary elevated pressure levels that arise from heavy work.

34. Du Shihua et al., *Gaoxueya bing* 21.

35. Xu Kaisen, "Shegencao zhilia gaoxueya bing de zhishi 蛇根草治疗高血压病的知识," *Dazhong Yixue* 2 (1958): 57–59; Zhou Guanhong, "Gaoxueya bing fangzhi changshi wenda (1) 高血压病防治常识问答 (1)," *Dazhong Yixue* 11 (1978): 25–27; Zhang Chongde 张崇德, "Yuanfaxing gaoxueya fabing jili de yanjiu dongxiang 原发性高血压发病机理的研究动向," *Zhonghua Yixue Zazhi* 1 (1983): 49–52.

36. Qian Qiyuan 钱启源, "Shouyhu zhiliao gaoxueya bing 手术治疗高血压病," *Dazhong Yixue* 5 (1984): 30.

37. Shen Zhonggui 沈仲圭, "Mantan gaoxueya 漫谈高血压," *Dazhong Yixue* 6 (1956): 244–45; Bertschnikov (伊 彼 柏钦柯), "Xueya gao de ren keyi canjia tiyu yundong ma 血压高的人可以参加体育运动吗," trans. Zou Shunhe 邹顺和, *Xintiyu* 11 (1956): 6–7; Xu Kaisen, "Shegencao zhilia gaoxueya bing de zhishi 蛇根草治疗高血压病的知识," *Dazhong Yixue* 2 (1958): 57–59; Zhang Chongde, "原发性高血压发病机理的研究动向," *Zhonghua Yixue Zazhi* 1 (1983): 49–52.

38. Bertschnikov, "Xueya gao de ren keyi canjia tiyu yundong ma 血压高的人可以参加体育运动吗," trans. Zou Shunhe, *Xintiyu* 11 (1956): 6–7.

39. Tong Etang, born in 1933, was a neurologist. He studied at Fudan University and Wuhan Medical School. He graduated in 1957 and went on to work and do research in the field of neurology. (See *Shijie dangdai wenhua mingren cidian* 世界当代文化名人辞典 [Beijing Yanshan chubanshe, 1992], 547.)

40. Tu Yuanshu and Tong Etang, "Gaoxueya yu Zhongfeng 高血压与中风," *Dazhong Yixue* 12 (1978): 5–7.

41. Liu Minying 刘民英, trans., "Gaoxueyabing huanzhe zhiliao de yiban changgui 高血压病患者治疗的一般常规," *Zhonghua Yixue Zazhi* 2 (1954): 125–30.

42. Dan Shouzhun 单守谆, *Gaoxueya* 高血压 (Harbin: Heilongjiang kexue jishu chubanshe, 1981), 2.

43. Systolic and diastolic pressure describe the pressures in the arteries throughout the heart movements. Systolic pressure is measured when the heart muscle contracts, diastolic pressure when it relaxes.

44. A rice diet mostly consisted of rice and vegetables with low amounts of salt, and was sometimes considered rather bland.

45. Low potassium blood levels were found to be indicative of hypertension so that a dietary increase was strongly suggested. See Liu Minying, trans., "Gaoxueyabing huanzhe zhiliao de yiban changgui 高血压病患者治疗的一般常规," *Zhonghua Yixue Zazhi* 2 (1954): 125–30; Xu Xinmin 徐新民, "Gaoxueya yu dixuejia 高血压与低血钾," *Dazhong Yixue* 6 (1983): 39–40.

46. Zhou Guanhong and Zhao Guangsheng 赵光胜, "Gaoxueyabing yu tiyuduanlian 高血压病与体育锻炼," *Xintiyu* 2 (1980): 36–38.

47. Du Shihua et al., *Gaoxueya bing*, 45; Dan Shouzhun, *Gaoxueya*, 2.

48. Dan Shouzhun, 7–8.

49. Dan Shouzhun, 2–3.

50. Dan Shouzhun, 75–76.

51. Liu Minying, trans., "Gaoxueyabing huanzhe zhiliao de yiban changgui 高血压病患者治疗的一般常规," *Zhonghua Yixue Zazhi* 2 (1954): 125–30; B. A. Kondratiev, "Gaoxueya bing huanzhe de shenghuo zhidu 高血压病患者的生活制度," trans. Wu Zhongbi, *Dazhong Yixue* 1 (1954): 17–19; Lea Bernaya (勒 阿柏娜娅), "Gaoxueya bingren de tiyuliaofa 高血压病人的体育疗法," *Xintiyu* 18 (1957): 27; Kuang Ankun 邝安坤, "Zai gaoxueya bing zhong yanjiu Qigong yuanli—dui Qigong pingheng yinyang, tiaohe qixue, shutong jingluo zuoyong de chubu tantao 在高血压病中研究气功原理——对气功平衡阴阳□调和气血□疏通经络作用的初步探讨," *Zhongyi Zazhi* 10 (1980): 7–9.

52. Zhou Guanhong, "Gaoxueya bing fangzhi changshi wenda (1) 高血压病防治常识问答（1）," *Dazhong Yixue* 11 (1978): 25–27; Zhou Guanhong and Zhao Guangsheng, "Gaoxueyabing yu tiyuduanlian 高血压病与体育锻炼," *Xintiyu* 2 (1980): 36–38; Li Bingcheng, "Kepa de wenmingbing 可怕的文明病," *Shandong tiyu keji* 1 (1984): 25–27.

53. Zhou Guanhong, "Gaoxueya bing fangzhi changshi wenda (1) 高血压病防治常识问答（1）," *Dazhong Yixue* 11 (1978): 25–27: people of 40-plus years are of greater risk of succumbing to hypertension. Shi Yongde 施永德 and Tang Zhensheng 唐镇生, "Naxie ren yihuan que xuexing Zhongfeng 哪些人易患缺血性中风," *Dazhong Yixue* 11 (1981): 2–4. The risk of stroke increases in old age: 14.5 percent at 52, 50 percent at 63, 88 percent at 74, 100 percent at 85. Song Baosen 宋宝森, trans., "Gaoxueya, dongmai yinghua, Zhongfeng, xinzangbing—zuijia duice (yi) 高血压，动脉硬化，中风，心脏病—最佳对策（一）," *Dazhong Yixue* 11 (1981): 10–13: 40-plus years also as a threshold for the risk group.

54. Guo Jinyuan, born in 1914, was an internist. He studied medicine at Tonji University and in 1939 he graduated from the Medical School at the University of Munich, Germany. He holds a doctorate and was a professor of medicine at Tongji University after his return to China in 1946. (See *Shijie dangdai wenhua mingren cidian*, 135.)

55. Guo Jinyuan, "Duzhong zhiliao gaoxueya bing de chubu baogao 杜仲治疗高血压病的初步报告," *Zhonghua Yixue Zazhi* 9 (1954): 704–7.

56. Hebei sheng yixue kexue yanjiusuo xinxueguanbing yanjiuzu, "Shijiazhuang chengxiang jumin gaoxueya bing fabinglü ji fabing yinsu de diaocha baogao 石家庄城乡居民高血压病发病率及发病因素的调查报告," *Zhonghua Yixue Zazhi* 1 (1975): 79; Zhou Guanhong, "Gaoxueya bing fangzhi changshi wenda (1) 高血压病防治常识问答（1）," *Dazhong Yixue* 11 (1978): 25–27; Zhou Guanhong and Zhao Guangsheng, "Gaoxueyabing yu tiyuduanlian 高血压病与体育锻炼," *Xintiyu* 2 (1980): 36–38; Song Baosen, trans., "Gaoxueya, dongmai yinghua, Zhongfeng, xinzangbing—zuijia duice (yi) 高血压，动脉硬化，中风，心脏病—最佳对策（一)," *Dazhong Yixue* 11 (1981): 10–13.

57. Tu Yuanshu and Tong Etang, "Gaoxueya yu Zhongfeng 高血压与中风," *Dazhong Yixue* 12 (1978): 5–7.

58. Zhou Guanhong, "Gaoxueya bing fangzhi changshi wenda (2) 高血压病防治常识问答（2)," *Dazhong Yixue* 12 (1978): 8–10.

59. On hereditary hypertension, see Li Guanglian 李广镰, "Zai gaoxueya bing jiazu zhong 在高血压病家族中," *Dazhong Yixue* 1 (1986): 24–25.

60. B. A. Kondratiev, "Gaoxueya bing huanzhe de shenghuo zhidu 高血压病患者的生活制度," trans. Wu Zhongbi, *Dazhong Yixue* 1 (1954): 17–19.

61. Bertschnikov, "Xueya gao de ren keyi canjia tiyu yundong ma 血压高的人可以参加体育运动吗," trans. Zou Shunhe, *Xintiyu* 11 (1956): 6–7. Zhou Guanhong emphasizes this circumstance as well, not only in his 1978 article, but also in his 1980 *Xintiyu* article: Zhou Guanhong, "Gaoxueya bing fangzhi changshi wenda (1) 高血压病防治常识问答（1）," *Dazhong Yixue* 11 (1978): 25–27; Zhou Guanhong and Zhao Guangsheng, "Gaoxueyabing yu tiyuduanlian 高血压病与体育锻炼," *Xintiyu* 2 (1980): 36–38.

62. Song Baosen, trans., "Gaoxueya, dongmai yinghua, Zhongfeng, xinzangbing—zuijia duice (liu) 高血压，动脉硬化，中风，心脏病—最佳对策（六)," *Dazhong Yixue* 4 (1982): 35–37.

63. See Bridie Andrews, "From Case Records to Case Histories: The Modernisation of a Chinese Medical Genre, 1912–1949," in *Innovation in Chinese Medicine*, ed. Elizabeth Hsu, 324–36 (Cambridge: Cambridge University Press, 2001); and Christopher Cullen, "*Yi'an* 醫案 (case statements): The Origins of a Genre of Chinese Medical Literature," in Hsu, *Innovation in Chinese Medicine*, 297–323.

64. Gong Maode 公茂德, "Gaoxueya bing de zhenjiu zhiliao chubu jingyan 高血压病的针灸治疗初步经验," *Zhonghua Yixue Zazhi* 7 (1955): 653–54.

65. Zhongguo renmin jiefangjun di er er yiyiyuan waike, "Gaoxueya naochuxue waike zhiliao de chubu jingyan 高血压脑出血外科治疗的初步经验," *Zhonghua Yixue Zazhi* 12 (1977): 748–50.

66. Li Runmin 李润民, "Huayuqingsantang zhiliao gaoxueya bing 41 lie 化瘀清散汤治疗高血压病41例," *Zhongyi Zazhi* 3 (1981): 30.

67. See, for example, I. Y. Sberianski, "Gaoxueya bing 高血压病," trans. Zheng Yiliu 郑依柳, *Dazhong Yixue* 12 (1957): 485–86; Zhou Guanhong, "Gaoxueya bing fangzhi changshi wenda (3) 高血压病防治常识问答（3）," *Dazhong Yixue* 1 (1979): 28–29; Zhou Guanhong and Zhao Guangsheng, "Gaoxueyabing yu tiyuduanlian 高

血压病与体育锻炼," *Xintiyu* 2 (1980): 36–38: this article also lists ringing ears (i.e., tinnitus), blurred eyesight, loss of sleep, palpitations, and numbness as symptoms of hypertension.

68. Sun Ke, "Wo you xupang biande jiankang le 我由虚胖变得健康了," *Xintiyu* 4 (1954): 34.

69. B. A. Kondratiev, "Gaoxueya bing huanzhe de shenghuo zhidu 高血压病患者的生活制度," trans. Wu Zhongbi, *Dazhong Yixue* 1 (1954): 17–19; B. A. Kondratiev, "Gaoxueya bing huanzhe de shenghuo zhidu (xuwan) 高血压病患者的生活制度 (续完)," trans. Wu Zhongbi, *Dazhong Yixue* 2 (1954): 103–6.

70. A short break may also take place in the resting room at work. B. A. Kondratiev, "Gaoxueya bing huanzhe de shenghuo zhidu 高血压病患者的生活制度," trans. Wu Zhongbi, *Dazhong Yixue* 1 (1954): 17–19.

71. B. A. Kondratiev, "Gaoxueya bing huanzhe de shenghuo zhidu (xuwan) 高血压病患者的生活制度 (续完)," trans. Wu Zhongbi, *Dazhong Yixue* 2 (1954): 103–6.

72. See, for example, I. Y. Sberianski, "Gaoxueya bing 高血压病," trans. Zheng Yiliu 郑依柳, *Dazhong Yixue* 12 (1957): 485–86. A 1982 translation from Japanese also emphasizes a stable lifestyle with good sleep hygiene and dietary habits as one way to keep blood pressure regulated. See Song Baosen, trans., "Gaoxueya, dongmai yinghua, Zhongfeng, xinzangbing—zuijia duice (liu) 高血压，动脉硬化，中风，心脏病—最佳对策（六)," *Dazhong Yixue* 4 (1982): 35–37. For the elderly, Cai Shibiao sets down similar rules in 1983: Cai Shibiao 蔡士标, "Laonianxing gaoxueya you shenme tezheng 老年性高血压有什么特征," *Dazhong Yixue* 8 (1983): 44.

73. Liu Minying, trans., "Gaoxueyabing huanzhe zhiliao de yiban changgui 高血压病患者治疗的一般常规," *Zhonghua Yixue Zazhi* 2 (1954): 125–30. Sleep as a regular habit was also meant to help in the consistent evening out of blood pressure, as the translation by Wu Zhongbi from 1954 postulates: B. A. Kondratiev, "Gaoxueya bing huanzhe de shenghuo zhidu (xuwan) 高血压病患者的生活制度 (续完)," trans. Wu Zhongbi, *Dazhong Yixue* 2 (1954): 103–6.

74. This group also includes patients with weak heart muscles who tire easily. Their blood pressure is low due to the weak muscle state.

75. Bertschnikov, "Xueya gao de ren keyi canjia tiyu yundong ma 血压高的人可以参加体育运动吗," trans. Zou Shunhe, *Xintiyu* 11 (1956): 6–7.

76. Lea Bernaya, 勒阿柏娜娅, "Gaoxueya bingren de tiyuliaofa 高血压病人的体育疗法," *Xintiyu* 18 (1957): 27.

77. Moskov (维 恩 莫史科夫), "Shiyi yu chuqi gaoxueya bingren de ticao 适宜于初期高血压病人的体操," trans. You Dajun 游达钧, *Xintiyu* 18 (1957): 28.

78. Ding Haochuan 丁浩川, "Wo zai zhiyu gaoxueya bing zhong de yixie tihui 我在治愈高血压病中的一些体会," *Xintiyu* 18 (1961): 5–7.

79. B. A. Kondratiev, "Gaoxueya bing huanzhe de shenghuo zhidu (xuwan) 高血压病患者的生活制度 (续完)," trans. Wu Zhongbi, *Dazhong Yixue* 2 (1954): 103–6.

80. Zhou Guanhong, "Gaoxueya bing fangzhi changshi wenda (2) 高血压病防治常识问答（2）," *Dazhong Yixue* 12 (1978): 8–10.

81. Zhou Guanhong, "Gaoxueya bing fangzhi changshi wenda (3) 高血压病防治常识问答（3）," *Dazhong Yixue* 1 (1979): 28–29. In 1986, Li Guanglian 李广镰 concurs with the observation by Zhou Guanhong that a low sodium diet was the way

to go for hypertension patients. His article "In Families with Hypertension" (Zai gaoxueyabing jiazu zhong 在高血压病家族中) was published in the *Dazhong Yixue*. He advocates a low-sodium diet of mild taste including a lot of fresh food. Canned foods should be avoided due to the high sodium contents used for preservation. See Li Guanglian 李广镰, "Zai gaoxueya bing jiazu zhong 在高血压病家族中," *Dazhong Yixue* 1 (1986): 24–25.

82. Cong Linzhong 丛林中, "Yingyangxuejia tan shanshi guocheng he nongye jiegou 营养学家谈膳食构成和农业结构," *Renmin Ribao* (August 30, 1979).

83. Gong Xianzhong 龚宪中, "Niunai yufang gaoxueya 牛奶预防高血压," *Dazhong Yixue* 1 (1985): 20.

84. Five to ten milligrams intravenously or 15–20 milligrams intramuscular of a 25 percent solution, see Liu Minying, trans., "Gaoxueyabing huanzhe zhiliao de yiban changgui 高血压病患者治疗的一般常规," *Zhonghua Yixue Zazhi* 2 (1954): 125–30.

85. O. H. Afanaseva, "Liusuanmei zhilia gaoxueya de jiliang yongfa 硫酸镁治疗高血压的剂量用法," trans. Ye Zhixiu 叶知修, *Zhonghua Yixue Zazhi* 12 (1954): 1001–3.

86. Chitarev (A.П. 希塔列夫), "Moshao quyuxing nufokayin fengbifa zhilian gaoxueya toutong 末梢区域性奴佛卡因封闭法治疗高血压头痛," trans. Teng Xiheng 滕锡衡, *Zhonghua Yixue Zazhi* 3 (1956): 279–80. Novocaine was an accidental find of medicine, just like Diuril was. See Greene, *Prescribing by Numbers*.

87. Mirikumova 米里库莫娃等 and Streitova 斯特莱里卓娃, "Gaoxueya bing fabing jizhan jiqi bingyin liaofa wenti de cailiao 高血压病发病机转及其病因疗法问题的材料," trans. Ye Zhixiu, *Zhonghua Yixue Zazhi* 3 (1956): 284–87.

Not only were new drugs introduced from outside China, but new drugs were also developed in China for the growing national market for pharmaceuticals. Some of these drugs also had the side effect of lowering blood pressure and helped in treating other accompanying conditions such as coronary heart disease, high blood lipids, or diabetes. One such pill was the *Qingshen jianfeipian* 轻身减肥片 produced in a production plant in Hangzhou (Hangzhou di'er zhongyaochang 杭州第二中药厂), as Huang Dingsong mentions in a 1984 *Renmin Ribao* issue (Huang Dingsong 黄定松, "Meiyou fuzuoyong de jianfeiyao 没有副作用的减肥药," *Renmin Ribao* [November 15, 1984]). The Second Plant for CM Medicine in Hangzhou (Hangzhou di'er zhongyaochang 杭州第二中药厂) had existed in its basic form since the Qing dynasty, when it was called the Huqingyutang zhiyaochang 胡庆余堂制药厂. It was opened in 1874 by the local hygiene department. In 1972, the plant was renamed Hangzhou di'er zhongyaochang.

88. Zhongguo renmin jiefangjun di er er yiyiyuan waike 中国人民解放军第二二一医院外科, "Gaoxueya naochuxue waike zhiliao de chubu jingyan 高血压脑出血外科治疗的初步经验," *Zhonghua Yixue Zazhi* 12 (1977): 748–50.

89. Luo Zuyi, "Gaoxueyaxing naochuxue de zhiliao 高血压性脑出血的治疗," *Zhonghua Yixue Zazhi* 5 (1978): 312–14.

90. Qian Qiyuan, "Shouyhu zhiliao gaoxueya bing 手术治疗高血压病," *Dazhong Yixue* 5 (1984): 30.

91. David A. Palmer stresses that the system of Qigong was part of the PRC's "project of developing the health of the masses and of extracting and transforming all

useful elements of traditional culture in the service of building a New China" (David A. Palmer, *Qigong Fever: Body, Science, and Utopia in China* [New York: Columbia University Press, 2007], 5). Palmer refers to Qigong as an "invented tradition," referencing Hobsbawm and Ranger: Qigong is perceived as a traditional practice, as based on old texts and movements, but the system itself came into being much later than is often claimed (Palmer, *Qigong Fever*, 5, 18; Eric Hobsbawm and Terence Ranger, *The Invention of Tradition* [Cambridge: Cambridge University Press, 1983]).

92. The same thing occurred with Chinese Medicine, which from the 1980s onward gained the label "traditional" and is nowadays referred to as TCM, traditional Chinese Medicine.

93. Palmer, *Qigong fever*, 4.

94. Palmer, 4.

95. Zhao Guangsheng, "Gaoxueya de 'ziwo liaofa' 高血压病的'自我治疗,'" *Dazhong Yixue* 8 (1978): 17–18.

Sustainable means that a person can incorporate this habit comfortably into their life without effort.

96. Jiang Minda 蒋敏达, "50 lie gaoxueya binghuanzhe Qigong huxi tuxing guancha 50例高血压病患者气功呼吸图形观察," *Zhongyi Zazhi* 8 (1980): 42–44; Kuang Ankun, "Zai gaoxueya bing zhong yanjiu Qigong yuanli—dui Qigong pingheng yinyang, tiaohe qixue, shutong jingluo zuoyong de chubu tantao 在高血压病中研究气功原理——对气功平衡阴阳□调和气血□疏通经络作用的初步探讨," *Zhongyi Zazhi* 10 (1980): 7–9; Wang Chongxing 王崇行, "Gaoxueya binghuanzhe Qigong guocheng zhong hongwai fushe xianxiang de guancha 高血压病患者气功过程中红外辐射现象的观察," *Zhongyi Zazhi* 12 (1982): 37–38; Xie Songwei 谢松炜, "Qigong dui gaoxueya bingren zhongshu he waizhou quya shenshangxiansu daixie chanqu de yingxiang 气功对高血压病人中枢和外周去甲肾上腺素代谢产物的影响," *Zhongyi Zazhi* 7 (1983): 64–65; Kuang Ankun, "Qigong yufang gaoxueyaxing naocuzhong de changqi duibi guancha—244 lie yuanfaxing gaoxueya bing 18–22 nian yuhou suifang 气功预防高血压性脑卒中的长期对比观察——244例原发性高血压病18–22年预后随访," *Zhongyi Zazhi* 10 (1983): 26–29.

97. From the Chinese Medicine perspective, Qigong helps in regulating the *qi* and *xue* and unblocks the meridians.

98. Shen Zhonggui, "Mantan gaoxueya 漫谈高血压," *Dazhong Yixue* 6 (1956): 244–45. Another article by Zhu Boqing from 1981 goes back to the *Huangdi Neijing Suwen* 黄帝内经素问 to establish a base of traditional thinking (Zhu Boqing 朱伯卿, "Xinzangbingren de yundong chufang 心脏病人的运动处方," *Dazhong Yixue* 12 [1981]: 4–6).

99. "Suoyi wo renwei zhongfeng de bingli he gaoxueya xiangtong 所以我认为中风的病理和高血压相同," Shen Zhonggui, "Mantan gaoxueya 漫谈高血压," *Dazhong Yixue* 6 (1956): 244–45. It remains debatable whether it is justifiable merely to equate symptoms and suggest that because of their similarity the pathologies of different systems are also equivalent.

100. Du Shihua et al., *Gaoxueya bing*, 51: Different manifestations of hypertension in Chinese Medicine: *yangkang xing* 阳亢型, *yinxu yangkang xing* 阴虚阳亢型, *yinyang liangxu xing* 阴阳两虚型, *tanshi yongcheng xing* 痰湿壅盛型, *xueyu zuluo*

xing 血瘀阻络型. Beijingshi gaoxueya bing naoxueguan bing fangzhi yanjiu xiezuo zu, *Gaoxueya bing Naoxueguan bing Guanxinbing de fangzhi* 高血压病 脑血管病 冠心病的防治 (Beijing: Renmin chubanshe, 1976), 37: Different manifestations of hypertension in Chinese Medicine: *ganrexing* 干热型, *yinxu yan kang xing* 阴虚阳亢型, *ganxian yinxu xing* 肝肾阴虚型, *yinyang liangxu xing* 阴阳两虚型.

101. See, for example, Lu Guangxin 陆广莘, "Gaoxueya bing zhongxiyi jiehe yanjiu zhong de bianbing he bianzheng wenti 高血压病中西医结合研究中的辨病和辩证问题," *Zhongyi Zazhi* 5 (1980): 10–14.

102. These groups were examined thoroughly. Factors that were measured clinically included vanillylmandelic acid (VMA), 17-hydroxide levels, and triglycerides levels.

103. Li Zhensheng 李震生, "Gaoxueya bing zhongyi bianzheng fenxing de bingli shengli jichu chubu tantao 高血压病中医辨证分型的病理生理基础初步探讨," *Zhongyi Zazhi* 5 (1980): 26–30.

104. For a thorough discussion of the "modernization" of Chinese Medicine, see Nathan Sivin, *Traditional Medicine in Contemporary China: A Partial Translation of* Revised Outline of Chinese Medicine *(1972) with an Introductory Study on Change in Present Day and Early Medicine* (Ann Arbor: Center for Chinese Studies, University of Michigan, 1987); Volker Scheid, *Chinese Medicine in Contemporary China: Plurality and Synthesis* (Durham: Duke University Press, 2002); and Hsiang-lin Lei, *Neither Donkey nor Horse: Medicine in the Struggle over China's Modernity* (Chicago: University of Chicago Press, 2014).

105. Gong Maode, "Gaoxueya bing de zhenjiu zhiliao chubu jingyan 高血压病的针灸治疗初步经验," *Zhonghua Yixue Zazhi* 7 (1955): 653–54.

106. Li Runmin, "Huayuqingsantang zhiliao gaoxueya bing 41 lie 化瘀清散汤治疗高血压病41例," *Zhongyi Zazhi* 3 (1981): 30. The drug here researched is a mixture of root of thorowax, root of kudzu vine, root of red-rooted salvia, Chrysanthemum morifolium, mulberry twig, root bark of the tree peony, root of herbaceous peony, safflower, earthworm, and peppermint.

107. Guo Jinyuan, "Duzhong keyi zhiliao gaoxueya zheng 杜仲可以治疗高血压症," *Dazhong Yixue* 11 (1953): 429.

108. Guo Jinyuan, "Duzhong zhiliao gaoxueya bing de chubu baogao 杜仲治疗高血压病的初步报告," *Zhonghua Yixue Zazhi* 9 (1954): 704–7.

109. This concoction was used in case of palpitation and insomnia, dreaming and amnesia.

110. This concoction was used in cases of headaches and dizziness, redness in the face, constipation, heavy-headedness, dizzy vision and ringing ears.

111. In elderly with renal depletion, amnesia, and insomnia, if the waist and the legs are painful and weak, if there is frequent urination, a feeling of depression, if they are heated and they display a red face.

112. This concoction was used if the condition was not very clear or barely had symptoms. Shen Zhonggui, "Mantan gaoxueya 漫谈高血压," *Dazhong Yixue* 6 (1956): 244–45.

113. Jia Qian 嘉千, "Zhiliao gaoxueya bing de yaowu 治疗高血压病的药物," *Dazhong Yixue* 11 (1957): 420–22.

114. There were different kinds of Rauwolfia products available on the Chinese market at the time from different places around the world, including India, Switzerland, and the United States. Xu Kaisen considered the foreign trade for Rauwolfia rather uneconomical, which is why he advocated that drug plants be built in the PRC.

115. Xu Kaisen, "Shegencao zhilia gaoxueya bing de zhishi 蛇根草治疗高血压病的知识," *Dazhong Yixue* 2 (1958): 57–59.

116. Chen Qiucheng 陈秋澄, "Laifuzi zhiliao gaoxueya bing 70 lie liaoxiao guancha 莱菔子治疗高血压病70例疗效观察," *Zhongyi Zazhi* 4 (1980): 12; Zhang Tingxin 张听新, "Ziqianli fufang jiangyapian zhiliao gaoxueya bing 56 lie linchuang liaoxiao baogao 滋潜利复方降压片治疗高血压病56例临床疗效报告," *Zhongyi Zazhi* 5 (1980): 31–33.

117. Acupoints used: 足三里， 曲池，肝俞，身柱，风池，鸠尾. Sometimes specific acupoints were used to counter the patients' symptoms. See Gong Maode, "Gaoxueya bing de zhenjiu zhiliao chubu jingyan 高血压病的针灸治疗初步经验," *Zhonghua Yixue Zazhi* 7 (1955): 653–54; Sun Mingyi 孙明一, "Yingyong 'xienan bubei' fa zhiliao gaoxueya bing 60 lie liaoxiao guancha 应用'泻南补北'法治疗高血压病60例疗效观察," *Zhongyi Zazhi* 5 (1983): 50–51.

118. Fan Xingfa 范兴发, "Gaoxueya bing de ziwo tuina 高血压病的自我推拿," *Dazhong Yixue* 10 (1985): 40–41.

Conclusion

Governmentality's Playground

The central question this book asks is, What constituted health in socialist China and beyond? By asking this question I did not mean to imply that "Chinese health" may have been something different to health anywhere else in the world; rather, I sought to recognize its peculiar centrality to the narrative of a strong nation. With this question comes the realization that the state was heavily involved in forming a health narrative that would modernize both the body and the nation so that they could compete with the developed world. The health practices introduced in pursuit of this modernization process aimed not only at the problem of weak physiques and the attached national trauma, but also sought to structure daily life according to the requirements of state planning and economic production. Rather than manifesting simply as a top-down undertaking controlled purely from above, the interlinked processes involved in this exercise turned out to be much more complex, involving actors from the top as well as the bottom end of the hierarchy. In fact, the examination of the discourse of health and the associated practices that were introduced has uncovered a process of negotiation between those actors, including the Chinese state and its population as well as the experts and institutions involved. Indeed, we have even seen a process of negotiation between the past and the present concerning which health practices were most fruitful for which ailments. Traditional medical thought was brought into these negotiations so as to become part of the new medical system of the PRC and to form a new approach to disease and health.

At the same time, a more complex picture of the body emerged, with the body becoming not only a tool and machine in the service of the socialist revolution, but an entity that had to be assessed both externally (by measuring and testing) and internally (by reflection upon comfort and discomfort) to provide optimal conditions for it to thrive. This was the basis for thinking and talking about it as part of the processes of economic production, the driving force behind the discourse of health in the socialist era. The body had to be strengthened both to fight against intruders, and also to fulfil the ambitious plans for economic growth postulated in the five-year plans of the PRC government. The striving for economic development permeated every aspect of daily life, as my discussion has shown. This encompassed not only the food that was eaten, but also the way a body was trained and how much rest it got and whether or not these activities had to be done in company or alone.

Though production was central to the push for better health in the population, it was also the reason for fatigue, exhaustion, and disbalance in the body: thus workers exhausted themselves in the effort for economic growth and so had to rest. Rest as a period of time spent doing nothing produces no output, so it had to be justified as a biological need of the hard-working body. Physical aches and pains that arose due to the labor environment also had to be fixed to ensure a smooth production process. These needs showed that the human body was not machinelike. Rest, physical activity, and nutrition were essential countermeasures to exhaustion, and so formed a trinity of health practices. They are the basis on which a healthy life was built, and defined what was required for economic productivity.

The coveted state of health is, nevertheless, an ideal that seemingly was never reached, although the practices intended to attain it were laid out for everyone to follow. Health threats change over time and depend on the circumstances, as we have seen regarding the transition from the era in which epidemics were the major health threat, to the new era marked by the prevalence of non-communicable threats such as obesity and hypertension or other cardiovascular diseases. This transition is not necessarily a linear process of change, and it induces a shift in health practices as well. What strikes me here as most interesting is the insight that there was a deep and widespread discussion of health in the narrative of the popular media during the Mao era and earlier, yet this still did not prevent what was to come in post-reform China. The new health and hygiene practices were able to eliminate the old infectious diseases, but could not prevent an increase in civilization diseases, which gained a firm foothold in the Chinese population. This shows how the potential threat of a sedentary lifestyle with too much food and too little physical activity was already discussed in the Mao era, and that there were actually cases of civilization diseases even at the time when the Great Famine devastated China. It also demonstrates that these seemingly new diseases could not be prevented by the mere knowledge of them. Today, obesity rates in China are skyrocketing, and cardiovascular diseases are just as common in the PRC as they are anywhere else in the world.

Apart from the recognition of civilization diseases, I found considerations in the literature concerning the care that factories and the state seemingly extended to the workers and peasants who suffered from the requirements of labor. The fitness programs designed for the populace show a clear perception of their physical plight, which was not at all taken lightly. The nutrition considerations speak to a scientific approach to their energy and micronutrient needs, although the effort to provide for the workers' food centrally was a failure. The acknowledgment of the need for resting as well as working time is another very caring gesture that was made with the aim of maintaining the existing bodies and not burning through them.

The central narrative of building a healthy body for the good of the nation was dominated by the state authorities, both in the form of the policies that were issued to promote a healthy lifestyle and in the form of the trained professionals who supplied not only translations of foreign expertise but also engaged in original research and offered their own interpretations of the new medical treatments. The state, predictably, emerges as the agent with all the power. Yet this power was curbed by the limits to the state's supposed omnipotence. The act of introducing health practices and protocols for eating, sleeping, and exercising is an act of control that pushes at those limits. Ideally, all these practices would occur in a controlled environment according to an ironclad plan with specific goals to be reached in a specific time. By tracing the concept of health and the health practices entwined with it, the impact on daily life and the structure of a healthy routine emerges and shows what healthy living was supposed to look like. As it turns out, total control of daily habits and individual bodies was hard for the Chinese authorities to achieve, despite their best efforts. The state and the individual first negotiated what can be called healthy and, especially in the context of labor, this negotiation displays the dynamics between state and individual bodies. While the state always tries to establish its dominance and power over the population, claiming to pursue the benefit of that population, it reaches its limits once it seeks to tackle the issue of a healthy body. The health discussion has thus uncovered the acknowledgment of these limits. Similar observations were made by James Watson in his research on the failure of public canteens. Watson asks, "Just how far can people be pushed before the social fabric begins to unravel?,"[1] referring to the severe infringements on daily life imposed by the CCP government.[2]

The negative backlash to this strict governmental control led to its loosening. This can be observed in many of the health topics examined in this book: the state tries to seep into every aspect of daily life and to infiltrate every part of a person's presence, for example through physical education at schools and factories, and the time and areas allotted for sleeping. And just like with the control of public eating spaces, in all of those fields the governance hits obstacles.

Undoubtedly, ideology plays a huge part in this discourse in which the individual was not controlled completely. It was the tool used to convince the population to participate in health practices, outside of physically forcing them to do so. I argue that ideology and scientification played a major part in establishing a sense of urgency for health in the Chinese population, but even with this conviction there were still some limits that the Chinese state could not completely overcome. The realization that there are limits to individual bodies that are not the same for the entire population led to a diversification in health practices and advice. Adjustments had to be made dependent on the sex, workload, age, and the state of health of the individual in question. This opened up the necessity for self-regulation and self-care—though, of course, this was according to government-sanctioned guidelines. People thus had to listen to their bodies as well as to the authorities. Listening to and acting upon the cues sent by their bodies was a way to prevent overexhausting the population further, as wrong choices would tire them out and lead to a decline in energy for labor. The mere necessity to talk about self-awareness while exercising, or regarding food choices and sleep, understood as an inherently non-violent action, gives rise to a decision space for the individual person, and proves that there seems to be no one-size-fits-all approach to health. This does not count as individualism, but instead is a cultivation of mindfulness of the body. The state could not look into people's heads to see their discomfort or physical limits. This is where control stops physically, and where mental control through ideology has to start.

David Palmer encountered this controversy in his work on Qigong, where he asked why an authoritarian state would allow such a space to come into existence.[3] The politically charged Qigong body techniques were much more heavily sanctioned than the health practices this book examines, due to the political affiliations of its participants. The participation in health practices for the Mao era, on the other hand, can be interpreted as a political statement of the socialist revolution. As health practices were embedded in the narrative of national strengthening and rejuvenation, they were also permanently loaded with ideological meaning and connected to the appeal to socialism and the common good. By binding the individual to the nation on an ideological level, the practices and everyday habits were all put into an ideological context. Ingraining them into people's minds as good habits of all classes was a prevention method designed to avoid diseases where possible. I have to stress one more time that these practices and the binding of the population to the health discourse did not discriminate between the different classes. The health discourse included mental and manual workers and offered both of them an array of health advice for living a good, socialist life.

A healthy life, in the end, was an ideal the population had to aspire to. It consisted of good rest (depending on individual need but for at least eight hours and with enough rest during the workday), physical activity (outside of work to strengthen and balance the body for the benefit of economic production), and adequate meals (adjusted to individual requirements). These practices are structured by work shifts and production and show how in turn everyday life was governed through this health discourse.

Another limitation that calls into question the omnipotence of the state and the success of governmentality are the diseases that still occur today. Their causes may have changed slightly, but they are still a problem in the PRC (and elsewhere). Diseases of affluence were not obviated by the health discussions and education of the population on proper health routines. French and Crabbe elaborate on the rising weight of the Chinese population, which shows how the discussion of civilization diseases in the Mao era was not able to prevent the PRC from suffering the same high rates of obesity, cardiovascular diseases, and so on, as the United States or the United Kingdom. Although we may ask for an answer to the question of why that should be, no satisfying reply seems to be at hand.

Further research is needed into whether the state today is more controlling and has more resources to direct toward the governing of its population's health. With the introduction of new technologies such as health apps and video cameras, and the thorough scientification of the population, a more thorough control seems possible. This also includes the rigorous admonition for self-control according to scientific standards. It remains to be seen whether the PRC can counter civilization diseases more efficiently than Western developed countries. Is it even possible for the PRC to really make their nation a healthy nation? The case of civilization diseases so far does not offer any promising solutions.

An area where the PRC government recently demonstrated its willingness to infringe heavily on its population's life, thus pushing the boundaries of governmentality once more, was the outbreak of COVID-19 in 2020. This showed just how far the authorities could control the Chinese population. Their ability to close down entire cities, nearly indeed the whole country, was first considered highly troubling by the international press and observers, although later their actions were mirrored globally albeit on a milder scale. This use of governing power demonstrates its reach into everyday life. While the need to fight against the virus is at the same time more pressing and may prove more successful in the long run, as experience has taught us in this case, the fight against civilization diseases still persists, although it may for the moment be overshadowed.

Another issue that needs to remain in the focus of the discussion is health and what it means to be healthy. For the case of China, further research needs to be fostered into the grassroot perception of health practices, their actual implementation, and their meaning to the population. The development of health practices and their democratization is another topic for future scholarship, especially regarding the turn toward external impulses that then lead the development of the practices, that is, generating a certain kind of "look." [4] A further possible question for future research is the health practices that are alternative to the state narrative of health. The diversification and individualization of health practices lends itself to the question of what alternative health practices look like, and how they were expressed and perceived in the traditional medical system.

All these practices and all this thinking about health was geared toward production, but also toward the well-being of the individual body, so as to alleviate suffering and to improve living standards. Through my discussion it has become clear that this is not an easy state to define, and neither is it easy to achieve. Perhaps it is simply not something anybody can obtain perfectly, at least not for the entirety of their lives. As Canguilhem noted: perfect health is actually the abnormal state. This makes disease and discomfort part of daily life.

NOTES

1. Watson, *Feeding the Revolution*, 316.
2. Watson, 316.
3. David A. Palmer, *Qigong Fever: Body, Science, and Utopia in China* (New York: Columbia University Press, 2007), 282.
4. Anett Dippner has engaged with concepts of happiness and beauty as regards Chinese women in the late twentieth century in her book *Miss Perfect—Neue Weiblichkeitsregime und die sozialen Skripte des Glücks in China* (Bielefeld: Transcript, 2016).

Bibliography

Ahlheim, Hannah. *Der Traum vom Schlaf im Zwanzigsten Jahrhundert*. Göttingen: Wallstein Verlag, 2018.

Amelung, Iwo, ed. *Discourses of Weakness in Modern China: Historical Diagnoses of the "Sick Man of East Asia."* Frankfurt: Campus Verlag, 2020.

Anderson, Eugene N. *The Food of China*. New Haven: Yale University Press, 1988.

Andreas, Joel. *Rise of the Red Engineers: The Cultural Revolution and the Origins of China's New Class*. California: Stanford University Press, 2009.

Andrews, Bridie. "From Case Records to Case Histories: The Modernisation of a Chinese Medical Genre, 1912–1949." In *Innovation in Chinese Medicine*, edited by Elizabeth Hsu, 324–36. Cambridge: Cambridge University Press, 2001.

Andrews, Bridie, and Mary Brown Bullock, eds. *Medical Transitions in Twentieth-Century China*. Indiana: Indiana University Press, 2014.

Atwater, Wilbur O. "Food as Building Material and Fuel." In *Principles of Nutrition and Nutritive Value of Food*, edited by Wilbur O. Atwater, 8–14. Washington, DC: U.S. Government Printing Office, 1910.

Babaeva, E. A. (Babayewa, Ye A 巴巴耶娃 叶·阿). *Shengchan ticao (Shangji)* 生产体操 (上集). Translated by Yibing 一兵. Beijing: Renmin tiyu chubanshe, 1955.

Beard, Robert. *1936 Constitution of the USSR, Chapter X*. Lewisburg, PA: Bucknell University, 1996. Accessed July 2, 2018. https://www.departments.bucknell.edu/russian/const/36cons04.html.

Beijingshi gaoxueya bing naoxueguan bing fangzhi yanjiu xiezuo zu, Beijing diqu guanxinbing fangzhi keyan xiezuo zu 北京市高血压病脑血管病防治研究协作组, 北京地区冠心病防治科研协作组. *Gaoxueya bing Naoxueguan bing Guanxinbing de fangzhi* 高血压病 脑血管病 冠心病的防治. Beijing: Renmin chubanshe, 1976.

Beijing yiyuan. *Laoren baojian bidu* 老人保健必读. Beijing: Renmin weisheng chubanshe, 1982.

Beller, Anne Scott. *Fat and Thin—A Natural History of Obesity*. New York: McGraw-Hill, 1977.

Bernstein, Thomas, and Hua-yu Li, eds. *China Learns from the Soviet Union, 1949–present*. Lanham: Lexington Books, 2010.

Bourdieu, Pierre, Patrick Champagne, Julien Duval, Franck Poupeau, Marie-Christine Rivière, Peter Collier, and Pierre Bourdieu. *Habitus and Field: General Sociology, Volume 2; Lectures at the Collège de France (1982–1983)*. Cambridge: Polity Press, 2020.

Bowers, H. J. W., J. Z. Bowers, J. W. Hess, and N. Sivin. *Science and Medicine in Twentieth-Century China: Research and Education*. Ann Arbor: Center for Chinese Studies, the University of Michigan, 1988.

Brazelton, Mary Augusta. *Mass Vaccinations: Citizens' Bodies and State Power in Modern China*. Ithaca, NY: Cornell University Press, 2019.

Brownell, Susan. *Training the Body for China: Sports in the Moral Order of the People's Republic*. Chicago: University of Chicago Press, 1995.

Brykin, A. T. (Bu Leijin 布雷金). *Ticao. Shang ji* 体操. 上集. Translated by Fang Bin方瑸, Li Guozhen 李国珍, and Liang Ziqing梁子勤. Beijing: Renmin tiyu chubanshe, 1954.

Bucharin, Nikolaj I. *Das ABC des Kommunismus*. Wien: Kommunist. Partei Deutschoesterreichs, 1920.

Bücher, Karl. *Arbeit und Rhythmus*. Leipzig: Teubner Verlag, 1902.

Bu, Liping. "Anti-Malaria Campaigns and the Socialist Reconstruction of China, 1950–80." *East Asian History* 39 (2014): 117–30.

Burke, Peter. *What is the History of Knowledge?* Cambridge: Polity Press, 2016.

Canguilhem, Georges. *The Normal and the Pathological*. New York: Zone Books, 1989.

"Cankao xiaoxi" bianjibu. *Shengming zaiyu yundong* 生命在于运动. Taiyuan: Shanxi renmin chubanshe, 1979.

Cao Wujun 曹武君, ed. *Yinshi yu jiankang* 饮食与健康. Guangzhou: Guangdong keji chubanshe, 1981.

Carden-Coyne, Ana. *Reconstructing the Body—Classicism, Modernism, and the First World War*. Oxford: Oxford University Press, 2009.

Carpenter, Kenneth J. "The History of Enthusiasm for Protein." *Journal of Nutrition* 116, no. 7 (July 1986): 1364–70.

Carrington, Ben, and Ian McDonald. *Marxism, Cultural Studies and Sport*. New York: Routledge, 2009.

Chen Feirun 陈费润, ed. *Zenyang banhao gonggong shanshi* 怎样办好公共膳食. Shanghai: Zhonghua shuju chuban, 1951.

[Chen] Feirun [陈]费润, ed. *Zenyang banhao gonggong shanshi* 怎样办好公共膳食. Beijing: Renmin weisheng chubanshe, 1954.

Chen Haifeng 陈海锋, ed. *Zhongguo weisheng baojianshi* 中国卫生保健史. Shanghai: Shanghai kexuejishu chubanshe, 1993.

Chen Meiyu 陈美愉. *Yingyang weisheng* 营养卫生. Beijing: Renmin weisheng chubanshe, 1954.

Chen Shuqi 陈叔骐. *Yingyang weisheng* 营养卫生. Beijng: Renmin weisheng chubanshe, 1954.

Chen Su 陈苏. *Tiyu yu jiankang* 体育与健康. Nanchang: Jiangxi renmin chubanshe, 1955.

Chen, Tina Mai. "Proletarian White and Working Bodies in Mao's China." *Positions: East Asia Cultures Critique* 11, no. 2 (2003): 361–93.

———. "The Human-Machine Continuum in Maoism: The Intersection of Soviet Socialist Realism, Japanese Theoretical Physics, and Chinese Revolutionary Theory." *Cultural Critique* 80 (Winter 2012): 151–81.

Chen Xuecun 陈学存. *Yingyong yingyang xue* 应用营养学. Beijing: Renmin weisheng chubanshe, 1984.

Chenguang chuban gongsi bianji 晨光出版公司编辑. *Laodong renmin xiuyang suo* 劳动人民休养所. Shanghai: Chenguang chuban gongsi, 1950.

———. *Xinzhongguo laodong renmin xiuyang suo* 新中国劳动人民休养所. Shanghai: Chenguang chuban gongsi, 1953.

Cherevkov, M. (Qiliefukefu 契列甫柯夫). *Sulian tiyu jiaocai* 苏联体育教材. Translated by Qiu Biao 仇标. Shanghai: Beixin shuju, 1952.

Cho, Ko, and Kyoko Iriye Selden. *The Search for the Beautiful Woman: A Cultural History of Japanese and Chinese Beauty*. Lanham, MD: Rowman & Littlefield, 2012.

Collingham, Lizzie. *The Taste of War*. London: Penguin Books, 2011.

Core, Rachel. "Tuberculosis Control in Shanghai: Bringing Health to the Masses, 1928–Present." In *Medical Transitions in Twentieth-Century China*, edited by Bridie Andrews and Mary Brown Bullock, 126–45. Bloomington: Indiana University Press, 2014.

Croizier, Ralph C. *Traditional Medicine in Modern China: Science, Nationalism, and the Tensions of Cultural Change*. Cambridge: Harvard University Press, 1968.

Cullather, Nick. "The Foreign Policy of the Calorie." *American Historical Review* 112, no. 2 (April 2007): 337–64.

Cullen, Christopher. "*Yi'an* 醫案 (case statements): The Origins of a Genre of Chinese Medical Literature." In *Innovation in Chinese Medicine*, edited by Elizabeth Hsu, 297–323. Cambridge: Cambridge University Press, 2001.

Dangdai Zhongguo shehui kexue xuezhe dacidian 当代中国社会科学学者大辞典. Hangzhou: Zhejiang Daxue chubanshe, 1990.

Dan Shouzhun 单守谆. *Gaoxueya* 高血压. Harbin: Heilongjiang kexue jishu chubanshe, 1981.

Dazhong caipu bianxiezu bian. *Dazhong caipu* 大众菜谱. Beijing: Qinggongye chubanshe, 1979.

Descartes, René. *A Discourse on Method (1637)*. Translated by John Veitch. Project Gutenberg, 2008. Accessed 19 April 2020. https://www.gutenberg.org/files/59/59-h/59-h.htm.

Deurenberg, P., M. Deurenberg-Yap, and S. Guricci. "Asians are Different from Caucasians and from Each Other in Their Body Mass Index/Body Fat per Cent Relationship." *Obesity Reviews*, no. 3 (2002): 141–46.

Dikötter, Frank. *Mao's Great Famine: The History of China's Most Devastating Catastrophe, 1958–1962*. New York: Walker & Co., 2010.

Dippner, Anett. *Miss Perfect—Neue Weiblichkeitsregime und die sozialen Skripte des Glücks in China*. Bielefeld: Transcript, 2016.

Dittmer, Lowell. Death and Transfiguration: Liu Shaoqi's Rehabilitation and Contemporary Chinese Politics." *The Journal of Asian Studies*, vol. 40, no. 3 (1981): 455–479.

Dubuque, N. E. (Qiubiyouke 裘毕尤克). *Yinshi yu jiankang* 饮食与健康. Translated by Huang Zhenhua黄振华 and Zhang Yujian 张与健. Shanghai: Xin zhishi chubanshe, 1956.

Du Shihua 席时华, Li Zhensheng 李震生, Lü Jingzhong 吕敬中, and Wang Rukun 王汝琨. *Gaoxueya bing* 高血压病. Henan: Renmin chubanshe, 1978.

Dutton, Michael. *Policing Chinese Politics: A History*. London: Duke University Press, 2005.

Du Xixian 杜希贤. *Yinshi yingyangxue* 饮食营养学. Jinan: Shandong kexue jishu chubanshe, 1980.

Eaton, S. B., M. Konner, and M. Shostak. "Stone Agers in the Fast Lane: Chronic Degenerative Diseases in Evolutionary Perspective." *American Journal of Medicine* 84, no. 4 (April 1988): 739–49.

Eisenman, Joshua. *Red China's Green Revolution: Technological Innovation, Institutional Change, and Economic Development under the Commune*. New York: Columbia University Press, 2018.

Engels, Friedrich. "The Part Played by Labour in the Transition from Ape to Man." In *Beyond the Body Proper*, edited by Margaret Lock and Judith Farquhar, 25–29. Durham, NC: Duke University Press, 2007 [1876].

Eyferth, Jacob. *Eating Rice from Bamboo Roots*. Cambridge: Harvard University Press, 2009.

———. "Less for More: Rural Women's Overwork and Underconsumption in Mao's China." *Clio. Women, Gender, History*, no. 41 (2015): 65–84.

———. "Women's Work and the Politics of Homespun in Socialist China, 1949–1980." *International Review of Social History* 57, no. 3 (December 2012): 365–91.

Fang, Xiaoping. *Barefoot Doctors and Western Medicine in China*. Rochester: University of Rochester Press, 2012.

Farquhar, Judith, and Zhang Qizheng. *Ten Thousand Things: Nurturing Life in Contemporary Beijing*. New York: Zone Books, 2012.

Feng Ailan 冯蔼兰. *Gonggong yingyang* 公共营养. Beijing: Qinggongye chubanshe, 1985.

Food and Agriculture Organization of the United Nations, World Health Organization, and United Nations University. *Human Energy Requirements*. Food and Nutrition Technical Report Series, vol. 1. FAO, 2001. Accessed November 10, 2017. http://www.fao.org/3/a-y5686e.pdf.

Forth, Christopher. *Fat—A Cultural History of the Stuff of Life*. London: Reaktion Books, 2019.

Foster, George McClelland, and Barbara G. Anderson. *Medical Anthropology*. New York: John Wiley, 1978.

Foucault, Michel. *Analytik der Macht*. Frankfurt: Suhrkamp Verlag, 2005.

———. *Die Sorge um sich* (*Sexualität und Wahrheit 3*) [*History of Sexuality*]. Frankfurt: Suhrkamp Verlag, 2012.

French, Paul, and Matthew Crabbe. *Fat China: How Expanding Waistlines Are Changing a Nation*. London: Anthem Press, 2010.

Friedman, Edward, Paul G. Pickowicz, and Mark Selden. *Revolution, Resistance, and Reform in Village China*. New Haven, CT: Yale University Press, 2005.

Fu, Jia-Chen. *The Other Milk: Reinventing Soy in Republican China*. Seattle: University of Washington Press, 2018.

Fu Qisheng 傅柒生, and Li Zhengang 李贞刚, eds. *Hongse jiyi* 红色记忆 [Red Memories]. Beijing: Jiefangjun chubanshe, 2011.

Fuzhou budui houqinbu weishengbu. *Minbing weishengyuan keben* 民兵卫生员课本. Beijing: Renmin weisheng chubanshe, 1975.

Gao, Hua. "Food Augmentation Methods and Food Substitutes during the Great Famine." In *Eating Bitterness*, edited by Kimberly E. Mannings and Felix Wemheuer, 171–96. Vancouver: UBC Press, 2011.

Gao, Xi. "Foreign Models of Medicine in Twentieth-Century China." In *Medical Transitions in Twentieth-Century China*, edited by Bridie Andrews and Mary Brown Bullock, 173–211. Bloomington: Indiana University Press, 2014.

Ghosh, Arunabh. *Making it Count*. Princeton: Princeton University Press, 2020.

Gilman, Sander L. *Obesity: The Biography*. Oxford: Oxford University Press, 2010.

Greenhalgh, Susan, and Edwin A. Winckler. *Governing China's Population: From Leninist to Neoliberal Biopolitics*. Stanford: Stanford University Press, 2005.

Greene, Jeremy A. *Prescribing by Numbers: Drugs and the Definition of Disease*. Baltimore: John Hopkins University Press, 2007.

Gross, Miriam. *Farewell to the God of Plague—Chairman Mao's Campaign to Deworm China*. Oakland: University of California Press, 2016.

Gross, Miriam, and Kawai Fan. "Schistosomiasis." In *Medical Transitions in Twentieth-Century China*, edited by Bridie Andrews and Mary Brown Bullock, 106–25. Bloomington: Indiana University Press, 2014.

Guo, Yuhua. "The Generation Gap at the Table." In *Feeding China's Little Emperors: Food, Children, and Social Change*, edited by Jing Jun, 94–113. Stanford: Stanford University Press, 2000.

Hanson, Marta. *Speaking of Epidemics in Chinese Medicine*. London: Routledge, 2011.

Hayhoe, Ruth. *Education and Modernization: The Chinese Experience*. Oxford: Pergamon Press, 1992.

Hebei shifan daxue tiyuxi bian. *Shengli weisheng* 生理卫生. Beijing: Renmin tiyu chubanshe, 1978.

Hebeisen, Walter, and Frederick W. Taylor. *F.W. Taylor und der Taylorismus: über das Wirken und die Lehre Taylors und die Kritik am Taylorismus*. Zürich: Vdf, Hochschulverlag an der ETH, 1999.

Heinrich, Larissa. *The Afterlife of Images: Translating the Pathological Body Between China and the West*. Durham, NC: Duke University Press, 2008.

Hikita and Oda. "*Qing ni yigeren paobu*" 请你一个人跑步. In *Shengming zaiyu yundong* 生命在于运动, edited by "Cankao xiaoxi" bianjibu, 29–31. Taiyuan: Shanxi renmin chubanshe, 1979.

Hinsch, Bret. *Masculinities in Chinese History*. Plymouth, UK: Rowman & Littlefield, 2013.

Hobsbawm, Eric, and Terence Ranger. *The Invention of Tradition*. Cambridge: Cambridge University Press, 1983.

Howell, Reet. "The USSR: Sport and Politics Intertwined." *Comparative Education* 11, no. 2 (1975): 137–45.

Hou Xiangchuan 侯祥川, ed. *Yingyangxue jinzhan* 营养学进展. Shanghai: Shanghai kexue jishu chubanshe, 1966.

Huang Chengguo 黄承国, ed. *Jianming yingyang xue* 简明营养学. Shanghai: Xinan yixue shushe, 1950.

Imamura Yoshio, Kinbara Isamu, Ishiko Toshihiro, and Kuroda Yoshio, eds. *Riben zhongxue baojian tiyu* 日本中学保健体育. Translated by Wang Deshen 王德深. Beijing: Wenhua jiaoyu chubanshe, 1982.

Jiaoyu dacidian zengding hebianben xia 教育大辞典 增订合编本 下. Shanghai jiaoyu chubanshe, 1998.

Jing, Jun, ed. *Feeding China's Little Emperors: Food, Children, and Social Change*. Stanford: Stanford University Press, 2000.

Jonsson, Urban. "The Rise and Fall of Paradigms in World Food and Nutrition Policy (Commentary)." *World Nutrition* 1, no. 3 (June 2010): 128–58.

Kaple, Deborah A. *Dream of a Red Factory*. New York: Oxford University Press, 1994.

———. "Soviet Advisors in China in the 1950s." In *Brothers in Arms: The Rise and Fall of the Sino-Soviet Alliance, 1945–1963*, edited by O. A. Westad. Washington, D.C.: Woodrow Wilson Center Press, 1998: 117–140.

Kasulis, Thomas P., Roger T. Aimes, and Wimal Dissanayake. *Self as Body in Asian Theory and Practice*. Albany: State University of New York, 1993.

Keller, Kathleen. *Encyclopedia of Obesity*. Los Angeles: Sage, 2008.

Kleinman, Arthur. *Social Origins of Distress and Disease*. London: Yale University Press, 1986.

———. *The Illness Narratives: Suffering, Healing, and the Human Condition*. New York: Basic Books, 1988.

Korzec, Michael. *Labour and the Failure of Reform in China*. New York: Macmillan Press, 1992.

Kraus, Willy. *Wirtschaftliche Entwicklung und sozialer Wandel in der Volksrepublik China*. Berlin: Springer-Verlag, 1979.

Kroker, Kenton. *The Sleep of Others and the Transformations of Sleep Research*. Toronto: University of Toronto Press, 2007.

Kubin, Wolfgang. "Warum und zu welchem Zweck geht ein Chinese (nicht) spazieren? Ein Versuch." In *Kopflandschaften, Landschaftsgänge: Kulturgeschichte und Poetik des Spaziergangs*, edited by Axel Gellhaus, Christian Moser, and Helmut J. Schneider, 83–97. Köln: Böhlau, 2007.

Kunze, Rui, and Marc A. Matten. *Knowledge Production in Mao-Era China: Learning Science from the Masses*. Lanham: Lexington Books, 2021.

Kuriyama, Shigehisa. *The Expressiveness of the Body and the Divergence of Greek and Chinese Medicine*. New York: Zone Books, 2002.

Kurtz, Joachim. "Translating the Vocation of Man: Liang Qichao (1873–1929), J. G. Fichte, and the Body Politic in Early Republican China." In *Why Concepts Matter*, edited by Martin J. Burke, 153–75. Leiden, Netherlands: Brill, 2012.

Labisch, Alfons. *Homo hygienicus: Gesundheit und Medizin in der Neuzeit*. Frankfurt am Main: Campus Verlag, 1992.

Lam, Tong. *A Passion for Facts*. London: University of California Press, 2011.

Lan Ding 蓝宁. *Zenyang zaineng shenti hao* 怎样才能身体好. Beijing: Zhongguo qingnian chubanshe, 1964.

Landwehr, Achim. *Historische Diskursanalyse*. Frankfurt: Campus Verlag, 2018.

Larson, Wendy. *From Ah Q to Lei Feng*. Stanford: Stanford University Press, 2009.

Leder, Drew. *The Absent Body*. Chicago: University of Chicago Press, 1990.

———. *The Body in Medical Thought and Practice*. Dordrecht: Kluwer Academic Publishers, 1992.

———. *The Distressed Body: Rethinking Illness, Imprisonment, and Healing*. Chicago: University of Chicago Press, 2016.

Lee, Seung-Joon. "The Patriot's Scientific Diet: Nutrition Science and Dietary Reform Campaigns in China, 1910s–1950s." *Modern Asian Studies* 6, no. 49 (February 2015): 1–32.

Lei, Hsiang-lin. *Neither Donkey nor Horse: Medicine in the Struggle over China's Modernity*. Chicago: University of Chicago Press, 2014.

———. "Moral Community of *Weisheng*: Contesting Hygiene in Republican China." *East Asian Science, Technology and Society* 3 (2009): 475–504.

———. "*Weisheng, shentishi, yu shenfen rentong: yi minguo shiqi de feijiehe yu weisheng cantai wei lie* 卫生，身体史，与身分认同：以民国时期的肺结核与卫生餐台为例." In *Jiankang yu shehui* 健康与社会, edited by Zhu Pingyi, 119–44. Taibei: Lianjing chubangongsi, 2013.

Levent, Nina S. *Healthy Spirit in a Healthy Body: Representations of the Sports Body in Soviet Art of the 1920s and 1930s*. New York: P. Lang, 2004.

Liu, He Lydia. *Translingual Practice: Literature, National Culture, and Translated Modernity—China, 1900–1937*. Stanford: Stanford University Press, 1999.

Liu Lin 刘林, ed. *Shipin weisheng* 食品卫生. Beijing: Renmin weisheng chubanshe, 1957.

Liu, Michael Shiyung. "Diet for War: Military Nutrition in Republican China." *Journal of Modern Chinese History* 14, no. 2 (2020): 240–54.

Liu, Shaoqi. "How to Be a Good Communist." In *Sources of Chinese Tradition*, vol. 2, edited by William Theodore de Bary, 427–31. New York: Columbia University Press, 1960.

Li, Yi. "Discourse of Mid-Day Napping—a Political Windsock in Contemporary China." In *Night-Time and Sleep in Asia and the West: Exploring the Dark Side of Life*, edited by Brigitte Steger and Lodewijk Brunt, 45–64. New York: Routledge Curzon, 2003.

Lucas, AnElissa. "Changing Medical Models in China: Organizational Options or Obstacles?" In *The China Quarterly*, no. 83 (September 1980): 461–89.

Luesink, David. "Anatomy and the Reconfiguration of Life and Death in Republican China." In *Journal of Asian Studies* 76, no. 4 (November 2017): 1009–34.

Luesink, David, William Schneider, and Daqing Zhang, eds. *China and the Globalization of Biomedicine*. Rochester, NY: University of Rochester Press, 2019.

Lukyanov. *Jiankang yu laodong nengli de baohu* 健康与劳动能力的保护. Translated by Li Guangcheng 李广成. Beijing: Renmin weisheng chubanshe, 1955.

Luo, Pinghan. *"Daguofan": Nongcun gonggong shitang shimo* "大锅饭": 农村公共食堂始末. Nanming: Sichuan renmin chubanshe, 2015.

Lu, Xiaoning. "Promote Physical Culture and Sport, Improve the People's Constitution." In *Words and Their Stories—Essays on the Language of Chinese Revolution*, edited by Ban Wang, 171–84. Leiden, Netherlands: Brill, 2011.

Mallory, Walter H. *China—Land of Famine*. New York: American Geographical Society, 1926.

Manning, Kimberly E., and Felix Wemheuer. *Eating Bitterness: New Perspectives on China's Great Leap Forward and Famine*. Vancouver: UBC Press, 2011.

Mao Zedong. "Guanyu bantian wenzhang de tanhua" 关于坂田文章的谈话. In *Mao Zedong sixiang wansui; zhongwen makesi zhuyi wenku* 毛泽东思想万岁; 中文马克色主义文库, 158–60. 1969. Accessed August 12, 2021. https://www.marxists.org/chinese/pdf/08/01210804.pdf.

———. "Guanyu gongzuo, shenghuo tongshi bingzhong fangzhen de piyu" 关于工作，生活同时并重方针的批语. In *Jianguo yilai Mao Zedong wengao. Diqice, yi jiu wu ba nian yi yue—yi jiu wu ba nian shi'er yue* 建国以来毛泽东文稿. 第七册, 一九五八年一月—一九五八年十二月, edited by Zhongyang wenxian yanjiushi. Beijing: Zhongyang wenxian chubanshe, 1992.

———. "On the Correct Handling of Contradictions among the People [1957]." In *Selected Works of Mao Tsetung*, Vol. 5 (1977), 384–42.

———. "Shijianlun" 实践论 [On Practice]. In *Mao Zedong xuanji* 毛泽东选集, Vol. 1, 259–73. Beijing: Renmin chubanshe, 1968.

———. "Tiyu zhi yanjiu" 体育之研究 [A Study of Physical Education]. In *Xin Qingnian* (April 1917).

———. "Where Do Correct Ideas Come From? [1963]" In *Selected Readings from the Works of Mao Tsetung*, 502–4. Beijing: Foreign Language Press, 1971.

Mauss, Marcel. "Techniques of the Body." *Economy and Society* 2 (1973): 70–88.

Matten, Marc A. "Coping with Invisible Threats: Nuclear Radiation and Science Dissemination in Maoist China." *East Asian Science, Technology and Society* 12, no. 3 (2018): 235–56.

Morehouse, Laurence E., and Leonard Gross. *Total Fitness in 30 Minutes a Week*. Granada: St Albans, 1977.

Morris, Andrew D. *Marrow of the Nation: A History of Sport and Physical Culture in Republican China*. Berkeley: University of California Press, 2004.

Needham, Joseph, and Gwei-Djen Lu. "A Contribution to the History of Chinese Dietetics." *Isis* 42, no. 1 (April 1951): 13–20.

Ng, Brady. "Obesity: The Big, Fat Problem with Chinese Cities." *The Guardian*, January 9, 2017. https://www.theguardian.com/sustainable-business/2017/jan/09/obesity-fat-problem-chinese-cities.

O'Mahony, Mike. *Sport in the USSR—Physical Culture—Visible Culture*. London: Reaktion Books, 2006.

Ott, Christine. *Identität geht durch den Magen*. Frankfurt: S. Fischer Verlag, 2017.

Oxfeld, Ellen. *Bitter and Sweet: Food, Meaning, and Modernity in Rural China*. Oakland: University of California Press, 2017.

Packard, Randall. "The Fielding H. Garrison Lecture: 'Break Bone' Fever in Philadelphia, 1780; Reflections on the History of Disease." *Bulletin of the History of Medicine* 90, no. 2 (Summer 2016): 193–221.

Palmer, David A. *Qigong Fever: Body, Science, and Utopia in China*. New York: Columbia University Press, 2007.

Pickering, George. "Hypertension—Definitions, Natural Histories and Consequences." In *Hypertension Manual*, edited by John H. Laragh, 3–30. New York: Yorke Medical Books, 1974.

Plügge, Herbert, and Rolf Kohn. "Wohlbefinden und Missbefinden." *Psyche* 12, no. 1 (1959): 33–49.

Porter, Theodore M. *Trust in Numbers: The Pursuit of Objectivity in Science and Public Life*. Princeton: Princeton University Press, 1995.

Postel-Vinay, Nicolas. *A Century of Arterial Hypertension 1896–1996*. Chichester: John Wiley, 1996.

Qiu Keping邱科平. *Shijie dabaike quanshu disanjuan keji tianwen shengwu renti yixue* 世界大百科全书 第三卷 科技 天文 生物 人体 医学. Beijing: Guangming ribao chubanshe, 2003.

Qu Huiqing 区慧清. *Jiating yingyang shipu* 家庭营养食谱. Beijing: Kexue puji chubanshe, 1959.

Qu Mianyu 曲绵域, Gao Yunqiu 高云秋, Pu Junzong 浦钧宗, and Chen Jidi 陈吉棣. *Shiyong yundong yixue* 实用运动医学. Beijing: Beijing daxue yixue chubanshe, 1965.

Rabinbach, Anson. *The Human Motor: Energy, Fatigue, and the Origins of Modernity*. Berkeley: University of California Press, 1992.

Rapoport, A. (Lapopo'ertuo 拉波波尔脱, A.). *Heli de xiuxi* 合理的休息. Translated by Miao Lanqing 苗兰卿. Shanghai: Shanghai weisheng chubanshe, 1952.

Rguibi, Mohamed, and Rekia Belahsen. "Fattening Practices among Moroccan Saharawi Women." *Eastern Mediterranean Health Journal* 12, no. 5 (2006): 619–24.

Richter, Antje. *Das Bild des Schlafes in der altchinesischen Literatur*. Hamburg: Hamburger Sinologische Gesellschaft, 2001.

———. "Der Schlaf in der medizinischen Literatur des Alten China." *Chinesische Medizin* 17, no. 4 (2002): 154–67.

———. "Sleeping Time in Early Chinese Literature." In *Night-Time and Sleep in Asia and the West: Exploring the Dark Side of Life*, edited by Brigitte Steger and Lodewijk Brunt, 24–44. New York: Routledge Curzon, 2003.

Riordan, James. *Sport in Soviet Society: Development of Sport and Physical Education in Russia and the USSR*. New York: Cambridge University Press, 1977.

Rogaski, Ruth. *Hygienic Modernity: Meanings of Health and Disease in Treaty-Port China*. Berkeley: University of California Press, 2004.

Rosenberg, Charles. "Introduction." In *Framing Disease*, edited by Charles Rosenberg and Janet Golden, xiii–xxvi. New Brunswick, NJ: Rutgers University Press, 1997.

Ruskin, Arthur. *Classics in Arterial Hypertension*. Springfield, IL: Charles C. Thomas, 1956.

Scheid, Volker. *Chinese Medicine in Contemporary China: Plurality and Synthesis*. Durham, NC: Duke University Press, 2002.

Schillinger, Nicolas. *The Body and Military Masculinity in Late Qing and Early Republican China: The Art of Governing Soldiers*. Lanham, MD: Lexington Books, 2016.

Schmalzer, Sigrid. "Beyond Bias: Critical Analysis and Layered Reading of Mao-Era Sources." *Positions: Asia critique* 29, no. 4 (November 2021): 759–781.

———. "Labor Created Humanity: Cultural Revolution Science on Its Own Terms." In *The Chinese Cultural Revolution as History*, edited by Joseph W. Esherick, Paul G. Pickowicz, and Andrew G. Walder, 185–210. Stanford: Stanford University Press, 2006.

———. *The People's Peking Man: Popular Science and Human Identity in Twentieth-Century China*. Chicago: University of Chicago Press, 2008.

———. *Red Revolution, Green Revolution*. Chicago: University of Chicago Press, 2016.

Schneider, Helen M. *Keeping the Nation's House*. Vancouver: UBC Press, 2011.

Scrinis, Gyorgy. "On the Ideology of Nutritionism." In *Contemporary Transitions*, edited by Jeffrey M. Pilcher, 405–21. Vol. 4 of *Food History: Critical and Primary Sources*. London: Bloomsbury, 2015.

Seeberg, Vilma. *The Rhetoric and Reality of Mass Education in Mao's China*. Lewiston: E. Mellen Press, 2000.

Sewell, William. "A Theory of Structure: Duality, Agency, and Transformation." *American Journal of Sociology* 98, no. 1 (July 1992): 1–29.

Shanghai yixue zhuankexuexiao weishengxue jiaoyanzu. *Yingyang weisheng xue* 营养卫生学. Beijing: Renmin weisheng chubanshe, 1961.

Sharp, Lesley A. "The Commodification of the Body and its Parts." *Annual Review of Anthropology* 29 (2000): 287–328.

Shen Zhihua, and Guy Alitto. "A Historical Examination of the Issue of Soviet Experts in China: Basic Situation and Policy Changes." *Russian History* 29, no. 2 (2000): 377–400.

Shijie dangdai wenhua mingren cidian 世界当代文化名人辞典. Beijing Yanshan chubanshe, 1992.

Shobert, Benjamin. "China's Growing Obesity Problem." *Forbes*, January 22, 2017. https://www.forbes.com/sites/benjaminshobert/2017/01/22/chinas-growing-obesity-problem/#7f8b3ca86ecf.

Shuman, Amanda. "Elite Competitive Sport in the People's Republic of China 1958–1966: The Games of the New Emerging Forces (GANEFO)." *Journal of Sport History* 40, no. 2 (2013): 258–83.

———. "The Politics of Socialist Athletics in the People's Republic of China, 1949–1966." PhD Thesis, University of California, 2014.

Shu Xincheng 舒新城. *Wo zenyang huifu jiankangde* 我怎样恢复健康的. Beijing: Zhonghua shuju chubanshe, 1956.

Simoons, Frederick J. *Food in China: A Cultural and Historical Inquiry*. Boca Raton: CRC Press, 1991.

Sivin, Nathan. *Traditional Medicine in Contemporary China: A Partial Translation of* Revised Outline of Chinese Medicine *(1972) with an Introductory Study on Change in Present-Day and Early Medicine*. Ann Arbor: Center for Chinese Studies, University of Michigan, 1987.

Smith, Hillary A. *Forgotten Disease: Illness Transformed in Chinese Medicine*. Stanford: Stanford University Press, 2017.

Staley, Seward C. *Geren yu tuanti zhi jingzhi yundong* 个人与团体之竞技运动. Translated by Wang Yicheng 王毅诚 and Jin Feijun 金非均. Shanghai: Shanghai renwen yinshuguan, 1930.

Sterzel, Julia. *Vom Genossen Lei Feng lernen? Eine Analyse von 50 Jahren Kampagnengeschichte in der VR China*. Bochum: Projektverlag, 2015.

Strauss, Julia. "Morality, Coercion and State Building by Campaign in the Early PRC: Regime Consolidation and After, 1949–1956." *The China Quarterly*, no. 188 (2006): 891–912.

Summers-Bremner, Eluned. *Insomnia—A Cultural History*. London: Reaktion Books, 2008.

Swislocki, Mark. *Culinary Nostalgia: Regional Food Culture and the Urban Experience in Shanghai*. Stanford: Stanford University Press, 2009.

———. "Nutritional Governmentality—Food and the Politics of Health in Late Imperial and Republican China." *Radical History Review*, no. 110 (Spring 2011): 9–35.

Taylor, Frederick W. *The Principles of Scientific Management*. New York: Harper & Brothers Publishing, 1911.

Taylor, Kim. *Chinese Medicine in Early Communist China, 1945–63: A Medicine of Revolution*. London: Routledge, 2011.

Ticao dacidian 体操大辞典. Beijing: Renmin tiyu chubanshe, 1999.

Tiyu yu jiankang bianxie xiaozu. *Tiyu yu jiankang—yundong shengli weisheng changshi* 体育与健康—运动生理卫生常识. Beijing: Renmin tiyu chubanshe, 1976.

True, A. C. "Wilbur Olin Atwater, 1844–1907." In *Proceedings of the Washington Academy of Sciences* 10 (1908): 194–198.

United Nations Children's Fund. *Obesity Report on China*. UNICEF, 2019, http://www.unicef.cn/en/uploadfile/2018/0423/20180423114400165.pdf. Accessed February 25, 2019.

Unschuld, Paul U. *Medicine in China: A History of Ideas*. Berkeley: University of California Press, 1985.

Vernon, James. *Hunger—A Modern History*. London: Belknap Press, 2007.

Wagner, Rudolph. "China 'Asleep' and 'Awakening.' A Study in Conceptualizing Asymmetry and Coping with It." *Transcultural Studies* 1 (2011): 4–139.

Washburn, John N. "Sport as a Soviet Tool." *Foreign Affairs* 34, no. 3 (April 1956): 490–99.

Watson, James L. "China's Big Mac Attack." In *The Cultural Politics of Food and Eating*, edited by James L. Watson and Melissa Caldwell, 70–79. Oxford: Blackwell Publishing, 2005.

———. "Feeding the Revolution: Public Mess Halls and Coercive Commensality in Maoist China." In *The Handbook of Food and Anthropology*, edited by Jakob Klein and James L. Watson, 308–22. London: Bloomsbury Academic, 2016.

———. "Food as a Lens: The Past, Present, and Future of Family Life in China." In *Feeding China's Little Emperors: Food, Children, and Social Change*, edited by Jun Jing, 199–212. Stanford: Stanford Universtiy Press, 2000.

Weber, Max. "Die protestantische Ethik und der Geist des Kapitalismus." *Archiv für Sozialwissenschaften und Sozialpolitik* 21, no. 1 (1904): 1–96.

Wei Mingyan 魏铭炎. *Jiankang. Yukuai. Changshou* 健康· 愉快· 长寿. Guangzhou: Kexuepuji chubanshe guangzhou fenshe, 1980.

Weishengbu bangongshi ting, ed. *Weishengbu lishi kaoji 1949–1996 nian* 卫生部历史考记1949–1996年. Beijing: Renmin weisheng chubanshe, 2013.

Will, Pierre Etienne. *Nourish the People: The State Civilian Granary System in China, 1650–1850*. Ann Arbor: Center for Chinese Studies, 1991.

Wilson, Adrian. "On the History of Disease-Concepts: The Case of Pleurisy." *History of Science* 38, no. 3 (2000): 271–319.

WHO [World Health Organization]. *Constitution of the World Health Organization*, 1948, https://www.loc.gov/law/help/us-treaties/bevans/m-ust000004-0119.pdf. Accessed March 22, 2020.

———. *Obesity in the Pacific: Too Big to Ignore*. Noumea, New Caledonia: Graphoprint, 2002.

WHO and IASO [World Health Organization (Regional Office for the Western Pacific), International Diabetes Institute, International Association for the Study of Obesity, and International Obesity Task Force]. *The Asia-Pacific Perspective: Redefining Obesity and its Treatment*. Melbourne: Health Communications Australia, 2000.

Wu Bangwei 吴邦伟. *Tiyu lilun jiben zhishi* 体育理论基本知识. Beijing: Renmin tiyu chubanshe, 1957.

Wu Mengchao 吴孟超, and Wu Zaide 吴在德. *Bainian yixue Tongji ren: bainian lai woguo yixue shiye fazhan zhong de Tongji he Tongjiren* 百年医学同济人: 百年来我国医学事业发展中的同济和同济人. Shanghai: Tongji daxue chubanshe, 2009.

Xinjiaoyu shebian. *Xintiyu de lilun he shixian* 新体育的理论和实践. Shanghai: Huadong renmin chubanshe, 1951.

Xu Shengwen 许胜文, ed. *Feipangbing de yiliao ticao* 肥胖病的医疗体操. Shanghai: Shanghai kexue jishu chubanshe, 1959.

Yang, Jisheng. *Grabstein—Mùbei: Eine Dokumentation der großen chinesischen Hungerkatastrophe 1958–1962*. Frankfurt am Main: Fischer Verlag, 2012.

Yang, Nianqun 杨念群. "Disease Prevention, Social Mobilization and Spatial Politics: The Anti Germ-Warfare Incident of 1952 and the 'Patriotic Health Campaign.'" *Chinese Historical Review* 11 (2004): 155–82.

———. *Zaizao "bingren"* 再造 "病人." Bejing: Zhongguo renmin chubanshe, 2012.

Yang Shouyi 杨守义. *Gaoxueya* 高血压. Beijing: Renmin tiyu chubanshe, 1983.

Yu Lishuang 于丽爽. "Guangbo ticao, bange shiji de quanmin jianshen jiyi 广播体操，半个世纪的全民健身记忆." In *Lishi de beijing* 历史的背景, edited by Beijing ribao jishi caixiezu, 230–49. Beijing: Jiefangjun wenyi chubanshe, 2009.

Yu, Miin-ling. "'Labour is Glorious': Model Labourers in the PRC." In *China Learns from the Soviet Union, 1949–Present*, edited by Thomas P. Bernstein, 231–58. Lanham, MD: Lexington Books, 2010.

Yundong jiepouxue, yundingyixue dacidian 运动解剖学、运动医学大辞典. Beijing: Renmin tiyu chubanshe, 2000.

Yu, Xinzhong. "Epidemics and Public Health in Twentieth-Century China: Plague, Smallpox, and AIDS." In *Medical Transitions in Twentieth-Century China*, edited by Bridie Andrews and Mary Brown Bullock, 91–105. Bloomington: Indiana University Press, 2014.

Zhang, Daqing. "Changing Patterns of Diseases and Longevity: The Evolution of Health in Twentieth-Century Beijing." In *Medical Transitions in Twentieth-Century China*, edited by Bridie Andrews and Mary Brown Bullock, 32–50. Bloomington: Indiana University Press, 2014.

Zhang, Libin. "A Multilevel Study of Effects of Socioeconomic Status, Income Equality, and the Built Environment on Adult Obesity in China." PhD diss., University of Illinois, 2012.

Zheng Ji 郑集. *Shiyong yingyangxue* 实用营养学. Shanghai: Huadong yiwu shenghuoshe, 1952.

———. "Xiandai Zhongguo yingyang xue (1920–1953) shiliao" 现代中国营养学(1920–1953) 史料. *Acta Nutrimenta Sinica* 17, no. 1 (March 1995): 96–111.

Zheng Qiming 郑启明. *Changjian jibing minjian yinshi liaofa* 常见疾病民间饮食疗法. Nanning: Guangxi tongzu zizhiqu renmin chubanshe, 1964.

Zhonggong Henan sheng weishuji shenghuofuli bangongshi. *Yingyang tiaoji jiben changshi* 营养调剂基本常识. Zhengzhou: Henan renmin chubanshe, 1959.

Zhongguo dangdai wenhua mingren xiaozhuan 中国当代文化名人小传. Shenyang: Liaoning renmin chubanshe, 1993.

Zhongguo gongchangdan lishi dacidian zonglun. renwu 中国共产党历史大辞典 总论·人物. Zhonggong zhongyang dangxiao chubanshe, 2001.

Zhongguo kexuejia cidian. Xiandai disi fence 中国科学家辞典. 现代第四分册. Jinan: Shandong kexue jishu chubanshe, 1984.

Zhongguo renmin daxue fajiao yanshi bian. *Zhonghua renmin gongheguo laodong fa ziliao huibian* 中华人民共和国劳动法资料汇编. Beijing: Zhongguo renmin daxue chubanshe, 1954.

Zhongguo renminjiefangjun Nanjingjunqu junyi xuexiao. *Yinshi yingyang weishengxue jiangyi* 饮食营养卫生学讲义. Nanjing: Nanjing junqu junyi xuexiao, 1976.

Zhongguo tiyu baike quanshu 中国体育百科全书. Beijing: Renmin tiyu chubanshe, 2001.

Zhongguo wushu renming cidian 中国武术人名辞典. Beijing: Renmin tiyu chubanshe, 1993.

Zhongguo yixue kexueyuan weisheng yanjiusuo, ed. *Shiwu chengfen biao* 食物成分表. Beijing: Renmin weisheng chubanshe, 1977.

Zhongguo Zhongyi renming cidian 中国中医人名辞典. Zhongyi guji chubanshe, 1991.

Zhonghua renmin gongheguoshi cidian. Edited by Zhu Jianhua 朱建华 and Guo Binwei 郭彬蔚. Guilin 吉林文史出版社, 1989.

Zhou Chao 周超. *Yingyang changshi jianghua* 营养常识讲话. Xi'an: Shanxi renmin chubanshe, 1958.

Zhou Mian 周棉, ed. *Zhongguo liuxuesheng dacidian* 中国留学大辞典. Nanjing: Nanjing daxue chubanshe, 1999.

Zhou, Xun. *The Great Famine in China, 1958–1962: A Documentary History*. New Haven, CT: Yale University Press, 2012.

Zhu Pingyi 祝平一, ed. *Jiangkang yu shehui* 健康与社会. Taipei: Linking Books, 2013.

Zito, Angela, and Tani E. Barlow, eds. *Body, Subject and Power in China*. Chicago: University of Chicago Press, 1994.

Ziegler, Mildred. "The History of the Calorie in Nutrition." *Scientific Monthly* 15 (1922): 520–6.

JOURNALS AND PAPERS

Dazhong Yixue 大众医学 (*Popular Medicine*)

Hubei tiyu keji 湖北体育科技 (*Hubei Sports Science*)

Jiankangbao 健康报 (*Health News*)

Laodong 劳动 (*Labor*)

Liaoning Zhongyi 辽宁中医 (*Liaoning Journal of Traditional Chinese Medicine*)

*Renmin Ribao*人民日报 (*People's Daily*)

Shandong tiyu keji 山东体育科技 (*Shandong Sports Science*)

Shengwuxue tongbao 生物学通报 (*Bulletin of Biology*)

Tiyu jiaoxue yu keyan 体育教学与科研 (*Sports Instruction and Research*)

Wenhua Yicong 文化译丛 (*Collections of Translation on Culture*)

Xintiyu 新体育 (*New Sports*)

Yixue yu Zhexue 医学与哲学 (*Medicine and Philosophy*)

Yunnan Zhongyi Zazhi 云南中医杂志 (*Yunnan Journal of Traditional Chinese Medicine*)

Zhi he Zaozhi 纸和造纸 (*Paper and Papermaking*)

Zhonghua Yixue Zazhi 中华医学杂志 (*Chinese Medical Journal*)

Zhongyi Zazhi 中医杂志 (*Journal of Traditional Chinese Medicine*)

Index

About the Author

Renée Krusche holds a PhD in Chinese studies from the Friedrich-Alexander-University Erlangen-Nürnberg, where she is a postdoctoral research fellow and lecturer.

www.ingramcontent.com/pod-product-compliance
Ingram Content Group UK Ltd.
Pitfield, Milton Keynes, MK11 3LW, UK
UKHW012118150926
475560UK00002B/166

9 781793 65455